Soft Tissue Surgery

Editor

NICOLE J. BUOTE

VETERINARY CLINICS OF NORTH AMERICA: SMALL ANIMAL PRACTICE

www.vetsmall.theclinics.com

March 2022 • Volume 52 • Number 2

ELSEVIER

1600 John F. Kennedy Boulevard • Suite 1800 • Philadelphia, Pennsylvania, 19103-2899
http://www.vetsmall.theclinics.com

VETERINARY CLINICS OF NORTH AMERICA: SMALL ANIMAL PRACTICE Volume 52, Number 2
March 2022 ISSN 0195-5616, ISBN-13: 978-0-323-98699-1

Editor: Stacy Eastman
Developmental Editor: Axell Ivan Jade Purificacion

Veterinary Clinics of North America: Small Animal Practice (ISSN 0195-5616) is published bimonthly by Elsevier Inc., 360 Park Avenue South, New York, NY 10010-1710. Months of issue are January, March, May, July, September, and November. Business and Editorial Offices: 1600 John F. Kennedy Blvd., Ste. 1800, Philadelphia, PA 19103-2899. Customer Service Office: 3251 Riverport Lane, Maryland Heights, MO 63043. Periodicals postage paid at New York, NY and additional mailing offices. Subscription prices are $369.00 per year (domestic individuals), $980.00 per year (domestic institutions), $100.00 per year (domestic students/residents), $465.00 per year (Canadian individuals), $1029.00 per year (Canadian institutions), $503.00 per year (international individuals), $1029.00 per year (international institutions), $100.00 per year (Canadian students/residents), and $220.00 per year (international students/residents). To receive student/resident rate, orders must be accompanied by name of affiliated institution, date of term, and the *signature* of program/residency coordinator on institution letterhead. Orders will be billed at individual rate until proof of status is received. Foreign air speed delivery is included in all *Clinics* subscription prices. All prices are subject to change without notice. **POSTMASTER:** Send address changes to *Veterinary Clinics of North America: Small Animal Practice,* Elsevier Health Sciences Division, Subscription Customer Service, 3251 Riverport Lane, Maryland Heights, MO 63043. Customer Service (orders, claims, online, change of address): Elsevier Periodicals Customer Service, Elsevier Health Sciences Division Subscription **Customer Service 3251 Riverport Lane Maryland Heights, MO 63043. Tel: 1-800-654-2452 (U.S. and Canada); 314-447-8871 (outside U.S. and Canada). Fax: 314-447-8029. E-mail: journalscustomerservice-usa@elsevier.com (for print support); journalsonlinesupport-usa@elsevier.com (for online support).**

Reprints. For copies of 100 or more of articles in this publication, please contact the Commercial Reprints Department, Elsevier Inc., 360 Park Avenue South, New York, NY 10010-1710. Tel.: 212-633-3874; Fax: 212-633-3820; E-mail: reprints@elsevier.com.

Veterinary Clinics of North America: Small Animal Practice is also published in Japanese by Inter Zoo Publishing Co., Ltd., Aoyama Crystal-Bldg 5F, 3-5-12 Kitaaoyama, Minato-ku, Tokyo 107-0061, Japan.

Veterinary Clinics of North America: Small Animal Practice is covered in *Current Contents/Agriculture, Biology and Environmental Sciences, Science Citation Index, ASCA, MEDLINE/PubMed (Index Medicus), Excerpta Medica, and BIOSIS.*

Contributors

EDITOR

NICOLE J. BUOTE, DVM
Diplomate, American College of Veterinary Surgeons - Small Animal; Associate Professor, Department of Clinical Sciences–Small Animal Surgery Section, Soft Tissue Service, Cornell University School of Veterinary Medicine, Ithaca, New York, USA

AUTHORS

JUDITH BERTRAN, DVM, MSc
Diplomate, American College of Veterinary Surgeons; ACVS Fellow Surgical Oncology, Assistant Professor, Small Animal Clinical Sciences, Veterinary Clinical Sciences, University of Florida, Gainesville, Florida, USA

NICOLE J. BUOTE, DVM
Diplomate, American College of Veterinary Surgeons - Small Animal; Associate Professor, Department of Clinical Sciences–Small Animal Surgery Section, Soft Tissue Service, Cornell University School of Veterinary Medicine, Ithaca, New York, USA

KATHLEEN M. HAM, DVM, MS
Diplomate, American College of Veterinary Surgeons - Small Animal; Associate Clinical Professor, Small Animal Surgery, Department of Small Animal Clinical Sciences, University of Florida, Gainesville, Florida, USA

GALINA HAYES, PhD, DVSc, BVSc
Diplomate, American College of Veterinary Emergency Critical Care; Diplomate, American College of Veterinary Surgeons; Associate Professor, Cornell University, Ithaca, New York, USA

SARAH J. MARVEL, DVM, MS
Diplomate, American College of Veterinary Surgeons - Small Animal; ACVS Fellow, Surgical Oncology, Assistant Professor, Clinical Sciences, Colorado State University, Fort Collins, Colorado, USA

MEGAN ANN MICKELSON, DVM
Diplomate, American College of Veterinary Surgeons - Small Animal; University of Missouri, College of Veterinary Medicine, Department of Veterinary Medicine and Surgery, Columbia, Missouri, USA

HEIDI PHILLIPS, VMD
Diplomate, American College of Veterinary Surgeons - Small Animal; Associate Professor, Small Animal Surgery, Department of Veterinary Clinical Medicine, University of Illinois College of Veterinary Medicine, Urbana, Illinois, USA

PENNY J. REGIER, DVM, MS
Diplomate, American College of Veterinary Surgeons - Small Animal; ACVS Fellow, Minimally Invasive Surgery (Small Animal Soft Tissue), Assistant Professor, Small Animal Surgery, University of Florida, Gainesville, Florida, USA

DESIREE ROSSELLI, DVM
Diplomate, American College of Veterinary Surgeons - Small Animal; VCA West Los Angeles Animal Hospital, Los Angeles, California, USA

VALERY FAIRFAX SCHARF, DVM, MS
Diplomate, American College of Veterinary Surgeons; Assistant Professor of Soft Tissue and Oncologic Surgery, Department of Clinical Sciences, NC State University, Raleigh, North California, USA

PAMELA SCHWARTZ, DVM, CCRP
Diplomate, American College of Veterinary Surgeons; Surgeon and Department Chair, The Animal Medical Center, New York, New York, USA

ALEXANDER C.S. THOMSON, DVM
Diplomate, American College of Veterinary Anesthesia and Analgesia; City University of Hong Kong Veterinary Medical Centre, Kowloon, HKSAR

KATY L. TOWNSEND, BVSc(hons), MS
Diplomate, American College of Veterinary Surgeons; Associate Professor, Small Animal Surgery, Veterinary Clinical Sciences, Carlson College of Veterinary Medicine, Oregon State University, Corvallis, Oregon, USA

MANDY L. WALLACE, DVM, MS
Diplomate, American College of Veterinary Surgeons - Small Animal; Assistant Professor, Small Animal Surgery, Department of Small Animal Medicine and Surgery, University of Georgia, Athens, Georgia, USA

Contents

> Wound healing is a complex process that traverses 4 main phases which overlap and are interdependent. Many patient-related factors can impede healing by disrupting the normal pathways from one phase to the next. Wound-related factors also determine the best techniques or dressings for each patient. Species differences between cats and dogs must be understood for the successful treatment of cats. New techniques such as fish skin graft application, photobiomodulation, and bioelectric dressings hold promise as an addition to our armamentarium against wounds. NPWT, hyperbaric oxygen, regenerative medicine techniques, and low-level laser therapies yield mixed results and large-scale controlled studies are needed.

> Gastric dilatation and volvulus (GDV) is an acute, life-threatening syndrome of dogs, particularly large and giant breeds with a deep chest conformation. Rapid diagnosis is important for prompt initiation of stabilization therapy and surgical correction. Negative prognostic factors include hyperlactatemia not responding to fluid therapy, gastric perforation, or need for splenectomy or gastric resection. Gastropexy is essential for all dogs affected by GDV, following correct gastric repositioning. Prophylactic gastropexy for at-risk breeds can be performed via minimally invasive laparoscopic surgery.

> This article discusses updates in brachycephalic and other upper respiratory surgery of dogs and cats, including schemata for classifying brachycephalic dogs in terms of severity of disease and indications for monitoring and treatment, new characterizations of the primary and secondary components of brachycephalic obstructive airway syndrome (BOAS), and updates to traditional brachycephalic airway surgical procedures as well as novel surgeries to treat BOAS, including laser-assisted turbinectomy, the cardiopulmonary effects of brachycephaly on some feline breeds, epiglottic entrapment and retroversion, and upper airway syndrome in Norwich terriers.

> Advances regarding surgical treatment of hepatobiliary diseases over the past 5 years have resulted in improved outcomes and decreased mortality in veterinary patients. Options for minimally invasive treatment of intrahepatic portosystemic shunts and gallbladder disease have led to decreased morbidity with similar outcomes to open procedures. For extrahepatic portosystemic shunts, studies evaluating long-term outcome between surgical attenuation and medical management, as well as between options for surgical attenuation, are being used to direct evidence-based treatment of this congenital anomaly. In addition, evaluation of timing in surgical intervention for gallbladder mucoceles has led to an opportunity for decreased mortality rates after cholecystectomy.

 Video content accompanies this article at http://www.vetsmall. theclinics.com.

> Management of canine and feline ureteral obstructions and urinary incontinence can be both controversial and frustrating. There has been a movement toward minimally invasive procedures, which in certain cases, can be used to both confirm the diagnosis as well as treat the condition. This chapter focuses on the advancements in urologic surgery associated with ureteral obstruction and urinary incontinence with primary focus on ureteral stenting, subcutaneous ureteral bypass systems, transurethral bulking agents, and hydraulic occluders.

> The topic of surgical sterilization in companion animals is evolving. Although early spay and neuter has been advocated to prevent overpopulation of unwanted pets, recent research has focused on the timing of gonadectomy in relation to risk of various neoplasms, orthopedic conditions, and miscellaneous conditions. Many of these studies are breed-specific or draw from large veterinary medical databases, making it difficult to guide recommendations on the timing of sterilization across various breeds and mixed-breeds. This article attempts to synthesize the data and help guide decision making on the type and timing of sterilization procedures performed, including gonad sparing sterilization surgeries.

 Video content accompanies this article at http://www.vetsmall. theclinics.com.

> Both handsewn and stapled anastomosis techniques are performed commonly in veterinary medicine. This article discusses variations and

comparisons of these techniques with different suture patterns, suture materials, types of stapling equipment, and staple sizes along with benefits of surgical reinforcement techniques and leak testing. In addition, a minimally invasive surgical approach for gastrointestinal surgery is discussed briefly. This article also briefly highlights current research under way in determining more accurate means of assessing intestinal tissue viability, because determining when and where to resect compromised, and potentially devitalized, intestine is of utmost importance for patient outcomes.

This article provides a review with a focus on clinical updates in treating patients with surgical parathyroid or thyroid disease. Primary hyperparathyroidism is a common cause of hypercalcemia. Patients are older and often asymptomatic, and urinary stones and urinary tract infection are common. Surgical treatment is recommended with an excellent prognosis. Thyroid tumors in dogs are the most common endocrine neoplasm. Functional thyroid testing, laryngeal examinations, and regional lymphadenectomy should be considered during surgery, along with use of vessel-sealing devices to mitigate hemorrhage. Long-term outcomes for dogs with advanced disease can be reached, so surgical resection should be an option.

Surgical removal is the standard of care for adrenal tumors greater than 2.0 cm diameter. For tumors smaller than 2.0 cm, imaging techniques evaluating patterns of contrast washout may offer a promising avenue for early identification of adrenal malignancy. Pretreatment of pheochromocytoma with phenoxybenzamine is associated with reduced surgical mortality risk. Surgical technique can be laparoscopic or open, depending on tumor anatomy and the experience of the surgeon. Vascular invasion is a contraindication for a laparoscopic technique. This review provides a summary of minimally invasive and open adrenalectomy techniques, including a discussion of management of vascular invasion and partial cavectomy.

This article is intended to "brush up" on the literature updates for the management of head and neck surgeries, particularly mandibulectomy and maxillectomy. Few new techniques have been described in the past decade in dental and oral oncological surgery. A tendency of developing more aggressive surgical strategies to treat complex oral tumors is evident from the recent veterinary literature and the emerging novel techniques for bone regeneration of maxillofacial defects. In addition, this article also focuses on the basic oral surgical oncology principles, an important part of any maxillofacial surgery.

Minimally invasive surgery continues to be an active area of experimental and clinical research in veterinary medicine. The advances we make in this field correspond to multiple benefits for our patients. New MIS approaches (retroperitoneal, NOTES, robotics) continue to be investigated to provide better visualization and manipulation of important anatomic structures for specific procedures. Increasing the number of MIS techniques available to our patient population is of utmost concern for clinicians and owners and is encouraging exciting new clinical research. New technologies (near-infrared fluorescence, barbed suture, 3D printing) are at the forefront of these developments.

 Video content accompanies this article at http://www.vetsmall. theclinics.com.

Novel approaches and innovations in small animal thoracoscopy are being rapidly developed; this article aims to describe recent updates in commonly performed thoracoscopic procedures, including lung lobectomy, pericardiectomy and pericardial and cardiac neoplasia evaluation, chylothorax treatment, cranial mediastinal mass resection, persistent right aortic arch treatment, and management of pyothorax and primary spontaneous pneumothorax.

Advancements within the field of veterinary surgical oncology are constantly presenting themselves, especially with continued development of comprehensive cancer programs. With the use of more advanced imaging techniques within veterinary medicine, tumor staging is improving and techniques novel to veterinary medicine are being evaluated for potential clinical application. Recommended tumor staging and treatment approach for apocrine gland anal sac adenocarcinoma in dogs has evolved, with the anticipation of good long-term patient outcomes. Preoperative staging for mast cell tumors and recommendations for surgical margins to obtain for wide surgical excision is being reassessed by surgeons.

VETERINARY CLINICS OF NORTH AMERICA: SMALL ANIMAL PRACTICE

FORTHCOMING ISSUES

May 2022
Hot Topics in Small Animal Medicine
Lisa Powell, *Editor*

July 2022
Small Animal Orthopedic Medicine
Felix Duerr and Lindsay Elam, *Editors*

September 2022
Telemedicine
Aaron Smiley, *Editor*

RECENT ISSUES

January 2022
Veterinary Dentistry and Oral Surgery
Alexander M. Reiter, *Editor*

November 2021
Diagnostic Imaging: Point-of-Care Ultrasound
Gregory R. Lisciandro, Jennifer M. Gambino, *Editors*

September 2021
Effective Communication in Veterinary Medicine
Christopher A. Adin, Kelly D. Farnsworth, *Editors*

SERIES OF RELATED INTEREST

Veterinary Clinics of North America: Exotic Animal Practice
https://www.vetexotic.theclinics.com/

Preface

Soft Tissue Surgery: Techniques and Topics for Every Practice and Experience Level

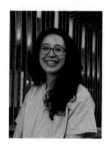

Nicole J. Buote, DVM
Editor

Soft tissue surgery includes topics from every body system and techniques doctors must master and use daily in practice. During my almost 2 decades in veterinary surgery, the complexity of soft tissue cases always appealed to me. It is with these cases that a doctor must meld the skills of a thorough physical examination, diagnostic test interpretation, surgical procedure decision making, and postoperative care management. Clinicians of all experience levels (new graduates to board-certified clinicians) and working in every type of practice (general practice to universities) require updated information on these surgical subjects to ensure the best clinical practice; however, the volume of information published on a yearly basis can be overwhelming. This is why updated issues are so important. The last Soft Tissue issue in 2015 highlighted surgical concerns, including oncologic principles, hepatobiliary surgery, wound management, and minimally invasive procedures, but new data, instruments, and techniques are constantly being generated.

This issue of *Veterinary Clinics of North America: Small Animal Practice* brings together experts in their fields on topics that will resonate with clinicians at all stages of their career, across species and practice types. Wound management and updates in gastrointestinal surgery are just two of the articles in this issue that illustrate significant updates that are far-reaching. Another relevant article concerns new concepts in sterilization that affect not only general practitioners but also specialists as well. This article delves into ovary-sparing procedures and the latest information regarding the effects of timing of sterilization for male and female patients. We also present information on open and minimally invasive surgical procedures, allowing the reader the flexibility to choose the best procedures for their clients as these procedures become more available.

Vet Clin Small Anim 52 (2022) xi–xii
https://doi.org/10.1016/j.cvsm.2021.12.009
0195-5616/22/© 2021 Published by Elsevier Inc.

vetsmall.theclinics.com

Building on the foundation of the previous issue, we provide updates on hepatobiliary, endocrine, and oncologic subjects as well. Specifically, these articles describe and illustrate surgical procedures, compare outcomes wherever possible between surgical techniques, and help guide clinicians through discussions with owners. Risk factors for positive and negative outcomes for Gastric Dilatation and Volvulus (GDV) and new scoring systems for respiratory diseases are also reviewed. The authors hope that this issue will be pulled from the shelf often and will aid clinicians in their daily practice.

I want to thank every contributor for their tireless work for this issue as well as the continual effort of the *Veterinary Clinics of North America: Small Animal Practice* staff, especially Axel, who was a most dedicated partner in creating this issue. These clinicians and staff members dedicated their valuable time to help clinicians, students, pets, and clients, and I am aware of the sacrifices they made regarding family and free time. We hope this issue helps you and your patients for years to come. Enjoy!

Nicole J. Buote, DVM, DACVS-SA
Department of Clinical Sciences–
Small Animal Surgery Section
Soft Tissue Service
Cornell University School of Veterinary Medicine
930 Campus Road
Ithaca, NY 14853, USA

E-mail address:
Njb235@cornell.edu

Updates in Wound Management and Dressings

Nicole J. Buote, DVM, DACVS-SA

KEYWORDS

- Wound healing • Wound management • Topical wound treatments
- Fish skin dressing • Bioelectric dressing • Leeches
- Regenerative medicine wound treatments • Bandaging

KEY POINTS

- Knowing the phases of wound healing and their typical progression are crucial in surveillance of progression and treating wounds with appropriate management strategies.
- Multiple patient and wound-related factors can complicate wound healing. If these factors are not considered, delays in healing may turn an uncomplicated wound into a chronic nonhealing wound.
- Negative pressure wound therapy improves wound healing by 5 known mechanisms and can be used by multiple different techniques for open and closed wounds.
- New treatments under investigation include fish skin application, photobiomodulation, and bioelectric dressings. Treatments such as low-level laser therapy, hyperbaric oxygen therapy, stem cell, and platelet-rich plasma injections continue to be studied with mixed results.

BACKGROUND

Introduction

Wound management is an ever-changing field in veterinary medicine with the advent of new cellular treatments and new topical dressings occurring all the time. The care of patients with wounds is performed by veterinarians of all experience levels and across the world with each locale enduring unique challenges. There are differences in wound healing depending on causation, comorbidities, and species that must always be taken into account and owners' finances and availability of care also play significant roles in management decisions. To choose the most beneficial treatment, a thorough understanding of the phases of wound healing is a necessity as each treatment is specifically tailored to benefit certain phases. While this chapter will not discuss the initial management of wounds (clipping, cleaning, flushing, debridement, and so forth), it will provide a brief review of the phases of wound healing, specific anatomic and patient considerations, and species differences. The majority of the chapter will then focus on innovative treatment modalities and dressings and when best to use them.

Department of Clinical Sciences, Small Animal Surgery Soft Tissue Section, Cornell University School of Veterinary Medicine, 930 Campus Road, Ithaca, NY 14853, USA

Vet Clin Small Anim 52 (2022) 289–315
https://doi.org/10.1016/j.cvsm.2021.12.001
0195-5616/22/© 2021 Elsevier Inc. All rights reserved.

BASIC PRINCIPLES OF WOUND HEALING

The phases of wound healing are a continuum with overlapping phases commonly occurring (**Table 1**). It is also important to note that within one wound there may be areas undergoing different phases at the same time. An exhaustive discussion of the phases can be found in other references[1–4] but a brief synopsis follows.

Inflammatory Phase

This phase begins at the time of wounding and continues until the debridement phase begins, usually at 6 to 12 hours postinitial injury. The first action in this phase is vaso-constriction due to the release by endothelial cells of catecholamines (epinephrine and norepinephrine) and prostaglandins.[5,6] The primary role of vasoconstriction is to decrease blood loss from the wound, but this is reversed to a vasodilatory state within minutes to allow for the influx of platelets, and white and red blood cells to fill and clean the wound. Increased vascular permeability allows for cytokine and growth factor release from activated platelets to encourage chemotaxis of inflammatory cells. The release of thromboplastin initiates the extrinsic pathway of the clotting cascade and platelet aggregation. Fibrin cross-linking leads to primary clot formation within the

Table 1
Phases of healing and the cell types involved

Phase	Cell Type	Action
Inflammatory phase	Injured endothelial cells	release of catecholamines → vasoconstriction → vasodilation
	Injured endothelial cells	release thromboplastin to initiate extrinsic clotting cascade
	Activated platelets	cytokine & growth factor release → migration of white blood cells into the wound
Debridement phase	Neutrophils	degeneration releases enzymes and free radicals that kill bacteria and break down debris
	Monocytes/Macrophages	synthesize and secrete growth factors for tissue formation Stimulate angiogenesis and matrix production
Repair/Proliferation phase		
Fibroplasia	Fibroblasts	migrate into fibrin clot and proliferate Collagen and elastin synthesis
	Macrophages	stimulate migration of fibroblasts
Angiogenesis	Existing vascular endothelial cells	migrate into wound behind fibroblasts giving tissue red color *granulation tissue = new capillaries, fibroblasts, fibrous tissue & extracellular matrix
Epithelialization	Basal epithelial cells keratinocytes	migrate from edges, proliferate, and differentiate to form the new basement membrane
	Myofibroblasts	contraction of the wound edges
Maturation/Remodeling	Epithelium	collagen becomes thicker and more cross-linked
	Myofibroblasts	continued contraction

wound bed. The end of this phase is generally considered when white blood cells begin to enter the wound to begin debridement.

Debridement Phase

In this phase, neutrophils and monocytes migrate into the wound bed due to increased vascular permeability and phagocytose organisms and debris contaminating the wound. When neutrophils degenerate, they release enzymes and free radicals that kill the bacteria and break down the debris. Monocytes transform into macrophages and synthesize and secrete growth factors necessary for tissue formation and remodeling. Macrophages also stimulate angiogenesis and matrix production in wounds.[7] Exudate is the hallmark of this phase and can be septic or nonseptic (**Fig. 1**).

Repair/proliferation Phase

This phase is typically considered to include 3 distinct processes all overlapping in time: fibroplasia, angiogenesis, and epithelialization. During fibroplasia, fibroblasts originating from undifferentiated mesenchymal cells at the border of the wound begin to migrate into the fibrin clot. Fibroblast proliferation is stimulated by macrophages, cytokines, growth factors, and wound environment factors such as pH and oxygen content. Fibroblasts are also responsible for collagen and elastin synthesis. Usually, around day 5 postinjury tension acting on the wound will begin to reorient the disorganized fibroblasts, new blood vessels, and matrix parallel to the wound edges. Collagen content continues to increase in the wound bed until 2 to 3 weeks postinjury.

Angiogenesis is stimulated by cytokines and growth factors such as fibroblast growth factor, vascular endothelial cell growth factor, endothelial growth factor,

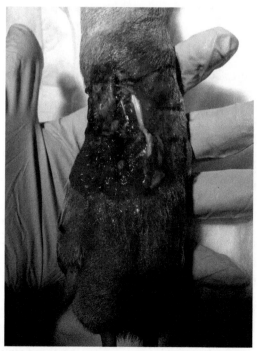

Fig. 1. Photograph of an exudative wound caused by self-trauma before cleaning.

and TGF-B. New capillaries give granulation tissue, its red color (**Fig. 2**). The formation of visible granulation tissue usually takes at least 4 to 5 days postinjury and is necessary for wound contraction as it acts as a scaffold for epithelial cell migration. Healthy granulation tissue is resistant to infection and has no nerve endings.

Epithelialization is the last component of this phase of healing and begins when keratinocytes begin to migrate across the granulation tissue. Epithelial cells are stimulated to proliferate by the secretion of cytokines and growth factors (endothelial growth factor, TGF-alpha) from platelets and macrophages. Epithelial migration continues until cells come in contact with each other across the wound bed (contact inhibition). Myofibroblasts play a central role in the contraction of the wound during this phase. Contraction is important as it is a principle factor in closing the wound but it can be associated with deleterious effects as well such as excessive scar tissue formation and contractures.[8] The newly formed epithelial tissue is devoid of hair follicles or glands and is usually quite thin and fragile (**Fig. 3**).

Maturation/Remodeling Phase

This phase begins approximately 1 week after the initial injury but lasts several months to years. During this time, the newly formed skin becomes stronger as the collagen fibers become thicker and more cross-linked. They orient along lines of tension of the body and myofibroblasts at the wound edges continue to contract to decrease the scar over time. The scar will eventually reach a strength that is 80% of the original tissue before injury.

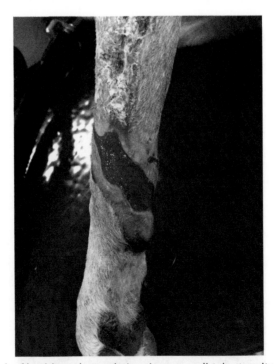

Fig. 2. Photograph of healthy red granulation tissue on a distal extremity wound on a dog. The wound had been managed to this point with NPWT.

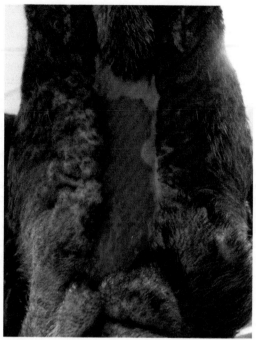

Fig. 3. Photograph of ventral chin wound in different phases of healing. Epithelialization (new skin formation) is seen at edges as light pink fragile skin. Granulation tissue is present in the middle of the wound. Contraction is occurring to slowly reduce the size of this wound.

CONSIDERATIONS FOR WOUND HEALING

It is important to not only consider the cause of the wound or visual findings but also the chronicity of the wound, patient comorbidities and the location as these factors will play a large role in the prognosis for the patient. The difference between acute and chronic wounds is not only the potential increase in bacterial load but also the change in inflammatory cytokines found in wound fluid.[9,10] An excess in matrix metalloproteinases and serine proteinases leads to a breakdown of the extracellular matrix and can halt the progression of the wound healing.

PATIENT COMORBIDITIES/FACTORS AFFECTING WOUND HEALING

Many different patient-related factors affect wound healing including age, preexisting medical conditions, and medications/treatments the patient has or is receiving (**Table 2**). While research is mixed regarding the effects of aging on wound healing, there is a reduction in dermal thickness and decreased microcirculation as aging progresses.[2,11] It is likely that most effects seen in elderly dogs are due to concurrent disease processes, but delayed healing should still be planned for and primary closure pursued whenever possible for patients in this category. Wound-related factors include the amount and type of tissue damage, the presence of infection and foreign debris, and anatomic location of the injury.

Metabolic Diseases

While veterinary patients do suffer from many metabolic diseases, they do not smoke cigarettes or drink alcohol which can account for serious complications in wound

Table 2 Patient considerations for wound healing	
Age	Reduction in dermal thickness, decreased microcirculation
Comorbidities	Diabetes, Cushings, Liver disease, Immune-mediated diseases (IMHA, ITP), malnutrition, kidney disease, neoplasia
Medications	Steroids, NSAIDs, chemotherapy
Radiation therapy to the site	fibrotic microangiopathy

healing in humans. We also do not see vascular diseases (atherosclerosis and thrombosis) as commonly in our pet population. The common metabolic disease we encounter include diabetes mellitus, hyperadrenocorticism, kidney, and liver disease.[2,12] These diseases are theorized to delay wound healing by decreasing the inflammatory response to wounds, which impairs chemotaxis of inflammatory cells and reduces bacterial destruction. However, clear causation has yet to be seen as wound healing is multifactorial. While malnutrition can easily affect wound healing, especially in patients with neoplasia, but this is not as common a phenomenon in veterinary medicine. Nutritional status is especially important for the healing of highly exudative wounds such as burns and all efforts should be made to keep patients' total protein above 2.0 g/dL.

Medications and Treatments

Many medications can affect wound healing; therefore, we will briefly mention the most relevant to veterinary medicine. The most common medication that can delay wound healing is steroids. Glucocorticoids cause epidermal and granulation tissue atrophy, impair macrophage activity, fibroblast proliferation, and collagen synthesis, and they inhibit the synthesis of matrix metalloproteinases. All of these actions delay wound healing and reduce wound tensile strength and are time and dose dependent.[2,13,14] Not surprisingly nonsteroidal antiinflammatory medications have also been shown to have an effect on wound healing because they suppress the inflammatory phase.[2,15] This class of medication is commonly used in veterinary medicine for pain relief from trauma and surgery but considerations to the potentially significant delay in wound healing should be weighed. Chemotherapeutic agents may also result in delays in wound healing owing to their mechanism of action. As they attack rapidly dividing cells, through cytotoxic (nitrogen mustards and methylating agents), antiproliferative (microtubule stabilizers, DNA synthesis inhibitors, and antiangiogenic agents), or antimetabolic (folic acid synthesis inhibitors) mechanisms, wound healing is inhibited. All of these pathways are executed by epithelial, fibroblast, and white blood cells during normal wound healing and therefore, wound strength and rate are affected.[16]

Radiation therapy affects tissue, fibroblasts, and growth factor production, as well as local vasculature.[17] The decrease in vasculature at a radiated site is due to a process called fibrotic microangiopathy. This is theorized to decrease oxygen content to below what is needed for normal wound healing.[18,19] Recommendations currently are to radiate before surgery if you can remove that region with your definitive procedure or to wait until incisions are well healing if we are planning to radiate the site postoperatively.

Immunosuppression/Cancer

Immune-mediated diseases such as immune-mediated hemolytic anemia, thrombocytopenia, and erosive polyarthritis have abnormal inflammatory responses and therefore, atypical wound healing responses, but it may also be that the treatments for these diseases (glucocorticoids and chemotherapeutic agents) are what truly delay wound healing. Delayed healing in patients with cancer may be seen with cancer related malnutrition or due to the chronic inflammation and dysregulation of proliferation and angiogenesis pathways seen with neoplastic processes.[2,20,21]

WOUND FACTORS

Wound-related considerations usually take center stage when assessing for treatment options and prognosis for healing (**Table 3**). Whereby on the body the wound occurred, how much damage was experienced, and the presence of infection or foreign material are the most relevant factors to consider.

Anatomic Considerations

When discussing anatomic considerations related to wound healing 3 factors are the most important for surgical planning and prognosis. The location of the wound on the body, the amount of motion the wound will undergo and the available skin in the region and its elasticity. Location is clearly significant as there is no extra skin or subcutaneous tissues overlying the limbs, head, or tail and the inguinal and axillary regions can be prone to complications due to inherent dead space and motion (**Fig. 4**). Motion is inherent in certain sites on the body, such as over joints, the tail, and the oral cavity. In areas whereby weight-bearing will be anticipated bandages are commonly used but motion can occur within the bandage if it is not applied properly. Tension of the skin in the area of the wound should be assessed preoperatively. Pinching and moving the available skin while the patient is anesthetized will allow the surgeon to determine whether a primary closure is even possible. Multiple tension-relieving suture patterns and techniques are available to aid in tricky closure, but some wounds are simply too large to close initially.[3,4] Different breeds and species have varied elasticity to their skin. Cats, for example, have very elastic skin that can be easily stretched to close large wounds. Certain dog breeds with thick nonelastic skin will be much more challenging to address surgically. Changes in tension during normal range of motion should always be assessed before definitive closure so that appropriate surgical steps or postoperative management strategies (bandages, hobbles, and so forth) can be used. Excessive motion and tension can lead to dehiscence, damaged blood supply, and eventual necrosis of the skin. If excessive tension is applied circumferentially (limbs, tail, and so forth), disruption in vascular supply and lymphatic drainage can occur causing congestion and swelling of the limb (**Fig. 5**). Advanced therapeutics such as negative pressure wound therapy (NPWT) (discussed later in this chapter) can be used to decrease tension and medicinal leech therapy can be effectively used for constrictive swelling.[22]

Table 3	
Wound-related consideration for wound healing	
Anatomic location	Extremities, head, tail, oral cavity, inguinal, axillary regions
Motion	Joints, tails, weight-bearing surfaces
Tension	Related to motion, dependent on patient skin elasticity and thickness
Extent of tissue damage	nonviable tissue, damage to perfusion
Infection	produce inflammatory mediators/cytokines, trigger cell death
Implants	sensitive to biofilm production

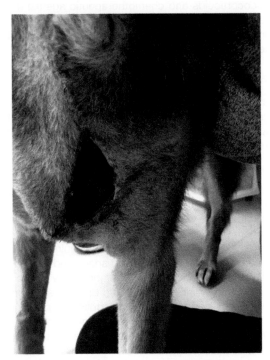

Fig. 4. Photograph of open wound at axilla. Due to constant motion, this wound dehisced multiple times after attempted closure and was eventually managed as an open wound and allowed to heal by second intention.

Tissue Damage

The severity of tissue damage is usually the first physical examination finding that doctors assess during the initial evaluation. Due to the complex nature of wounds and various injuries that can occur (crushing, degloving, puncture, and so forth), the full extent of damage is not always clear. This is easily described with the "tip of the iceberg" analogy. It is extremely important for client communications to include a discussion of the risk of ongoing tissue destruction due to damage to microcirculation or ongoing inflammatory mediators. The amount of damage can be assessed for the amount of tissue that is missing or clearly nonviable (black/gray, leather-like) and the amount that may have decreased or damaged perfusion. Clearly nonviable tissue **(Fig. 6)** must be debrided but tissue with reduced but present perfusion should be maintained if possible. A healthy blood supply is required for normal wound healing. Poor perfusion can be due to trauma to the vascular supply, systemic factors such as hypotension or hypovolemia, or comorbidities (diabetes).

Crush and wrenching injuries, most commonly seen with bite wounds, can severely compromise the blood supply to the region surrounding the obvious wound. In these cases, wounds can be addressed satisfactorily initially only to have ongoing tissue loss hours to days later as the true extent of the damage becomes evident. Oxygen delivery to wound beds and healing tissues is paramount to a smooth recovery and is affected by intercapillary distances and peripheral vasoconstriction more than the patients packed cell volume.[2] Because of this hyperbaric oxygen therapy (HBOT)

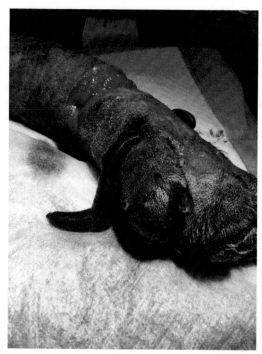

Fig. 5. Photographs of a constrictive wound from a bandage with distal limb swelling. Two leeches were applied to this patient's paw to aid in venous constriction.

has been recommended for various wounds in human and veterinary medicine. As we will discuss later in the chapter, the evidence is not consistent with regard to HBOT's efficacy.

Infection/Foreign Debris/Implants

The classifications of wound based on their contamination levels are thoroughly detailed elsewhere[1–3] but infection and debris within wounds are an important factor

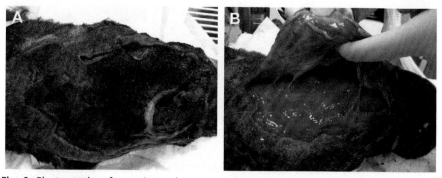

Fig. 6. Photographs of a patient who sustained a rattlesnake bit to ventral chin & neck weeks before presentation. Patient is anesthetized with nose to the right. (*A*) ventral surface of chin with clear demarcation of necrotic tissue. (*B*) when the tissue was gently lifted away from chin, thick exudate is present and visible muscle seen deep into the wound.

relating to treatment and prognosis. The appropriate treatment of wounds depends on differentiating between clean, contaminated, and infected. Clean and clean-contaminated wounds should heal routinely with no/minimal prophylactic antibiosis if the animal is otherwise healthy and tissue damage is minimal. Contaminated wounds have obvious debris and or presumed bacteria present in numbers lower than 10^5 per gram of tissue. Infected wounds (**Fig. 7**) have a higher bacterial load and usually illustrate a host response (redness, pain, swelling, exudate). Bacteria produce inflammatory mediators that interfere with multiple steps of the healing process as well trigger cell death in the surrounding tissue.[23–25] Any patient with visible debris or exudate should undergo thorough lavage and debridement before any attempt at closure is performed. The most common closure times for infected wounds are after the inflammatory and debridement phases when healthy granulation tissue is present. The presence of implants in wounds can complicate healing due to the possibility of biofilm production in the face of bacterial contamination. Successful healing of wounds with implants has been documented, however, but advanced and lengthy healing processes are necessary.[26]

SPECIES DIFFERENCES

Differences between cats and dogs are highly important with regards to wound healing (**Box 1**). If ever there was an aspect of veterinary medicine whereby the adage "Cats aren't small dogs" rings true it is with wound management. Dogs and cats have differences in their vascular anatomy with dogs having a greater density of collateral subcutaneous trunk vessels.[27–29] This increase in density leads to an increase in tissue perfusion and therefore faster healing. Studies have shown that primarily closed incisions on cats are only half as strong as dog wounds by day 7 postinjury and cats have decreased cutaneous perfusion compared with dogs during this time.[27] When second intention healing in cats was studied, less granulation tissue developed compared with dogs and it was located peripherally in the wound as compared centrally in dogs. Granulation tissue also seemed earlier for dogs (4.5 days vs 6.3 days) compared with cats with the complete granulation of the wound bed not occurring

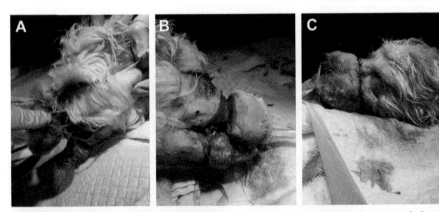

Fig. 7. Photographs of a patient who suffered from a malicious constrictive injury (a leash was placed for many weeks to muzzle the dog). (*A*) Patient anesthetized. Obvious exudate is present at the maxillary lip but the extent of wound is difficult to assess. (*B*) After clipping and cleaning the full extent is now visible. Full-thickness skin wound with evidence of some granulation tissue present on the maxillary lip and nasal skin defect. (*C*) Primary closure of maxillary/nasal skin wound.

Box 1	
Differences between dogs and cats in wound healing	
Anatomy	Dogs have higher density of collateral subcutaneous trunk vessels
Primary closure incisions	breaking strength 50% less at 7 d in cats (equal by 14 d)
	Decreased skin perfusion during the first week of healing in cats
Second intention healing	
Granulation	Cats: less granulation tissue, peripheral location, granulation tissue took a mean of 6.3 d to seem and a mean of 19 d to cover the wound
	Dogs: more granulation tissue, central location, granulation tissue took a mean of 4.5 d to appear and a mean of 7.5 to cover the wound
Epithelialization	Cats: only 13% of the wound bed area was re-epithelialized by day 14
	Dogs: 44% of the wound bed area was re-epithelialized by day 14

for cats until a mean of 19 days (compared with dogs 7.5 days). Effects on epithelialization and contraction were also seen with a marked difference between epithelialization at 14 days with a mean of 44% of the canine wound areas re-epithelialized compared with just 13% of the feline wounds. The slow rate of granulation tissue formation has been theorized to increase contraction and healing times in cats (**Fig. 8**). Another study determined the removal of subcutaneous tissue in either species was associated with a significant decrease in rates of granulation tissue formation and

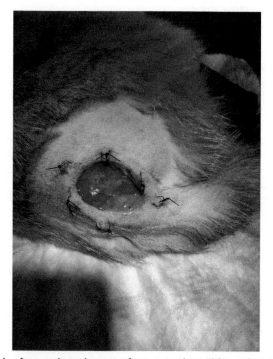

Fig. 8. Photograph of wound on dorsum of cat near the tail base that is being managed with a tie over bandage. Wound seems clean but no evidence of granulation tissue is yet present. This is 7 days after the initial presentation and debridement.

contraction, but this was seen more dramatically in cats.[28] Careful debridement of surrounding tissue, especially subcutaneous fat should be performed with cats to reduce the devitalization of the remaining skin.

UPDATE ON WOUND MANAGEMENT STRATEGIES

The following updates will summarize the mechanism of action and previous literature regarding each modality as well as new research and application advice. A brief outline of what phase of healing each modality can be found in **Table 4**.

NEGATIVE PRESSURE WOUND THERAPY

NPWT has been used in veterinary patients successfully for many years, especially in the realm of traumatic wounds and oncologic reconstructions. An exhaustive discussion of the mechanism of action of NPWT is beyond the scope of this article but can be found in numerous other veterinary resources.[2,30] Briefly, NPWT has 5 main effects which aid in wound healing:

1. withdraw wound exudate
2. improve the skins' elasticity by applying mechanical strain to bring edges together
3. increase perfusion to the wound as far as 3 cm away from the foam[31]
4. reduce interstitial edema
5. and decrease the inflammatory response to injury by removing detrimental cytokines such as matrix metalloproteinases.

NPWT typically requires an open-cell polyurethane or polyvinyl alcohol foam to be placed within or over the surface of a wound. The active suction device is attached to this foam and effectively seals the wound under an occlusive bandage (**Fig. 9**). In some cases, specialized tubing attaches this bandage to a vacuum pump to allow for either continuous or intermittent suction to be applied to the wound. Based on earlier studies, a pressure of 125 mm Hg at a continuous rate is the most common method. Commonly found suction tubing attached to surgical suction units can and is also used and in the authors, experience affords excellent outcomes with less expense.[32]

The clinical benefits of NPWT include reduced time to granulation tissue and healing compared with other topical dressings.[30] In humans studies have shown an increase in blood supply and granulation tissue formation, and a reduction in bacterial load (most likely due to the hypoxic environment).[33,34] NPWT has been used for open wounds, planned oncologic reconstructions (skin flaps or grafts) and incisional protection. One of the major benefits to NPWT is the reduction in required bandage changes for patients and clients and these bandages are typically well-tolerated by patients including cats and exotic animals when the pressure is at a continuous rate. NPWT is most appropriate during the inflammatory and debridement phases of healing when exudate is expected. These bandages should be kept in place for 2 to 3 days at a time which eliminates daily or twice daily bandage changes that can be necessary during this time to avoid the maceration of tissues due to.[35] While some veterinarians are able to send the vacuum units home with patients, other facilities do require hospitalization for NPWT management which can be considered a disadvantage. Application of an NPWT can be performed under moderate sedation if the wound has already been debrided or general anesthesia if surgical debridement is necessary. **Table 5** reviews the steps of application with different options highlighted at each step.

Table 4
Wound dressings, mechanisms, and best time to apply

Dressing Name	Proposed Mechanism of Action	Application times Tested
NWPT	1. withdraw wound exudate 2. improve the skin's elasticity 3. increase perfusion to the wound 4. reduce interstitial edema 5. removes detrimental cytokines (MMPs).	Contaminated/Infection open wounds in inflammatory or debridement phase Free skin grafts or flaps Primarily closed at-risk incisions
Tilapia/Cod Skin grafts	1. induction of epidermal growth factor and fibroblast growth factor expression 2. high levels of type 1 collagen 3. stimulate proliferation and differentiation of fibroblasts and keratinocyte	After debridement phase on healthy granulation tissue to stimulate epithelialization Must be used on clean wound
Low-level laser	1. photon activation of cytochrome oxidase leads to energy production and synthesis of proteins involved in cellular repair 2. possible effects of radiation on cellular differentiation and prostaglandin synthesis	After inflammatory phase to encourage granulation tissue or epithelialization Primary closed incisions
Photobio modulation	1. Stimulate cellular transduction pathways 2. activation of photoacceptors in cells/tissue	Primary closed incisions
HBOT	1. Increased dissolved O2 in blood 2. Increasing tissue oxygen perfusion 3. barometric effects 4. immunomodulation 5. Antioxidant effects	During all phases of healing Best during the repair phase Primary closed incisions
Stem cells	1. proliferate and differentiate into different cell lines 2. anti-inflammatory 3. pain modulation 4. immunomodulation	During all phases of healing Topical or Injections
Platelet-rich	1. stimulate fibroblast proliferation and migration 2. recruits mesenchymal cells 3. improves extracellular matrix synthesis 4. antimicrobial 5. anti-inflammatory 6. pain-modulating	During all phases of healing Topicals or Injections

(continued on next page)

Table 4 (continued)		
Dressing Name	**Proposed Mechanism of Action**	**Application times Tested**
Bioelectric	1. Mimics transepithelial resting electric potential stimulating cell migration and epithelialization 2. antibacterial properties 3. prevention of biofilm formation 4. optimization of the moist wound environment	After the inflammatory and debridement phase

Recent Investigations

Silver impregnated foam is available for use with and without NPWT devices and may decrease bacterial load and maceration of the peri-wound tissue.[36] A prospective randomized control trial by Nolff and colleagues reported on the outcomes of 26 clinical dogs treated with NPWT compared with a polyurethane silver-impregnated foam dressing.[37] In this study, dogs were matched by the underlying cause of wound, duration of wound presence, wound size, location, time to closure, bacterial load, and complications. Total time to closure was significantly shorter (14.2 days vs 28.6 days), wound size decreased significantly and there was less progression of infection in the NPWT group compared with the silver-impregnated foam group. The effective control of local infection in the NPWT was the most important factor associated with a decreased complication rate and an overall decreased cost for this group when compared with the silver-impregnated foam group. While the local effects of NPWT on bacterial load are controversial,[38] a study looking at the effects on antibiotic tissue or plasma concentrations under vacuum pressure in an experimental model did not illustrate a benefit.[39]

Incisional Negative Pressure Wound Therapy

The benefits of NPWT for traumatic wounds and reconstructive surgeries such as skin grafts and flaps are well documented but studies investigating the use with primary closure procedures have also been reported.[40] A case report in a dog with a history of chronic incisional complications and abscess formation reported the use of a

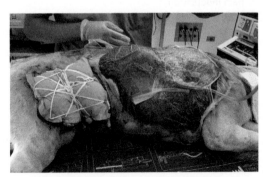

Fig. 9. Photograph of NPWT bandage applied to the lateral aspect of patient who sustained significant burns.

Table 5
Steps for Application of Negative Pressure Wound bandage.

Step	Guidelines	Tip
1	Prepare the skin and wound/flap/graft/ incision: Make sure the surrounding skin in clipped, clean and dry.	Consider alcohol application to the edges for better adherence of the occlusive dressing
2	Cut foam to the desired shape/size and apply directly to the wound. Foam comes in standard or silver-impregnated for added antibacterial properties.	You can place simple interrupted sutures (3–0 to 2–0 m onofilament nonabsorbable) or skin staples to the wound edge to secure the foam to the wound.
3	Place the impermeable dressing over the foam and cut a hole to attached specialized disc/tubing.	Alternative 1: Place specialized disc/tubing directly on the foam and then place the impermeable dressing over and around the tubing for extra security. Alternative 2: Place a red rubber catheter into the foam through a small incision and place impermeable dressing over and around the catheter.
4	Attach the tubing to the vacuum and set pressure. Watch for characteristic contraction of the foam and listen for any leaks.	Have additional strips impermeable dressing available to seal any leaks once vacuum pressure applied.
5	If desired, place additional soft padded bandage for patient comfort and security of the vacuum tubing.	Consider creating a window to assess the foam frequently for evidence of loss of pressure.

commercially available device (Prevena, 3M + KCI) after debridement and primary closure. This patient was managed in a staged procedure with open NPWT after abscess removal for 2 days and then INPWT for 7 days after primary closure.[41] A systematic review of the mechanism of action and outcomes of INPWT included 2 experimental prospective animal (pig) studies. Results reported a decrease of incisional infections, hematoma formation, and reoperation rates for human patients undergoing INPWT but data on dehiscence, skin necrosis, rehospitalization, and cost savings were inconclusive.

NPWT Without Foam or Gauze Dressing

NPWT is typically performed with filler dressings such as polyurethane and polyvinyl alcohol foams, or gauze as the contact layer. This layer is permeable allowing for airflow and suction to reach all areas of the wound, but tissue can grow into the material causing damage when it is removed, and fragments of the material can also break off becoming embedded. A recent study reported the development of a novel single-layer membrane dressing to deliver NPWT.[42] In this experimental porcine study, the novel device decreased wound area, and inflammation and increased viable granulation tissue after 4 days of use. Clinical studies must be performed before recommendations for this device can be made.

FISH SKIN DRESSINGS: TILAPIA/COD

One of the most promising treatments to be reported in few years is the use of fish skin grafts for the treatment of burns and other wounds (**Fig. 10**). First reported for the treatment of a burn in a pediatric patient, multiple randomized controlled studies

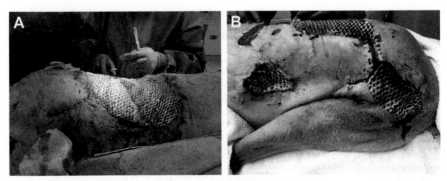

Fig. 10. Photographs of tilapia skin applied to open wounds created by unknown trauma. (A) Large wound on dorsum and right lateral flank. (B) Smaller wounds on the right lateral thigh and thorax.

have since been published describing multiple benefits.[43–46] In one study with 62 human burn patients randomized to tilapia skin graft dressing or conventional dressing with silver sulfadiazine cream 1%, faster re-epithelialization, reduced pain scores and therefore reduced pain medication administration and fewer bandage changes were required in the tilapia group.[44] Morphologic studies on tilapia skin found many similarities to human skin (a deep dermis of thick organized collagen fibers arranged in similar orientation) but with a higher amount of type I collagen and a high tensile strength.[47] One proposed mechanism of action of tilapia skin is the induction of epidermal growth factor and fibroblast growth factor expression from the tilapia collagen, stimulating the proliferation and differentiation of fibroblasts and keratinocytes.[48] Peptides found in tilapia skin (piscidin 3 and 4) have also been shown to have antimicrobial activity.[49,50] Another benefit to tilapia or fish skin is the excellent adherence it has to wound surfaces which allows for a moist environment and decreases the chance of bacterial colonization.[46]

The method for the application of tilapia grafts in veterinary medicine has not been published but based on human studies and the authors' experience using it steps are provided in **Box 2** and **Fig. 11**. There have been multiple human studies reporting different sterilization and storage techniques for fish skin.[45] The wound should not have active purulent or necrotic debris present at the time of graft placement. Specific preparation and sterilization techniques (glycerolization, irradiation) have been used in human studies on tilapia skin grafts, but less stringent techniques have been anecdotally utilized in veterinary medicine. These fish grafts seem to have a noninfectious microbiota which may allow their successful use without irradiation but experimental and clinical studies in veterinary medicine need to be performed. No adverse effects from tilapia grafts have been reported in people or in animal studies to date and decreased cost and anxiety in patients and medical professionals due to fewer hospital visits and bandage changes mean this treatment may be very useful for wound management. A study on the collagen hydrogels created from tilapia skin significantly accelerated wound healing in deep second degree burns in a mouse model.[51]

North Atlantic cod skin grafts (Kerecis) have also been reported to speed epithelialization in multiple human studies.[52,53] One prospective double-blind biopsy wound study compared these grafts to human amnionic/chorionic membrane dressings and found faster healing time with no difference in local inflammation or irritation.[53] These commercially available dressings have the benefit of being freeze-dried with a shelf life of 3 years. The advantages of these dressings according to earlier studies

---

Box 2
Steps for Application of Fish Skin to Wounds (Fig. 11)

1. Lavage and clean the wound to be treated. (No necrotic debris or active purulent exudate).

2. Place sterile hydrogel or wound gel in a thin layer on the wound to ensure adherence to the fish skin graft.

3. Place more hydrogel over the fish skin graft to ensure moisture is retained.

4. Place absorbent hydrophilic foam or gauze over the fish skin graft and then cover with a soft padded bandage.

5. Check bandage every 2 to 3 days. If excessive exudate is present, remove graft, cleanse and reapply new graft. If graft well-adhered and minimal exudate present at foam/gauze, reapply hydrogel over graft and new absorbent layer (foam/gauze) and rebandage.

6. To remove fish skin to evaluate wound/skin below saline or tap water can be used to gently break down material. Petrolatum jelly can also be used to loosen the graft from the wound/skin.

---

include the retention of Omega 3 fatty acids which have been shown to create a bacterial barrier and pain-modulating effects.[53] As more clinicians gain experience with these products future research needs to investigate the safety and efficacy of these grafts in veterinary medicine.

LOW-LEVEL LASER

Low-level laser therapy (LLLT) or cold laser therapy is considered any device which emits less than 10W of power when applied to the tissue. The use of these devices for accelerating wound healing has been investigated but the exact mechanism behind the cellular modulation is unknown.[54] A proposed mechanism posits photon activation of cytochrome oxidase leading to energy production and synthesis of proteins involved in cellular repair. Other possibilities include possible effects of the radiation on cellular differentiation and prostaglandin synthesis.[55,56] There are wide

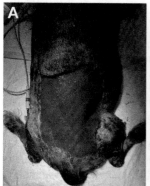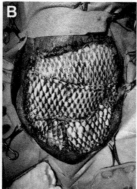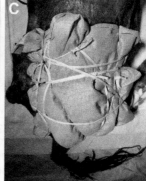

Fig. 11. Photographs of tilapia fish skin graft application. (*A*) Dorsum wound after debridement with NPWT in preparation for tilapia graft. (*B*) Application of thawed tilapia grafts. The grafts were sutured to the edges and sterile hydrogel was applied to keep them moist. (*C*) Tie over bandage applied with the layer of hydrophilic foam and a nonpermeable layer. (Photographs courtesy of Dr. Rosselli.)

disparities in the literature regarding the effects of LLLT for wound healing as the reports use varied machines, treatments, and outcome measures. There are differences between available commercial devices in laser class (I–IV), wavelength, and the energy density they can administer as well. The most commonly used wavelength in studies of LLLT that has shown improvement in wound healing is 635 nm (helium–neon) but an experimental randomized study using a class II He–Ne laser 3 times a week failed to show a benefit in an acute canine wound model over a 21 day period.[54]

A more recent experimental study in dogs prospectively created open and closed wounds that were treated with and without LLLT.[57] This study looked at bilateral flank ovariectomy incisions and bilateral open wounds created by a dermal punch in 10 healthy dogs. The treated sides received LLLT with a class IV laser (980 nm) once daily for 5 days. This study also failed to illustrate the effect of LLLT on the subjective wound healing assessment or wound measurements; however, the control group did have more necrosis and perivascular inflammation on day 7. An in vitro study on the effect of a class IV laser (helium–neon) on the cellular migration and proliferation of cultured canine keratinocytes did show a positive effect.[58] The lack of standardization of wavelength, energy density, and treatment regularity hinder a definitive answer regarding this modality of wound therapy. Future research must be performed to validate the use of LLLT in a clinical setting.

PHOTOBIOMODULATION

A recent addition to the long list of treatments used in veterinary medicine for wound healing is photobiomodulation (PBM) devices which consist of light-emitting devices (LED) that reportedly stimulate cellular transduction pathways. Biological processes are stimulated through the activation of photoacceptors present in many different cell types and tissues. A specific type of PBM called fluorescence photobiomodulation (FPBM) has recently been studied in veterinary medicine.[59] With FPBM, light-absorbing molecules convert the light emitted by the device to broader wavelengths and lower energy which in turn is reported to penetrate the skin and encourage healing.[60,61] When the chromophores in the topical photoconverter (gel) are activated by the LED light source, they release photons at varying wavelengths in the form of fluorescence.

In the study by Salvaggio and colleagues, a novel FPBM device comprised of a blue LED light and a carbopol-based amorphous hydrogel was used in a prospective blinded controlled clinical trial. Ten healthy dogs undergoing orthopedic procedures were enrolled and half of the length of their incisions was treated with the FPBM device, and the other half acted as an internal control. The incisions were treated with the Phovia device (KT-V lamp; Klox Technologies, Laval, Quebec, Canada) for 2 minutes on the first postoperative day and every 3 days after that until day 13. This device delivers a blue light with wavelengths between 440 and 460 nm and a power density ranging between 55 and 129 mW/cm^2. Biopsies performed from each section of the healed incisions on day 13 revealed less inflammation of the dermal layer, complete re-epithelialization, and a larger amount of collagen in the Phovia treated section. No adverse reactions were reported to the photoconverter gel. While other studies have looked at PBM treatments for pyoderma and otitis[62,63] this is the first to look at wound healing. Future studies will need to address the ability of this technology to improve open traumatic and chronic wounds.

HYPERBARIC OXYGEN THERAPY

HBOT necessitates the patient to breath 100% oxygen at an atmospheric pressure greater than 1 atm absolute (ATA) in an airtight room. By inhaling pure oxygen in this environment, the dissolved oxygen in the bloodstream is reported to be up to 15 times that of normal room air (Fio_2 21%). This treatment has been touted for a wide variety of diseases according to the Undersea and Hyperbaric Medical Society but recently several studies have attempted to prospectively investigate its safety and use in veterinary medicine (**Fig. 12**).[64–68] A recent clinical trial of 78 dogs and 12 cats suffering from neurologic, gastrointestinal, hemopoietic, cardiorespiratory and integumentary diseases reported a 33% (76/230) rate of minor adverse effects including head shaking, panting, and swallowing but no major adverse effects associated with HBOT.[65] No comments could be made regarding HBOTs efficacy in this population. The proposed mechanisms of the action of HBOT in these diseases include but are not limited to improving oxygen-carrying capacity in the plasma, increasing tissue oxygen perfusion, barometric effects, immunomodulation, and antioxidant effects. The increase in oxygen perfusion is especially helpful in wounds as it is reported to produce antibacterial effects, increase angiogenesis and growth factor synthesis, and decreases interstitial edema according to different human and animal model studies.

A thorough review on the scientific basis, proposed physiologic mechanisms and possible clinical indications in veterinary wound and trauma patients has been published recently.[66] The varied case reports and retrospective series highlighted in this review and elsewhere are interesting but controlled data objectively comparing outcomes in patients are lacking. A prospective controlled study on HBOT in dogs compared daily HBOT treatments for 7 days after controlled wounds and incisions were created.[67] No differences were seen between control and HBOT groups with regards to wound contraction, epithelialization, subjective wound assessment, histopathology, or culture results. A new area of research is lower pressure lower oxygen hyperbaric treatments (1500 hPa pressure and 26% oxygen concentration in the chamber). A clinical study of 6 dogs compared with 6 controls undergoing hemimastectomy reported subjectively faster healing and fewer complications in dogs treated for 5 consecutive days after surgery.[68] Future research should focus on randomized controlled trials with standardized methodologies to better characterize the true effects of HBOT on clinical patients.

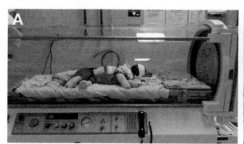 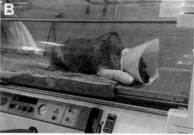

Fig. 12. (HBOT pics Jake, Sissy): Photographs of patients within a hyperbaric oxygen chamber. (*A*) Patient suffering from multiple wounds after being drug behind a truck accident. HBOT was used in this case due to questionable healing and severe edema all over the body. (*B*) Patient sustained a 360° slough of the antebrachium after tumor removal and closure with tourniquet effect. HBOT was used to maximize all chances for healing to avoid amputation and for potential improvement in antibiotic penetration due to ongoing infection. Most patients tolerate the chamber well with light sedation or pain medication administration. (Photographs courtesy of Dr. Lux.)

REGENERATIVE MEDICINE TECHNIQUES
Mesenchymal Stem Cells

Mesenchymal stem cell (MSC) therapy has been the focus of in vitro and in vivo research in both human and veterinary medicine for decades. The proposed benefits to these cells center on their ability to proliferate and differentiate into different cell lines, their antiinflammatory and pain-modulating properties, and immunomodulation. As with much of the data on the other treatments discussed in this chapter, MSC research in veterinary medicine was historically plagued by inconsistent methodologies between studies and anecdotal evidence.[69–72] Recently, however, there have been studies on the safety and efficacy of MSC's on wound healing in dogs.[73,74] One study by Encisco and colleagues, in 24 dogs with acute and chronic wounds compared conventional wound therapy to intradermal (3×10^7 allogeneic adipose MSC in phosphate-buffered saline) and intra-wound (3×10^7 allogeneic adipose MSC in phosphate-buffered saline) injections.[74] Patients received 2 injection treatments 7 days apart as well antibiotics during treatment. The control group had a neomycin/pennywort ointment applied as their wound treatment until healed. Wound size and epithelialization were measured at 7, 30, 90 days postinitiation of treatment and biopsies were performed on day 7 for histologic assessment and gene expression. Serum was also surveyed for both treatment and control patients on days 7 and 30 for cytokine secretion as an indication of an adverse event. Results of this study revealed improved epithelialization at 90 days of the MSC treated wounds, reduced inflammation, and the presence of hair follicles at 7 days in the MSC treated group, upregulation of genes relating to GM-CSF, and appropriate safety as evidenced by the lack of cytokine response.

Platelet-Rich Plasma

Platelet-rich plasma (PRP) has also been investigated in both veterinary and human medicine as a treatment of a range of disease processes including wound healing. PRP is created by the centrifugation of whole blood in a double centrifugation tube/syringe device. Currently, there are no specific veterinary standards regarding the concentration of platelets, amount of white blood cells, or red blood cells allowed in each aliquot or treatment protocol. There are multiple companies with devices on the veterinary market (Arthrex, VetStem Biopharma, ReBound, and so forth) all with different cell preparation techniques. PRP is known to contain cytokines and growth factors that stimulate fibroblast proliferation and migration, recruitment of mesenchymal cells, and extracellular matrix synthesis.[75–77] There have also been studies displaying antimicrobial, anti-inflammatory, and pain-modulating properties to PRP.[77,78] The literature has examples of both improved healing and no difference in the healing of wounds.[76,79] The variation is most likely due to differences in PRP preparation, wound models, treatment protocols and outcome endpoints. The proposed advantages of PRP over other regenerative medicine treatments (MSC's) are the ease of collection and cost-effectiveness of treatment.

Multiple experimental wound studies have been performed in veterinary medicine comparing the results of PRP injections or topical application to conventionally treated wounds in dogs.[75–79] Iacopetti and colleagues, in 2020 reported increased epithelialization and contraction in 6 dogs undergoing 2 topical applications of PRP 15 days apart. While they saw no evidence of adverse effects, there was no control group and the wounds.[76] An experimental study in 5 dogs in which 3 mLs of autologous PRP was injected subcutaneously in one of the 2 wounds created in each dog reported increased epithelialization in the treated wounds at 3 weeks and reduced scar tissue formation.[77] A follow-up study from the same group also reported the results of weekly subcutaneous PRP injections in experimentally created MRSA infected wounds in dogs and found that the treatment wounds had quicker re-epithelialization, more contraction, had decreased bacterial load, and decreased reactive oxidant stress compared with controls.[78]

BIOELECTRIC DRESSING

Bioelectric dressings designed for use in human medicine for diabetic ulcers, pressure sores, and burn injuries have also been used in veterinary medicine for acute and chronic wounds. When skin is injured a change in the transepithelial resting electric potential occurs stimulating cell migration and re-epithelialization.[80,81] Wound exudate provides the conduction medium for microcurrents (2–10 μA) created at the edges of the wound.[82] Because this microcurrent only extends 1–2 mm from the wound edge, large wounds can take a long time to heal. The dressing (**Fig. 13**) reportedly mimics the physiologic currents created at wound edges by generating microcurrents on the wound surface when in the presence of a conductive medium. Physiologic benefits to this dressing have been reported to include: antibacterial properties,[80–84] prevention of biofilm formation,[85] optimization of the moist wound environment, and increases in keratinocyte migration (galvanotaxis)[86] and epithelialization.[87,88] Similar to NPWT and fish skin grafts, these dressings are maintained for longer periods of time as well, decreasing the cost and stress to owners and patients. One bioelectric dressing available to veterinary professionals is the Procellera Antimicrobial wound dressing (Vomaris, Tempe, AZ, USA) consisting of a polyester substrate with embedded elemental silver and zinc microcell batteries.

A literature review of the use, effect, and mechanisms of electrical stimulation in experimentally created cutaneous wounds in animals reported the potential for improved healing with direct current and bioelectric dressings.[82] Some studies reviewed showed a variable effect with faster rates of re-epithelialization, increased wound collagen content and improved angiogenesis but other studies reported no improvement or even deleterious effects. Unsurprisingly, the methods, modality, and polarities in these experiments varied greatly. A case series in 10 client-owned equine patients reported improved wound healing and cosmesis without excessive granulation tissue with the use of a bioelectric dressing.[89] A recent case series in 4

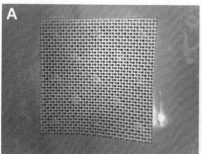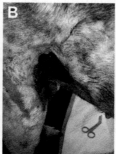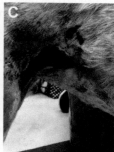

Fig. 13. (*A*) Photograph of commercially available bioelectric dressing with silver and zinc microbatteries embedded in a polyester backing. (*B*) Wound on flank fold before bioelectric dressing application. (*C*) Wound on flank fold after 4 days of bioelectric dressing. A considerable decrease in the width of the wound is seen and there is excessive granulation tissue at the edges which was debrided.

Box 3
Steps for Application of Bioelectric Dressing to Wounds

1. Clean and lavage wound as required by contamination level.

2. Moisten dressing on battery (dot) side with saline, sterile water, or sterile amorphous water-based hydrogel. Hydrogel will not evaporate as quickly, allows dressing to remain in place for 7 days, best for incisions and open wounds (according to company insert). Saline/water-excellent conductive medium but dries out more quickly and will require periodic remoistening, do not over saturate or wound maceration can occur.

3. Place dressing battery (dot) side down on wound. Ensure contact with the wound. If the wound is deep place filler material over the dressing in the wound to hold contact, be sure to include 1–2 cm of dressing overlap of the wound edge.

4. Cover with secondary dressing. If wound is mildly exudative a semiocclusive dressing can be placed (Tegaderm, Opsite, and so forth). If wound is highly exudative place absorptive layer (hydrocolloid foam, gauze, lap sponges, and so forth) as a secondary dressing.

5. Dressing change frequency is determined by the amount of wound exudate produced. The dressing can remain in place for up to 7 days if low-exudative wound. If the wound is highly exudative, dressings can be changed 2–3× a week.

6. To remove the bioelectric dressing if it is adhered to the wound moistens the dressing with sterile saline or water until it can be gently peeled away.

---

dogs and 1 cat also reported positive clinical outcomes in patients with severe traumatic or complex wounds treated with a bioelectric dressing.[83] The authors of this case series conclude the bioelectric dressing benefited wound healing in their case population by generating an electrical field at physiologic levels to induce galvanotaxis (thus improving re-epithelialization) and reduced the bacterial burden and potential for biofilm. Neither of these clinical studies was prospective or randomized and neither included control groups. The author has used these dressings on chronic and infected wounds in clinical cases with success in her practice and anecdotally agrees that epithelialization seems to occur at a faster rate when the dressing is applied to healthy granulation tissue. The steps and tips used for the application of this dressing can be found in **Box 3**.

With the data from experimental and anecdotal case series, bioelectric dressings seem a promising new tool in the treatment of veterinary wound but controlled clinical trials should be performed to determine the best timing (phase of healing) and methodology (dressing change frequency) for their use.

CLINICS CARE POINTS

- NPWT is best applied during the inflammatory and debridement phases of healing or to bolster closed at-risk incisions. This therapy can be applied with and without foam/dressings and with the use of commercial or common surgical suction devices.

- The use of fish skin grafts has been successfully used on veterinary patients for the treatment of large wounds, but an easily accessible preparation method of the fish skin grafts has yet to be published and risks associated with possible infection need to be considered.

- Platelet-rich plasma is a noninvasive treatment option for cutaneous wounds with mixed results. PRP can be injected subcutaneously or used topically and is easier to produce than stem cell therapies with commercially available kits and devices.

- Bioelectric dressings recreate the normal transepithelial potential to induce epithelialization and decrease bacterial contamination. These dressings need to be moistened before application to the wound but can be applied for 4 to 5 days at a time, decreasing the need for bandage changes during the repair phase.

DISCLOSURE

The author has nothing to disclose.

REFERENCES

1. Balsa IM, Culp WTN. Wound care. Vet Clin Small Anim 2015;45:1049–65.
2. Stanley BJ, Cornell K. Wound healing. In: Johnston SA, Tobias KM, editors. Veterinary surgery: small animal. 2nd edition. St. Louis: Elsevier Health Sciences; 2018. p. 132–48.
3. van Hengle T, ter Haar G, Kirpensteijn J. Wound management: a new protocol for dogs and cats. In: Kirpensteijn J, ter Haar G, editors. Reconstructive surgery and wound management of the dog and cat. 1st edition. London: Manson Publishing Ltd; 2013. p. 21–48.
4. Pavletic M. Basic principles of wound management. In: Pavletic M, editor. Atlas of small animal wound management and reconstructive surgery. 3rd edition. West Sussex, UK: Wiley-Blackwell; 2010. p. 31–50.
5. Teller P, White TK. The physiology of wound healing: injury through maturation. Surg Clin North Am 2009;89:599–610.
6. Kanji S, Das H. Advances of stem cell therapeutics in cutaneous wound healing and regeneration. Mediators Inflamm 2017;2017:5217967. https://doi.org/10.1155/2017/5217967.e.
7. Snyder RJ, Lantis J, Kirsner RS, et al. Macrophages: a review of their role in wound healing and their therapeutic use. Wound Rep Reg 2016;24:613–29.
8. Chitturi RT, Balasubramaniam AM, Parameswar RA, et al. The role of myofibroblasts in wound healing, contraction and its clinical implications in cleft palate repair. J Int Oral Health 2015;7:75–80.
9. Widgerow AD. Chronic wound fluid—thinking outside the box. Wound Rep Reg 2011;19:287–91.
10. Dissemond J, Augustin M, Dietlein M, et al. Efficacy of MMP-inhibiting wound dressings in the treatment of chronic wounds: a systematic review. J Wound Care 2020;29:102–18.
11. Norman D. The effects of age-related skin changes on wound healing rates. Rev J Wound Care 2004;13:199–201.
12. Winkler KP. Factors that interfere with wound healing, the Merck veterinary manual. Whitehouse Station, NJ: Merck Sharp & Dohme Corp; 2012. Available at: http://www.merckmanuals.com/vet/emergency_medicine_and_critical_care/wound_management/factors_that_interfere_with_wound_healing.html. [Accessed 21 October 2021].
13. Stephens FO, Hunt TK, Jawetz E, et al. Effect of cortisone and vitamin A on wound infection. Am J Surg 1971;121:569–71.
14. de Almeida TF, de Castro Pires T, Monte-Alto-Costa A. Blockade of glucocorticoid receptors improves cutaneous wound healing in stressed mice. Exp Biol Med (Maywood) 2016;241:353–8.
15. Fairweather M, Heit YI, Buie J, et al. Celecoxib inhibits early cutaneous wound healing. J Surg Res 2015;194:717–24.

16. Laing EJ. Problems in wound healing associated with chemotherapy and radiation therapy. Probl Vet Med 1990;2:433–41.
17. Amsellem P. Complications of reconstructive surgery in companion animals. Vet Clin North Am Small Anim Pract 2011;41:995–1006.
18. Seguin B, McDonald DE, Kent MS, et al. Tolerance of cutaneous or mucosal flaps placed into a radiation therapy field in dogs. Vet Surg 2005;34:214–22.
19. Beyene RT, Derryberry SL, Barbul A. The effect of comorbidities on wound healing. Rev Surg Clin North Am 2020;100:695–705.
20. McCaw DL. The effects of cancer and cancer therapies on wound healing. Rev Semin Vet Med Surg Small Anim 1989;4:281–6.
21. Singh K, Singh K. Carcinogenesis and diabetic wound healing: evidences of parallelism. Rev Curr Diabetes Rev 2015;11:32–45.
22. Buote NJ. The use of medical leeches for venous congestion. A review and case report. Vet Comp Orthop Traumatol 2014;27:173–8.
23. Phan HH, Montero P, Stefanidis D. Non-Healing Wounds. Medical Student Core Curiculum. American College of Surgeons Division of Education Blended Surgical Education and Training for Life® p.1-36. https://www.facs.org/-/media/files/education/core-curriculum/nonhealing_wounds.ashx
24. Anderson K, Hamm RL. Factors that impair wound healing. J Am Coll Clin Wound Spec 2014;4:84–91.
25. Punjataewakupt A, Napavichayanun S, Aramwit P. The downside of antimicrobial agents for wound healing. Eur J Clin Microbiol Infect Dis 2019;38:39–54.
26. Bertran J, Farrell M, Fitzpatrick N. Successful wound healing over exposed metal implants using vacuum-assisted wound closure in a dog. J Small Anim Pract 2013;54:381–5.
27. Bohling MW, Henderson RA, Swaim SF, et al. Cutaneous wound healing in the cat: a macroscopic description and comparison with cutaneous wound healing in the dog. Vet Surg 2004;33:579–87.
28. Bohling MW, Henderson RA, Swaim SF, et al. Comparison of the role of the subcutaneous tissues in cutaneous wound healing in the dog and cat. Vet Surg 2006;35:3–14.
29. Bohling MW, Henderson RA. Differences in cutaneous wound healing between dogs and cats. Vet Clin North Am Small Anim Pract 2006;36:687–92.
30. Stanley BJ. Negative pressure wound therapy. Vet Clin Small Anim 2017;47:1049–65.
31. Nolff MC, Albert R, Reese S, et al. Comparison of negative pressure wound therapy and silver-coated foam dressings in open wound treatment in dogs: a prospective controlled clinical trial. Vet Comp Orthop Traumatol 2018;31:229–38.
32. Buote NJ, Having ME. The use of vacuum-assisted closure in the management of septic peritonitis in six dogs. J Am Anim Hosp Assoc 2012;48:164–71.
33. Morykwas MJ, Argenta LC, Shelton-Brown EI, et al. Vacuum-assisted closure: a new method for wound control and treatment: animal studies and basic foundation. Ann Plast Surg 1997;38:553–62.
34. Morykwas MJ, Faler BJ, Pearce DJ, et al. Effects of varying levels of subatmospheric pressure on the rate of granulation tissue formation in experimental wounds in swine. Ann Plast Surg 2001;47:547–51.
35. Pitt KA, Stanley BJ. Negative pressure wound therapy: experience in 45 dogs. Vet Surg 2014;43:380–7.
36. Kotz P, Fisher J, McCluskey P, et al. Use of a new silver barrier dressing, ALLEVYN Ag in exuding chronic wounds. Int Wound J 2009;6(03):186–94.

37. Nolff MC, Fehr M, Bolling A, et al. Negative pressure wound therapy, silver coated foam dressing and conventional bandages in open wound treatment in dogs. A retrospective comparison of 50 paired cases. Vet Comp Orthop Traumatol 2015; 28:30–8.

38. Nolff MC, Fehr M, Reese S, et al. Retrospective comparison of negative pressure wound therapy and silvercoated foam dressings in open-wound treatment in cats. J Feline Med Surg 2017;19:624–30.

39. Coutin JV, Lanz OI, Magnin-Bissel GC, et al. Cefazolin concentration in surgically created wounds treated with negative pressure wound therapy compared to surgically created wounds treated with nonadherent wound dressings. Vet Surg 2015;44:9–16.

40. Scalise A, Calamita R, Tartaglione C, et al. Improving wound healing and preventing surgical site complications of closed surgical incisions: a possible role of Incisional Negative Pressure Wound Therapy. A systematic review of the literature. Int Wound J 2016;13:1260–81.

41. Nolf MC, Flatz KM, Meyer-Lindenberg A. Preventive incisional negative pressure wound therapy (Prevena®) for an at-risk-surgical closure in a female Rottweiler. Schweiz Arch Tierheilkd 2015;157:105–9.

42. Nuutila K, Eriksson E. Moist wound healing with commonly available dressings. Adv Wound Care 2021;10:685–98.

43. Costa BA, Lima Júnior EM, de Moraes Filho MO, et al. Use of tilapia skin as a xenograft for pediatric burn treatment: a case report. J Burn Care Res 2019;40: 714–7.

44. Lima Júnior EM, de Moraes Filho MO, Costa BA, et al. Innovative burn treatment using tilapia skin as a Xenograft: a phase II randomized controlled trial. J Burn Care Res 2020;41:585–92.

45. Lima Júnior EM, de Moraes Filho MO, Costa BA, et al. Lyophilised tilapia skin as a xenograft for superficial partial thickness burns: a novel preparation and storage technique. J Wound Care 2020;29:598–602.

46. Lima Júnior EM, de Moraes Filho MO, Costa BA, et al. Nile tilapia fish skin–based wound dressing improves pain and treatment-related costs of superficial partial-thickness burns: a phase III randomized controlled trial. Plast Reconstr Surg 2021;147:1189–98.

47. Alves APNN, Lima Júnior EM, Piccolo NS, et al. Study of tensiometric properties, microbiological and collagen content in nile tilapia skin submitted to different sterilization methods. Cell Tissue Bank 2018;19:373–82.

48. Chen J, Gao K, Liu S, et al. Fish collagen surgical compress repairing characteristics on wound healing process in vivo. Mar Drugs 2019;17:1–12.

49. Peng KC, Lee SH, Hour AL, et al. Five different piscidins from Nile tilapia, Oreochromis niloticus: Analysis of their expressions and biological functions. PLoS One 2012;7:e50263.

50. Pan CY, Tsai TY, Su BC, et al. Study of the antimicrobial activity of tilapia piscidin 3 (TP3) and TP4 and their effects on immune functions in hybrid tilapia (Oreochromis spp.). PLoS One 2017;12:e0169678.

51. Ge B, Wang H, Li J, et al. Comprehensive assessment of nile tilapia skin (Oreochromis niloticus) collagen hydrogels for wound dressings. Mar Drugs 2020; 18:178.

52. Fiakos G, Kuang Z, Lo E. Improved skin regeneration with acellular fish skin grafts. Engin Regen 2020;1:95–101. https://doi.org/10.1016/j.engreg.2020. 09.002.

53. Kirsner RS, Margolis DJ, Baldursson BT, et al. Fish skin grafts compared to human amnion/chorion membrane allografts: a double-blind, prospective, randomized clinical trial of acute wound healing. Wound Rep Reg 2020;28:75–80.

54. Kurach LM, Stanley BJ, Gazzola KM, et al. The Effect of low-level laser therapy on the healing of open wounds in dogs. Vet Surg 2015;44:988–96.

55. da Silva JP, da Silva MA, Almeida AP, et al. Laser therapy in the tissue repair process: a literature review. Photomed Laser Surg 2010;28:17–21.

56. Kushibiki T, Hirasawa T, Okawa S, et al. Regulation of miRNA expression by low-level laser therapy (LLLT) and photodynamic therapy (PDT). Int J Mol Sci 2013; 14:13542–58.

57. Gammel JE, Biskup JJ, Drum MG, et al. Effects of low-level laser therapy on the healing of surgically closed incisions and surgically created open wounds in dogs. Vet Surg 2018;47:499–506.

58. Gagnon D, Gibson TWG, Singh A, et al. An in vitro method to test the safety and efficacy of low-level laser therapy (LLLT) in the healing of a canine skin model. BMC Vet Res 2016;12:73.

59. Salvaggio A, Magi GE, Rossi G, et al. Effect of the topical Klox fluorescence biomodulation system on the healing of canine surgical wounds. Vet Surg 2020;49: 719–27.

60. Nikolis A, Grimard D, Pesant Y, et al. A prospective case series evaluating the safety and efficacy of the Klox BioPhotonic System in venous leg ulcers. Chron Wound Care Manag Res 2016;3:101–11.

61. Romanelli M, Piaggesi A, Scapagnini G, et al. EUREKA study—the evaluation of real-life use of a biophotonic system in chronic wound management: an interim analysis. Drug Des Devel Ther 2017;11:3551–8.

62. Marchegiani A, Cerquetella M, Laus F, et al. The Klox Biophotonic System, an innovative and integrated approach for the treatment of deep pyoderma in dogs: a preliminary report. In: Proceedings of the 29th ESVD-ECVD annual congress; September 7–9, 2017, Lausanne, Switzerland.

63. Tambella AM, Cerquetella M, Attili AR, et al. Klox Biophotonic System, a promising innovative approach to canine chronic otitis externa: preliminary report of a randomized controlled clinical trial. Vet Surg 2017;46(6):E50–1.

64. Elam L. Diving in: hyperbaric oxygen therapy in veterinary medicine. In: Today's veterinary practice. 2020. p. 69–72. Available at: https://mydigitalpublication.com/publication/?i=641969&article_id=3559489&view=articleBrowser.

65. Birnie GL, Fry DR, Best MP. Safety and tolerability of hyperbaric oxygen therapy in cats and dogs. J Am Anim Hosp Assoc 2018;54:188–94.

66. Levitan DM, Hitt M, Geiser DR, et al. Rationale for hyperbaric oxygen therapy in traumatic injury and wound care in small animal veterinary practice. J Small Anim Pract 2021;62:719–29.

67. Latimer CR, Lux CN, Roberts S, et al. Effects of hyperbaric oxygen therapy on uncomplicated incisional and open wound healing in dogs. Vet Surg 2018;47: 827–36.

68. Lunkiewicz W, Kiełbowicz Z, Kalisiak K, et al. Effect of hyperbaric oxygen therapy on the healing of postoperative wounds in bitches after hemimastectomy. Pol J Vet Sci 2020;23:495–9.

69. Kang MH, Park HM. Challenges of stem cell therapies in companion animal practice. J Vet Sci 2020;21:e42. https://doi.org/10.4142/jvs.2020.21.e42.

70. Hall MN, Rosenkrantz WS, Hong JH, et al. Evaluation of the potential use of adipose-derived mesenchymal stromal cells in the treatment of canine atopic dermatitis: a pilot study. Vet Ther 2010;11(2):E1–14.

71. Black LL, Gaynor J, Gahring D, et al. Effect of adipose-derived mesenchymal stem and regenerative cells on lameness in dogs with chronic osteoarthritis of the coxofemoral joints: a randomized, double-blinded, multicenter, controlled trial. Vet Ther 2007;8:272–84.

72. Kim JW, Lee JH, Lyoo YS, et al. The effects of topical mesenchymal stem cell transplantation in canine experimental cutaneous wounds. Vet Dermatol 2013; 24:242.

73. Enciso N, Avedillo L, Fermín ML, et al. Regenerative potential of allogeneic adipose tissue-derived mesenchymal cells in canine cutaneous wounds. Acta Vet Scand 2020;62:13–8.

74. Enciso N, Avedillo L, Fermín ML, et al. Cutaneous wound healing: canine allogeneic ASC therapy. Stem Cell Res Ther 2020;11:261–74.

75. Jee CH, Eom NY, Jang HM, et al. Effect of autologous platelet-rich plasma application on cutaneous wound healing in dogs. J Vet Sci 2016;17:79–87.

76. Iacopetti I, Patruno M, Melotti L, et al. Autologous platelet-rich plasma enhances the healing of large cutaneous wounds in dogs. Front Vet Sci 2020;7:575449. https://doi.org/10.3389/fvets.2020.575449.

77. Farghali HA, AbdElKader NA, Khattab MS, et al. Evaluation of subcutaneous infiltration of autologous platelet-rich plasma on skin-wound healing in dogs. Biosci Rep 2017;37. https://doi.org/10.1042/BSR20160503. BSR20160503.

78. Farghali HA, AbdElKader NA, AbuBakr HO, et al. Antimicrobial action of autologous platelet-rich plasma on MRSA-infected skin wounds in dog. Sci Rep 2019;9: 12722. https://doi.org/10.1038/s41598-019-48657-5.

79. Karayannopoulou M, Psalla D, Kazakos G, et al. Effect of locally injected autologous platelet-rich plasma on second intention wound healing of acute full-thickness skin defects in dogs. Vet Comp Orthop Traumatol 2015;28:172–8.

80. McCaig CD, Rajnicek AM, Song B, et al. Controlling cell behavior electrically: current views and future potential. Physiol Rev 2005;85:943–78.

81. Foulds IS, Barker AT. Human skin battery potentials and their possible role in wound healing. Br J Dermatol 1983;109:515–22.

82. Ashrafi M, Alonso-Rasgado T, Baguneid M, et al. The efficacy of electrical stimulation in experimentally induced cutaneous wounds in animals. Vet Dermatol 2016;27:235–e257.

83. Maijer A, Gessner A, Trumpatori B, et al. Bioelectric dressing supports complex wound healing in small animal patients. Top Companion Anim Med 2018;33:21–8.

84. Kim H, Makin I, Skiba J, et al. Antibacterial efficacy Tes7ng of a bioelectric wound dressing against clinical wound pathogens. Open Microbiol J 2014;8:15–21.

85. Banerjee J, Ghatak PD, Roy S, et al. Silver-zinc redox-coupled electroceutical wound dressing disrupts bacterial biofilm. PLoS One 2015;10(3):e0119531. https://doi.org/10.1371/journal.pone.0119531.

86. Sheridan DM, Isseroff RR, Nucitelli R. Imposition of a physiologic DC electric current alters the migratory response of human keratinocytes on extracellular matrix molecules. J Invest Dermatol 1996;106:642–6.

87. Blount AL, Foster S, Rapp DA, et al. The use of bioelectric dressings in skin graft harvest sites: a prospective case series. J Burn Care Res 2012;33:354–7.

88. Harding AC, Gil J, Valdes J, et al. Efficacy of a bio-electric dressing in healing deep, partial-thickness wounds using a porcine model. Ostomy Wound Manage 2012;58:50–5.

89. Varhus JD. A novel bioelectric device enhances wound healing: an equine case series. J Equine Vet Sci 2014;34:421–30.

Updated Information on Gastric Dilatation and Volvulus and Gastropexy in Dogs

Desiree Rosselli, DVM

KEYWORDS

- Gastric dilatation and volvulus • Gastropexy • Bloat • Gastric dilation • Canine

KEY POINTS

- Gastric dilatation and volvulus is life threatening; treatment aims at stabilization including fluid resuscitation and gastric decompression, followed by emergency surgery
- Lactate clearance (improvement in hyperlactatemia with treatment) is a positive prognostic indicator for reduced incidence of gastric necrosis and improved patient survival postoperatively
- Prophylactic gastropexy should be considered for at-risk breeds; minimally invasive techniques reduce surgical time and patient morbidity
- The use of barbed, knotless suture material shortens surgical time compared with traditional suture with knots

INTRODUCTION

Gastric dilatation and volvulus (GDV) is a life-threatening condition in dogs and is characterized by acute twisting of the stomach on its mesenteric axis, typically in a clockwise direction. This twisting causes obstruction of the pylorus and cardia of the stomach and subsequent gastric distention and gas accumulation. As a consequence, the following problems can develop: decreased venous return to the heart from compression of the vena cava and portal vein, hypovolemia and obstructive shock, gastric ischemia and necrosis, myocardial injury, gastrointestinal bacterial translocation and sepsis, systemic inflammatory response syndrome, disseminated intravascular coagulation (DIC), and death. Rapid diagnosis and institution of emergency stabilization followed by surgical correction is necessary.

DISCUSSION
Signalment and Presentation

Dogs presenting with acute GDV are usually middle-aged to older large breeds. Many breeds with a deep chest conformation are commonly described, including the Great

VCA West Los Angeles Animal Hospital, 1900 South Sepulveda Boulevard, Los Angeles, CA 90025, USA
E-mail address: ddrosselli@gmail.com

Vet Clin Small Anim 52 (2022) 317–337
https://doi.org/10.1016/j.cvsm.2021.11.004
0195-5616/22/© 2021 Elsevier Inc. All rights reserved.

vetsmall.theclinics.com

Dane, German shepherd, standard poodle, Weimaraner, and Setter breeds.[1–4] Typical clinical signs are pacing or restlessness, retching or nonproductive vomiting, ptyalism, abdominal distention, and weakness or collapse. Clinical signs at presentation can range from dogs that are mildly affected and otherwise stable and alert, to collapsed, in decompensated shock, or even dead.[5]

Risk Factors

Specific published patient risk factors associated with development of GDV include

- Large or giant breed of dog[3,5]
- Increased thoracic depth-to-width ratio (deep chest conformation)[4,6]
- Family history of GDV[6,7]
- Increasing age[3,6,8,9]
- Preexisting gastrointestinal disease such as gastric foreign material or inflammatory bowel disease[10,11]
- Various factors related to feeding or diet including large volume of food fed once daily, eating a meal quickly, and eating from a raised food bowl[7,12]

It has been hypothesized that large splenic masses or splenic torsion may increase the laxity of perigastric ligaments, and therefore increase the risk for GDV.[13] Some studies show no increased risk for GDV after splenectomy,[14–16] whereas one study showed a 5.3 times higher risk of GDV in dogs with previous splenectomy.[17]

Genetics

Genetics likely plays a role in the development of GDV. Dogs with a relative with GDV, particularly a parent, have an increased risk of developing GDV. Study of 5-generation pedigrees of Irish Setters suggested that certain genetic lines have an increased risk of GDV.[6] A genomic analysis was used to identify genetic susceptibility for GDV in 10 breeds of dogs: 27 significant single nucleotide polymorphisms were identified that could be associated with GDV or gastrointestinal tone and motility.[18] Three specific alleles of genes have been identified in Great Danes, which suggests a predisposition to GDV through alteration of the intestinal microbiome.[19,20] Further genetic research will help direct preventative efforts as well as more targeted treatment options for GDV.

Diagnostic Tests

Radiography

The diagnosis of GDV can be confirmed with abdominal radiography: a right lateral projection will show a gas-dilated stomach, compartmentalization of the stomach ("double bubble" sign), and craniodorsal displacement of the pylorus. **Fig. 1** shows a right lateral radiographic projection of a dog with GDV. A gas-dilated esophagus may also be seen. An orthogonal projection should ideally be obtained. The radiograph should be evaluated for evidence of pneumoperitoneum and gastric rupture.

Thoracic radiography should be considered. A small vena cava and microcardia are commonly identified. Although often recommended to screen for metastatic disease, thoracic radiographs may have more prognostic utility in screening for cardiac size, because a negative association between survival and the presence of cardiomegaly has been shown.[21]

Blood pressure

Monitoring trends in blood pressure along with changes in other perfusion parameters (heart rate, mentation, peripheral pulse quality, mucous membrane color and capillary

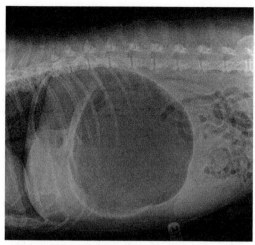

Fig. 1. The right lateral abdominal radiograph from an 11-year-old male neutered German Shepherd dog with GDV. Note the gas distention and compartmentalization of the stomach and craniodorsal displacement of the pylorus.

refill time) is useful for ongoing assessment of patient stability and monitoring effectiveness of fluid resuscitation.

Electrocardiography

Continuous electrocardiography should be monitored: approximately 40% of dogs with GDV have ventricular arrhythmias, most commonly occurring within 12 to 36 hours after the onset of GDV.[1,22] In one study, 18% of patients were noted to have ventricular arrhythmias at presentation, whereas 68% of patients developed ventricular arrhythmias during hospitalization.[23] Treatment is initiated when ventricular arrhythmias risk decreasing cardiac output or there is concern for development of fibrillation. Initial treatment is intravenous (IV) lidocaine as 2 mg/kg boluses, followed by a constant rate infusion 0.05 to 0.07 mg/kg/min if the rhythm is successfully converted to a sinus rhythm. Procainamide (2–4 mg/kg IV as a slow bolus, followed by 0.01–0.03 mg/kg as a constant rate infusion) or sotalol (1-2 mg/kg orally twice daily) can be considered for refractory ventricular arrhythmias.[24] Lidocaine may have secondary beneficial functions in reducing ischemic reperfusion injury, as a prokinetic, and as an analgesic medication. Initiating early lidocaine treatment can decrease the occurrence of cardiac arrhythmia, as well as kidney injury[25] but was not associated with differences in mortality rate.[2]

Blood analysis

Ideally, a complete blood cell count, serum chemistry, and coagulation profile would be performed. Results from these diagnostics may not be available efficiently in an emergency room setting, however, so point-of-care testing is more common including packed cell volume, total solids, blood glucose, and venous blood gas including creatinine, lactate, and electrolytes.

Lactate

Lactate has been associated with GDV prognosis. Lactate is a product of anaerobic metabolism and can accumulate in conditions associated with decreased oxygen delivery to tissues. Interestingly, a statistical difference was not observed between lactate concentrations collected from saphenous versus cephalic veins in dogs with GDV.[26] Both presenting lactate and lactate clearance (or improvement in hyperlactatemia from presentation to postfluid resuscitation) have been studied.[23,26–33] Not all reports show a prognostic utility for lactate measurements with GDV,[34,35] and comparison between studies is difficult because of difference in treatment protocols and intervals between lactate measurements. However, there is considerable evidence that a lower lactate at presentation as well as improvement in hyperlactatemia with treatment is associated with less morbidity and mortality (**Table 1**).

Other potential biomarkers

- Quantification of cytokines through the course of GDV treatment is the subject of ongoing research. No prognostic data are currently identified. Proinflammatory reactions peak after surgery for up to 24 hours, in addition to a systemic anti-inflammatory response both at admission and postsurgery, characterized by interlukin-10.[36]
- Cardiac troponin I levels were significantly higher in dogs with a higher arrhythmia grade.[23] Dogs that died had significantly higher serum cardiac troponin I and cardiac troponin T concentrations than those that survived.[37]
- Presenting myoglobin concentration may have some prognostic utility: only 50% of dogs survived when presenting myoglobin was greater than 168 ng/mL.[38]
- Higher procalcitonin concentrations at presentation were associated with nonsurvival.[32]
- Concentration of serum pepsinogen A was positively associated with severity of lesions on the gastric wall.[39]
- There is conflicting evidence regarding the prognostic value of C-reactive protein, canine pancreatic lipase immunoreactivity, and high mobility group box 1 (HMGB1).[34,39,40]
- pH and bicarbonate concentrations warrant further investigation as markers for gastric necrosis as well as outcome predictors.[31]

Coagulation assessment

Prolongation in clotting times can be seen with GDV.[41] In one study, prothrombin time (PT) was prolonged in 44% of dogs and activated partial thromboplastin time (aPTT) in 31% of dogs presenting with GDV.[26] Although prolongation of PT and aPTT at admission may not be a significant risk factor for death,[2] coagulation assessment may be useful for decision making regarding administration of blood products and monitoring for DIC.

Preoperative Therapy and Stabilization

Stabilization therapies should be performed before or in conjunction with the diagnostics listed earlier. Fluid resuscitation and gastric decompression are the most important immediate treatment goals.

Vascular access and fluid administration

Placement of large-gauge IV catheters in the cranial half of the body (usually cephalic or jugular veins) is necessary due to the reduced blood flow from the caudal half of the body. Balanced isotonic crystalloids are bolused for initial volume resuscitation at intervals of one-quarter shock volume (20–25 mL/kg up to 90 mL/kg). Depending on response to therapy, intervals of one-quarter boluses of synthetic colloid solutions (5 mL/kg up to 20 mL/kg) or hypertonic saline (4 mL/kg over 10 minutes) may be used.

Table 1
Studies showing a statistically significant prognostic utility for lactate

	Listed by Study Year and Number of Dogs in Each Study	
Presenting lactate and survival	1999[27] 102 dogs	Lactate >6.0 mmol/L: 58% survival Lactate <6.0 mmol/L 99% survival • Sensitivity 68%, specificity 86%
	2010[28] 64 dogs	Lactate >9.0 mmol/L: 54% survival Lactate <9.0 mmol/L: 90% survival • Sensitivity 74%, specificity 73%
	2011[29] 84 dogs	Lactate >4.1 mmol/L: 79% survival Lactate <4.1 mmol/L: 98% survival • Sensitivity 60%, specificity 91%
	2013[30] 78 dogs	Lactate >7.4 mmol/L: 70% survival Lactate <7.4 mmol/L: 95% survival • Accuracy 88% for predicting survival
	2018[26] 45 dogs	Median cephalic lactate in survivors: 3.8 mmol/L Median cephalic lactate in nonsurvivors: 11.4 mmol/L
	2020[31] 75 dogs	Survivors median lactate 3.35 mmol/L, nonsurvivors median 9.68 mmol/L Lactate ≤5.62 mmol/L predictive for survival • Sensitivity 75%, specificity 86%
Presenting lactate and gastric necrosis	1999[27] 102 dogs	Mean lactate 6.6 mmol/L with gastric necrosis, 3.3 mmol/L without Lactate >6.0mml/L predictive for gastric necrosis • Sensitivity 61%, specificity 88%
	2011[29] 84 dogs	Lactate >2.9 mmol/L predictive for gastric necrosis • Sensitivity 94%, specificity 43%
	2013[30] 78 dogs	Lactate >7.4 mmol/L predictive for gastric necrosis • Sensitivity 50%, specificity 88%, accuracy 82%
	2017[23] 22 dogs	Significantly higher lactate in dogs with gastric necrosis compared with those without
	2018[32] 29 dogs	Median lactate 3.36 mmol/L without gastric necrosis Median lactate 5.84 mmol/L with gastric necrosis
	2020[31] 75 dogs	Median lactate 9.7 mmol/L with gastric necrosis, 2.5 mmol/L without lactate >4.65 mmol/L predictive for gastric necrosis • Sensitivity 76%, specificity 67%
Lactate clearance and survival	2010[28] 64 dogs	For dogs presenting with lactate >9.0 mmol/L: Survival rates higher where • Final lactate improved to ≤6.4 mmol/L • Final lactate improved overall more than 4 mmol/L • Percentage change >42.5% 23% survival where posttreatment lactate >6.4 mmol/L • Sensitivity 77%, specificity 91% 15% survival where percentage change in lactate was >42.5% • Sensitivity 85%, specificity 100%
	2011[29] 84 dogs	Decrease in presenting lactate ≥50% within 12 h was a good indicator for survival
	2021[33] 41 dogs	Larger percentage decreases in lactate were associated with higher likelihood of survival to discharge
Lactate clearance and gastric necrosis	2021[33] 41 dogs	Larger percentage decreases in lactate were associated with better gastric health at surgery

Gastric decompression

Gastric decompression is performed as soon as possible. Trocharization, orogastric intubation, and temporary percutaneous gastrostomy catheter placement are described. Gastric decompression may need to be repeated depending on the timing between presentation and surgery and the technique chosen.

Trocharization. Percutaneous trocharization is performed with a large-gauge needle or over-the-needle catheter after clipping of the fur and aseptic skin preparation and can be performed in an awake patient. To choose the best site for decompression, clinicians may use abdominal radiography, ultrasonography, or most commonly palpation of the area of greatest distention or tympany on examination.

Oral gastric intubation. Passing a smooth orogastric tube requires general anesthesia or heavy sedation because it will not be tolerated in an awake patient. General anesthesia is recommended because it reduces complications such as the patient biting the tube, and the presence of an endotracheal tube also reduces the chance for inadvertent aspiration of gastric fluid. Gentle pressure should be used when passing the tube: pushing too firmly past areas of resistance (most commonly the lower esophageal sphincter) risks tearing or perforating the esophagus.

Ultrasound-guided temporary percutaneous gastrostomy catheter placement. This technique allows for sustained gastric decompression, and procedure duration is comparable to traditional trocharization.[42] Three T-fastener devices are placed percutaneously into the gastric lumen using ultrasound guidance; the T-fasteners provide temporary fixation of the stomach to the right body wall. A 5F self-retaining pigtail gastrostomy catheter is then placed between the T-fasteners into the gastric lumen and the pigtail is locked; initial placement of the pigtail catheter is facilitated by guidewire placement through a 21-gauge needle. This technique was developed for patients that may experience delay between stabilization and surgery and is demonstrated to be safe and effective for gastric decompression in patients with GDV.[42]

Analgesia

GDV is expected to be very painful, and administration of analgesic medications is strongly recommended. Full μ-agonist opioids are recommended and can be reversed if needed if a patient decompensates.

Antibiotics

GDV results in gastric mucosal compromise and increased permeability, as well as poor hepatic perfusion and compromise to reticuloendothelial function. These present a risk for bacterial translocation, and administration of antibiotics is warranted. Although bacterial translocation could not be proved via blood cultures,[43] evaluation of the CO_2 composition of intraluminal gastric gas suggests bacterial fermentation.[44] For straightforward GDV without gastric rupture, a first-generation cephalosporin, for example, cefazolin 22 mg/kg IV every 8 hours, can be administered preoperatively and for 2 to 3 days following surgery.

Oxygen

Oxygen supplementation should be provided to patients with evidence of hypoxia, including tachypnea, cyanosis, prolonged capillary refill time, poor pulse quality, oxygen saturation as measured by pulse oximetry less than 95%, and Pao_2 less than 80 mm Hg.

Blood products

Fresh frozen plasma may be beneficial for patients with prolonged coagulation times, and whole blood or packed red blood cell transfusion can be administered to dogs with anemia.

Surgery

Surgical intervention should be performed as soon as possible, to help limit the duration of tissue ischemia.[2,31,45,46] There is not definitive literature on the optimal timing of surgery in relation to medical stabilization, and spending some time on stabilization before surgery is warranted.[1,47] Even if time to surgery is necessarily delayed, one study showed gastric decompression and medical stabilization before surgery was still worthwhile and mortality rates were not significantly affected.[33] However, surgery should not be delayed where possible, because complete normalization of perfusion parameters may not be possible without surgical intervention. **Table 2** outlines the major surgical goals. Adjusting fluid therapy and monitoring perfusion parameters is still critical during surgery and anesthesia.

Gastric derotation

Correctly repositioning the stomach is the immediate primary goal following a ventral midline celiotomy. The greater omentum is gently retracted off the stomach, and the gas distention of stomach may need to be decompressed (by passing an orogastric tube or by intraoperative needle decompression) to aid in repositioning. The typical volvulus of the stomach is in a 180° to 270° clockwise direction. To reposition the stomach, the surgeon can gently pull the pylorus from the left, to the right and ventral direction in the dog's abdomen, while simultaneously pushing the fundus dorsally and to the dog's left. Verification of correct gastric position via observation and palpation of the gastroesophageal junction is critical, because other directions/configurations of volvulus are possible.

Evaluation of abdominal viscera

Following gastric repositioning, time should be allowed for reperfusion of organs. If there is ongoing hemorrhage from avulsion of short gastric arteries and veins, these vessels can be ligated. The stomach should be palpated for any foreign material.[10] The stomach should also be evaluated for evidence of gastric necrosis, particularly the greater curvature, fundus, and dorsal aspect of the stomach. **Fig. 2** is an intraoperative photograph of a dog with gastric necrosis.

Gastric necrosis is reported in 10.5% to 41% of patients.[1,26–31,46–49] Partial gastrectomy should be performed for areas of the stomach that are necrotic or nonviable: as indicated by gray, white, black, or green serosal discoloration, thin texture, or lack of capillary perfusion. Evaluation with IV fluorescein dye, scintigraphy, or laser Doppler

Table 2 Goals of surgical correction of GDV	
Gastric derotation	To reposition a typical clockwise volvulus, the fundus of the stomach can be pushed dorsally, whereas the pylorus is pulled ventrally and to the right of the dog's abdomen
Evaluation of abdominal viscera	Give time for reperfusion of organs and confirm correct gastric positioning. If necessary, splenectomy or partial gastrectomy can be performed
Right-sided gastropexy	Create a permanent adhesion between the pyloric antrum and the body wall

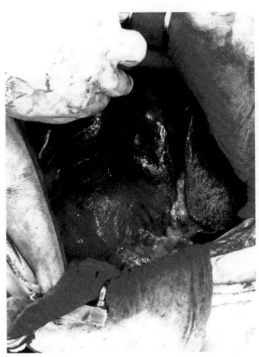

Fig. 2. Intraoperative photograph of the stomach of a dog affected by gastric necrosis. The cranial aspect of the abdomen is at the top of the image. The patient had GDV, and the stomach has been derotated. Note the demarcation across the body of the stomach between vascularized (pink) gastric tissue, and necrotic (dark purple) gastric tissue. (*Photograph courtesy of* Chad Schmiedt and Jacob Helmick.)

flowmetry have also been used to assess gastric viability and help guide decision making for gastric resection.[48,50,51] Resection is followed by two-layer hand-sewn closure or use of surgical stapling equipment.[48,52] Reinforcement of stapled closures with an inverting suture line is recommended to improve resistance to leakage.[53] Invagination techniques have been reported but may risk severe gastric ulceration.[54] If necrotic areas involve the cardia or esophagus, the ability to perform resection may be limited by available healthy tissue and esophageal lumen diameter.

The need for splenectomy is reported in 8.9% to 22.6% of patients.[26,46,47,49] Splenectomy is recommended if evidence of thrombosis, such as a lack of palpable splenic artery pulse, gray or black coloration, or spongy texture, is present. Suture ligation, surgical stapling equipment, or vessel sealant devices can be used. No significant presurgical biomarkers have been identified for dogs receiving or not receiving splenectomy.[23]

Right-sided gastropexy
Gastropexy is surgical creation of a permanent adhesion between the pyloric antrum of stomach and the body wall and is essential in patients following correction of gastric volvulus. Without gastropexy, the recurrence rate of GDV is more than 75%.[55] Anatomically correct gastropexy is important to prevent complications such as creation of partial pyloric outflow obstruction.[56] Computed tomographic (CT) imaging has been used to help describe the normal location of the pylorus in dogs, and future

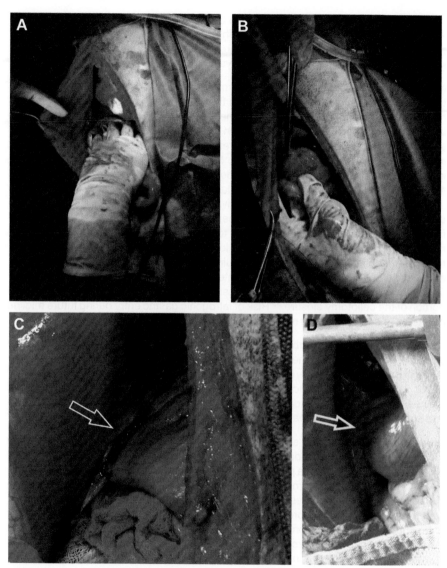

Fig. 3. Steps for right incisional gastropexy. In each image, the cranial aspect of the abdomen is at the top of the image. *A.* creation of an incision on the right lateral body wall through the transversus abdominis muscle *B.* a seromuscular incision of equal length is created in the pyloric antrum of the stomach, and the suturing is started on the dorsal aspect of the incision *C.* The yellow arrow highlights the completion of the dorsal line of suturing the edge of the body wall incision to the edge of the seromuscular incision. *D.* The yellow arrow highlights the completed gastropexy.

studies may be of value in defining the most anatomic location for gastropexy in individuals.[57]

Although there is not a direct comparison between all the different techniques for gastropexy, where different techniques are evaluated, there are no statistically significant differences in survival rates (88.3%–90.3%)[45] or recurrence of GDV (0%–4.3%),[5,45,58] and all result in permanent adhesion formation.[58] Strength of gastropexy differs between techniques,[59] and although the optimal strength for gastropexy is not known, strength is thought to be supraphysiologic for all the common techniques.

Incisional gastropexy. Although there are many techniques reported, incisional gastropexy is the most commonly reported in the literature; this is likely due to the technical ease, low risk of morbidity, effectiveness for inducing permanent adhesion, and lack of need for specialized instrumentation. An incision is made through the transversus abdominis muscle and sutured to the respective sides of a similar incision created in the seromuscular layer of the stomach. **Fig. 3** demonstrates a technique for right incisional gastropexy. In a cadaveric model, incisional gastropexies performed with 4-cm-long incisions had higher load to failure compared with 2-cm-long incisions[60]

Other techniques for creating an effective right-sided gastropexy include circumcostal gastropexy and belt-loop gastropexy, where a seromuscular flap elevated from the pyloric antrum is sutured back to the stomach, after passing behind the most caudal complete rib or behind a belt loop created in the right body wall, respectively.[61] A modification that does not require a seromuscular flap is described.[62] An automatic stapler can also be used to create a gastropexy.[63] An incorporating gastropexy technique is also described, which sutures the pyloric antrum into the cranial portion of the celiotomy closure.[55] Risk of iatrogenic gastric entry during future midline celiotomy is considered but not documented.[64]

Barbed suture material. Barbed suture material has circumferential barbs along the suture length that prevent the suture from backing out once placed in tissue. Advantages of barbed suture material over conventional knotted suture include: even distribution of tension along the incision, reduced surgical suturing times, and elimination of the need for knot tying. In cadaveric incisional gastropexy, unidirectional barbed knotless suture had similar or greater load to failure compared with monofilament suture.[65]

Tube gastropexy. A Foley or silicone mushroom-tipped catheter is introduced through the right abdominal wall caudal to the last rib, into the lumen of the stomach through a preplaced purse-string in the pyloric antrum region. Interrupted sutures are placed between the body wall and stomach. The catheter is removed 2 weeks after surgery. The surface area of the final adhesion was found to be less than for incisional and circumcostal gastropexy, with more incorporation of omentum.[59] The tube allows early enteral feeding; complications include soft tissue wounds or premature removal of the tube by the patient.[66] Percutaneous endoscopic gastrostomy is not recommended due to inconsistent formation of a weak gastropexy.[67]

Gastrocolopexy. Seromuscular sutures are placed between the transverse colon and the greater curvature of the stomach, after serosal scarification of each. Although not statistically significant, a recurrence rate of GDV of 20% was reported.[68]

Postsurgical Treatment

Treatment after surgery is a continuum of the therapeutics and monitoring instituted preoperatively and intraoperatively. Maintenance of volume resuscitation includes IV isotonic crystalloids and may include colloids or blood products depending on the needs of the patient. Repeated blood analysis including electrolyte monitoring will help guide fluid therapy. Injectable opioids are continued for analgesia. Nonsteroidal anti-inflammatory medications are avoided after GDV due to decreased gastric perfusion and concern for gastric ulceration. Antacid medications such as histamine-2 receptor antagonists, sucralfate, or proton pump inhibitor medications are typically administered. Antibiotic medications may be indicated after surgery due to the presumed risk for bacterial translocation. Antiemetic and promotility medications can be administered for nausea and regurgitation. Food and water can be offered to an awake and alert patient; nutritional support is considered for inappetent patients. Blood pressure and arrhythmia monitoring continues postoperatively.

Prognosis

In a study of 492 dogs with a presumptive diagnosis of GDV, 49.7% of overall patients survived to discharge and approximately 80% of surgically managed patients survived to discharge.[8] Overall mortality rates after surgery for GDV were 10% to 23%.[1,2,31,39,46,47,49] Similarly, studies report that survival to discharge following surgery is 77% to 88%.[26,28–30]

Poor prognostic indicators include

- Hyperlactatemia, especially with minimal response to fluid therapy (see **Table 1**)
- Splenectomy
  - 15% to 32% mortality[47,49]
- Gastric necrosis and need for partial gastrectomy[5,31]
  - 10% to 46% mortality[1,27,47,49,52]
  - Significantly longer hospitalization times for dogs with gastric necrosis[30]
- Partial gastrectomy with splenectomy[46]
  - 20% to 55% mortality[47,49]
- Cardiac arrhythmias: preoperative[49] and postoperative[47]
  - Not a risk factor in some studies[1,2]
- Decreased rectal temperature at admission
  - 40% mortality rate when T < 100.4°F[2]
- Severity of systemic affectedness at the time of presentation[2]
  - Depressed or comatose mentation on admission were 3 times and 36 times more likely to die than those that presented alert[5]
- Gastric perforation or sepsis[46,48]
- Increased time between clinical signs and admission[46]
  - 46% mortality rate when time between clinical signs and admission was greater than or equal to 5 hours, compared with 11.3%[2]

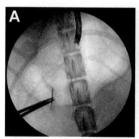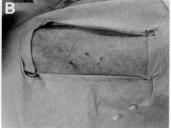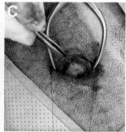

Fig. 4. Steps for radiologic-assisted incisional gastropexy. (*A*) A ventrodorsal fluoroscopic image shows a percutaneous needle being passed into the gastric lumen to facilitate T-fastener placement. (*B*) The T-fasteners are deployed in the gastric lumen and provide a guide for where to create the incision through the skin and the right body wall. The cranial aspect of the dog is located to the left of the image. (*C*) Following creation of the incision, the suture attached to the T-fasteners is used to elevate the pyloric antrum to the skin surface, to facilitate gastric seromuscular incision and gastropexy. The forceps denote the gastric serosal surface. (*Images courtesy of* William Culp.)

Recurrence

With medical management alone, the rate of recurrence of GDV can be more than 75%, with significantly shorter median survival times.[5,55] Recurrence of GDV following gastropexy is 0% in many studies,[55,69,70] but GDV recurrence has been documented rarely.[5,71] Ultrasonography is a simple and noninvasive technique to assess permanency of gastropexy if clinically warranted.[72]

Gastric dilatation without volvulus (or food engorgement) is reported in 3.3% to 11% of patients after GDV and gastropexy and is typically medically managed.[55,68–70,73] Gastric contractions and coordination of gastric motility are mediated through myoelectrical activity. This myoelectrical activity can be disrupted after GDV.[74] Delayed gastric emptying of solid particles was seen in dogs recovering from GDV and gastropexy and alterations of gastric motility are more likely related to the disease process rather than the surgical intervention, because healthy dogs did not show altered gastric emptying after open gastropexy.[75]

Prophylactic Gastropexy

Lifetime risk for development of GDV in at-risk breeds is estimated from 3.9% to 36.7,[9,76] and prophylactic gastropexy should be considered in at-risk breeds, or in dogs with other predisposing risk factors such as previous splenic disease or family history of GDV.[7,13,17] Numerous techniques are described for prophylactic gastropexy, including the open techniques described previously, and the less invasive techniques described here.

Grid approach

Blunt dissection through the muscle fibers of the body wall is performed caudal to the 13th rib. The stomach is isolated through visualization and palpation, and a seromuscular incision over the pyloric antrum allows suturing of the respective sides of the antrum and transversus abdominis incision. Surgical times can be faster compared with open laparotomy, and seroma formation is a described complication.[77]

Endoscopic or radiologic assisted

An endoscope passed to the level of the pyloric antrum helps visualize placement of temporary percutaneous stay sutures between the gastric wall and the right

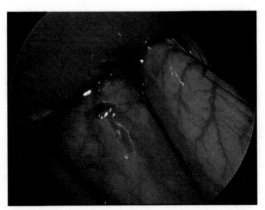

Fig. 5. Laparoscopic image of a completed gastropexy performed via laparoscopic-assisted technique. The body wall is located to the left of the image, and the stomach is on the right of the image.

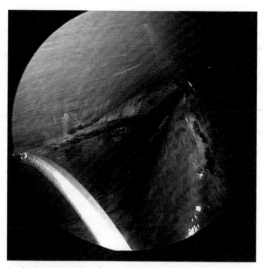

Fig. 6. Intra-abdominal photograph of total laparoscopic gastropexy. At this point in the procedure the stomach has been tacked to the body wall in the chosen location and a lapa-roscopic monopolar electrocautery instrument has been used to mark the peritoneum and serosa of the stomach. (*Photograph courtesy of* Nicole Buote.)

abdominal wall. The skin, abdominal muscles, and seromuscular layer of the stomach are incised, and simple continuous suture patterns are used to oppose the gastric and abdominal wall incisions.[78] The mean surgical time, incision length, and pain scores were significantly lower compared with open laparotomy.[79] A similar technique uses fluoroscopy to deploy temporary T-fasteners into the gastric lumen to facilitate creation of incision and suturing[80] (**Fig. 4**).

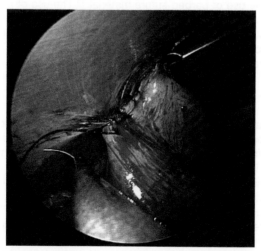

Fig. 7. Intra-abdominal photograph of total laparoscopic gastropexy. The stomach has been sutured to the body wall with barbed suture. The suture line will be ended with a backward needle pass out of the body wall. (*Photograph courtesy of* Nicole Buote.)

Laparoscopy

Both laparoscopic-assisted and total laparoscopic gastropexy have been described for prophylactic gastropexy in dogs. Compared with open techniques, laparoscopy is associated with lower postoperative pain and inflammation and shorter surgical times, with comparable strength of gastropexy.[81,82] Prophylactic laparoscopic gastropexy can be combined with sterilization,[83] although it is recommended for dogs to be skeletally mature, because rapid growth following gastropexy may result in mispositioning of the gastropexy.[56] Gastrointestinal transit times were not shown to be affected by laparoscopic-assisted or total laparoscopic gastropexy.[84–86]

Laparoscopic-assisted gastropexy uses a laparoscope through a ventral midline cannula to visualize placement of Babcock forceps through a cannula in the right body wall to exteriorize the pyloric antrum. Both sides of a seromuscular stomach incision are sutured to the respective sides of the lengthened incision in the transversus abdominis muscle (**Fig. 5**). Stomach positioning and emptying are normal after surgery, a strong fibrous adhesion is created, and recurrence of GDV is not reported.[83,87,88] A single port technique has also been described, but it is important to note that visualization of the final gastropexy is not possible with this technique.[89,90] A laparoscopic-assisted technique has even been used for treatment of select cases of GDV.[91] The most common complication is paramedian incision complications, including seroma formation in 12.4% to 23% of patients.[88,90]

Surgical time is longer for total laparoscopic gastropexy compared with laparoscopic-assisted gastropexy[92]; however, total laparoscopic gastropexy may provide superior patient comfort and avoids complications associated with the paramedian incision.[90,92] Total laparoscopic gastropexy can be performed using intracorporeal hand suturing (**Figs. 6** and **7**) or by use of a suture assist device, although device dysfunction has been reported.[92,93] Knotless, unidirectional barbed suture, sutured in 1 or 2 continuous lines, can be used to create a safe and effective gastropexy[82,94,95] with faster suturing times compared with conventional suture material.[95] An incision in the stomach and body wall are not necessary for creation of a permanent gastropexy with the use of barbed suture material.[96] The use of absorbable fixation straps have comparable load to failure as absorbable knotless barbed suture.[97,98] A technique for stapled laparoscopic gastropexy is also reported.[99] Three-dimensional laparoscopy imaging systems may represent a future direction for ease of teaching and learning.[100]

SUMMARY

GDV is a life-threatening emergency condition, in which pathologic gastric volvulus causes tissue hypoperfusion, hypovolemia, pain, and systemic inflammation. Treatment should be initiated immediately, including fluid resuscitation and gastric decompression. Surgery is performed in a timely manner to correct gastric positioning, allow for tissue reperfusion, and perform right-sided gastropexy; survival rates are around 80% after surgery.

Preoperative euthanasia accounts for most mortality in GDV,[101] although this is markedly decreased for owners with pet insurance,[102] which highlights the economic impact of decision making for owners. Ongoing research is aimed at identifying genetic factors and individual biomarkers that can help guide tailored treatment of those affected with GDV or prevention recommendations for at-risk individuals. Laparoscopic techniques provide a minimally invasive and effective prophylactic gastropexy.

CLINICS CARE POINTS

- A right lateral abdominal radiograph can confirm the diagnosis of GDV.
- Rapid diagnosis and stabilization are important to limit tissue hypoperfusion: immediate treatment goals are for gastric decompression and correction of hypovolemia.
- Trends in perfusion parameters can help guide fluid resuscitation. Prolonged hyperlactatemia can indicate a poorer prognosis; surgery should always be recommended
- Following surgery, patients have an approximately 80% survival rate. The need for splenectomy or gastric resection is associated with increased complications and increased mortality rates.
- Prophylactic gastropexy should be considered for at-risk breeds.

DISCLOSURE

The author has nothing to disclose.

REFERENCES

1. Brockman DJ, Washabau RJ, Drobatz KJ. Canine gastric dilatation/volvulus syndrome in a veterinary critical care unit: 295 cases (1986-1992). J Am Vet Med Assoc 1995;207(4):460–4.
2. Buber T, Saragusty J, Ranen E, et al. Evaluation of lidocaine treatment and risk factors for death associated with gastric dilatation and volvulus in dogs: 112 cases (1997-2005). J Am Vet Med Assoc 2007;230(9):1334–9.
3. Glickman LT, Glickman NW, Pérez CM, et al. Analysis of risk factors for gastric dilatation and dilatation-volvulus in dogs. J Am Vet Med Assoc 1994;204(9):1465–71.
4. Evans KM, Adams VJ. Mortality and morbidity due to gastric dilatation-volvulus syndrome in pedigree dogs in the UK. J Small Anim Pract 2010;51(7):376–81.
5. Glickman LT, Lantz GC, Schellenberg DB, et al. A prospective study of survival and recurrence following the acute gastric dilatation-volvulus syndrome in 136 dogs. J Am Anim Hosp Assoc 1998;34(3):253–9.
6. Schellenberg D, Yi Q, Glickman NW, et al. Influence of thoracic conformation and genetics on the risk of gastric dilatation-volvulus in Irish setters. J Am Anim Hosp Assoc 1998;34(1):64–73.
7. Glickman LT, Glickman NW, Schellenberg DB, et al. Non-dietary risk factors for gastric dilatation-volvulus in large and giant breed dogs. J Am Vet Med Assoc 2000;217(10):1492–9.
8. O'Neill DG, Case J, Boag AK, et al. Gastric dilation-volvulus in dogs attending UK emergency-care veterinary practices: prevalence, risk factors and survival. J Small Anim Pract 2017;58(11):629–38.
9. Glickman LT, Glickman NW, Schellenberg DB, et al. Incidence of and breed-related risk factors for gastric dilatation-volvulus in dogs. J Am Vet Med Assoc 2000;216(1):40–5.
10. de Battisti A, Toscano MJ, Formaggini L. Gastric foreign body as a risk factor for gastric dilatation and volvulus in dogs. J Am Vet Med Assoc 2012;241(9):1190–3.

11. Braun L, Lester S, Kuzma AB, et al. Gastric dilatation-volvulus in the dog with histological evidence of preexisting inflammatory bowel disease: a retrospective study of 23 cases. J Am Anim Hosp Assoc 1996;32(4):287–90.

12. Raghavan M, Glickman N, McCabe G, et al. Diet-related risk factors for gastric dilatation-volvulus in dogs of high-risk breeds. J Am Anim Hosp Assoc 2004; 40(3):192–203.

13. Millis DL, Nemzek J, Riggs C, et al. Gastric dilatation-volvulus after splenic torsion in two dogs. J Am Vet Med Assoc 1995;207(3):314–5.

14. Grange AM, Clough W, Casale SA. Evaluation of splenectomy as a risk factor for gastric dilatation-volvulus. J Am Vet Med Assoc 2012;241(4):461–6.

15. Goldhammer MA, Haining H, Milne EM, et al. Assessment of the incidence of GDV following splenectomy in dogs. J Small Anim Pract 2010;51(1):23–8.

16. Maki LC, Males KN, Byrnes MJ, et al. Incidence of gastric dilatation-volvulus following a splenectomy in 238 dogs. Can Vet J 2017;58(12):1275–80

17. Sartor AJ, Bentley AM, Brown DC. Association between previous splenectomy and gastric dilatation-volvulus in dogs: 453 cases (2004-2009). J Am Vet Med Assoc 2013;242(10):1381–4.

18. Piras IS, Perdigones N, Zismann V, et al. Identification of Genetic Susceptibility Factors Associated with Canine Gastric Dilatation-Volvulus. Genes (Basel) 2020; 11(11):1313.

19. Harkey MA, Villagran AM, Venkataraman GM, et al. Associations between gastric dilatation-volvulus in Great Danes and specific alleles of the canine immune-system genes DLA88, DRB1, and TLR5. Am J Vet Res 2017;78(8): 934–45.

20. Hullar MAJ, Lampe JW, Torok-Storb BJ, et al. The canine gut microbiome is associated with higher risk of gastric dilatation-volvulus and high risk genetic variants of the immune system. PLoS One 2018;13(6):e0197686.

21. Green JL, Cimino Brown D, Agnello KA. Preoperative thoracic radiographic findings in dogs presenting for gastric dilatation-volvulus (2000-2010): 101 cases. J Vet Emerg Crit Care 2012;22(5):595–600.

22. Muir WW. Gastric dilatation-volvulus in the dog, with emphasis on cardiac arrhythmias. J Am Vet Med Assoc 1982;180(7):739–42.

23. Aona BD, Rush JE, Rozanski EA, et al. Evaluation of echocardiography and cardiac biomarker concentrations in dogs with gastric dilatation volvulus. J Vet Emerg Crit Care (San Antonio) 2017;27(6):631–7.

24. Muir WW, Bonagura JD. Treatment of cardiac arrhythmias in dogs with gastric distention-volvulus. J Am Vet Med Assoc 1984;184(11):1366–71.

25. Bruchim Y, Itay S, Shira BH, et al. Evaluation of lidocaine treatment on frequency of cardiac arrhythmias, acute kidney injury, and hospitalization time in dogs with gastric dilatation volvulus. J Vet Emerg Crit Care (San Antonio) 2012;22(4): 419–27.

26. Oron LD, Klainbart S, Bruchim Y, et al. Comparison of saphenous and cephalic blood lactate concentrations in dogs with gastric dilatation and volvulus: 45 cases. Can J Vet Res 2018;82(4):271–7.

27. de Papp E, Drobatz KJ, Hughes D. Plasma lactate concentration as a predictor of gastric necrosis and survival among dogs with gastric dilatation-volvulus: 102 cases (1995-1998). J Am Vet Med Assoc 1999;215(1):49–52.

28. Zacher LA, Berg J, Shaw SP, et al. Association between outcome and changes in plasma lactate concentration during presurgical treatment in dogs with gastric dilatation-volvulus: 64 cases (2002-2008). J Am Vet Med Assoc 2010; 236(8):892–7.

29. Green TI, Tonozzi CC, Kirby R, et al. Evaluation of initial plasma lactate values as a predictor of gastric necrosis and initial and subsequent plasma lactate values as a predictor of survival in dogs with gastric dilatation-volvulus: 84 dogs (2003-2007). J Vet Emerg Crit Care 2011;21(1):36–44.

30. Beer KA, Syring RS, Drobatz KJ. Evaluation of plasma lactate concentration and base excess at the time of hospital admission as predictors of gastric necrosis and outcome and correlation between those variables in dogs with gastric dilatation-volvulus: 78 cases (2004-2009). J Am Vet Med Assoc 2013; 242(1):54–8.

31. Rauserova-Lexmaulova L, Vanova-Uhrikova I, Rehakova K. Acid-Base, Electrolyte and Lactate Abnormalities as Well as Gastric Necrosis and Survival in Dogs With Gastric Dilation-Volvulus Syndrome. A Retrospective Study in 75 Dogs. Top Companion Anim Med 2020;39:100403.

32. Troia R, Giunti M, Calipa S, et al. Cell-Free DNA, High-Mobility Group Box-1, and Procalcitonin Concentrations in Dogs With Gastric Dilatation-Volvulus Syndrome. Front Vet Sci 2018;5:67.

33. White RS, Sartor AJ, Bergman PJ. Evaluation of a staged technique of immediate decompressive and delayed surgical treatment for gastric dilatation-volvulus in dogs. J Am Vet Med Assoc 2021;258(1):72–9.

34. Spinella G, Dondi F, Grassato L, et al. Prognostic value of canine pancreatic lipase immunoreactivity and lipase activity in dogs with gastric dilatation-volvulus. PLoS One 2018;13(9):e0204216.

35. Grassato L, Spinella G, Musella V, et al. Pre- and post-surgical evaluation of plasma lactate concentration in 45 dogs with gastric dilatation-volvulus: A preliminary study. Heliyon 2020;6(1):e03307.

36. Brunner A, Schuller S, Hettlich B, et al. Kinetics of Plasma Cytokines, Angiopoietin-2, and C-Reactive Protein in Dogs With Gastric Dilatation Volvulus. Front Vet Sci 2021;8:652479.

37. Schober KE, Cornand C, Kirbach B, et al. Serum cardiac troponin I and cardiac troponin T concentrations in dogs with gastric dilatation-volvulus. J Am Vet Med Assoc 2002;221(3):381–8.

38. Adamik KN, Burgener IA, Kovacevic A, et al. Myoglobin as a prognostic indicator for outcome in dogs with gastric dilatation-volvulus. J Vet Emerg Crit Care (San Antonio) 2009;19(3):247–53.

39. Israeli I, Steiner J, Segev G, et al. Serum pepsinogen-A, canine pancreatic lipase immunoreactivity, and C-reactive protein as prognostic markers in dogs with gastric dilatation-volvulus. J Vet Intern Med 2012;26(4):920–8.

40. Uhrikova I, Rauserova-Lexmaulova L, Rehakova K, et al. C-reactive protein and high mobility group box 1 in dogs with gastric dilatation and volvulus. J Vet Emerg Crit Care (San Antonio) 2015;25(4):488–94.

41. Millis DL, Hauptman JG, Fulton RB Jr. Abnormal hemostatic profiles and gastric necrosis in canine gastric dilatation-volvulus. Vet Surg 1993;22(2):93–7.

42. Fox-Alvarez WA, Case JB, Lewis DD, et al. Evaluation of a novel technique involving ultrasound-guided, temporary, percutaneous gastropexy and gastrostomy catheter placement for providing sustained gastric decompression in dogs with gastric dilatation-volvulus. J Am Vet Med Assoc 2019;255(9): 1027–34.

43. Winkler KP, Greenfield CL, Schaeffer DJ. Bacteremia and bacterial translocation in the naturally occurring canine gastric dilatation-volvulus patient. J Am Anim Hosp Assoc 2003;39(4):361–8.

44. Van Kruiningen HJ, Gargamelli C, Havier J, et al. Stomach gas analyses in canine acute gastric dilatation with volvulus. J Vet Intern Med 2013;27(5): 1260–1.

45. Song KK, Goldsmid SE, Lee J, et al. Retrospective analysis of 736 cases of canine gastric dilatation volvulus. Aust Vet J 2020;98(6):232–8.

46. Beck JJ, Staatz AJ, Pelsue DH, et al. Risk factors associated with short-term outcome and development of perioperative complications in dogs undergoing surgery because of gastric dilatation-volvulus: 166 cases (1992-2003). J Am Vet Med Assoc 2006;229(12):1934–9.

47. Mackenzie G, Barnhart M, Kennedy S, et al. A retrospective study of factors influencing survival following surgery for gastric dilatation-volvulus syndrome in 306 dogs. J Am Anim Hosp Assoc 2010;46(2):97–102.

48. Matthiesen DT. Partial gastrectomy as treatment of gastric volvulus results in 30 dogs. Vet Surg 1985;14(3):185–93.

49. Brourman JD, Schertel ER, Allen DA, et al. Factors associated with perioperative mortality in dogs with surgically managed gastric dilatation-volvulus: 137 cases (1988-1993). J Am Vet Med Assoc 1996;208(11):1855–8.

50. Berardi C, Wheaton LG, Twardock AR, et al. Use of a nuclear imaging technique to detect gastric wall ischemia. Am J Vet Res 1991;52(7):1089–96.

51. Monnet E, Pelsue D, MacPhail C. Evaluation of laser Doppler flowmetry for measurement of capillary blood flow in the stomach wall of dogs during gastric dilatation-volvulus. Vet Surg 2006;35(2):198–205.

52. Clark GN, Pavletic MM. Partial gastrectomy with an automatic stapling instrument for treatment of gastric necrosis secondary to gastric dilatation-volvulus. Vet Surg 1991;20(1):61–8.

53. Duffy DJ, Cocca CJ, Chang YJ, et al. Evaluation of staple line reinforcement after partial gastrectomy closure in an ex vivo canine model. Vet Surg 2021;50(2): 435–43.

54. Parton AT, Volk SW, Weisse C. Gastric ulceration subsequent to partial invagination of the stomach in a dog with gastric dilatation-volvulus. J Am Vet Med Assoc 2006;228(12):1895–900.

55. Meyer-Lindenberg A, Harder A, Fehr M, et al. Treatment of gastric dilatation-volvulus and a rapid method for prevention of relapse in dogs: 134 cases (1988-1991). J Am Vet Med Assoc 1993;203(9):1303–7.

56. Sutton JS, Steffey MA, Bonadio CM, et al. Gastric malpositioning and chronic, intermittent vomiting following prophylactic gastropexy in a 20-month-old great Dane dog. Can Vet J 2015;56(10):1053–6.

57. Tomlinson AW, Lillis SM, German AJ, et al. Pyloric localisation in 57 dogs of breeds susceptible to gastric dilatation-volvulus in the UK using computed tomography. Vet Rec 2016;179(24):626.

58. Tanno F, Weber U, Wacker C, et al. Ultrasonographic comparison of adhesions induced by two different methods of gastropexy in the dog. J Small Anim Pract 1998;39(9):432–6.

59. Fox SM, Ellison GW, Miller GJ, et al. Observations on the mechanical failure of three gastropexy techniques. J Am Anim Hosp Assoc 1985;21(6):729–34.

60. Webb RJ, Monnet E. Influence of length of incision and number of suture lines on the biomechanical properties of incisional gastropexy. Vet Surg 2019;48(6): 933–7.

61. Fallah AM, Lumb WV, Nelson AW, et al. Circumcostal Gastropexy in the Dog A Preliminary Study. Vet Surg 1982;11:19–22.

62. Formaggini L, Degna MT. A Prospective Evaluation of a Modified Belt-Loop Gastropexy in 100 Dogs with Gastric Dilatation-Volvulus. J Am Anim Hosp Assoc 2018;54(5):239–45.

63. Belandria GA, Pavletic MM, Boulay JP, et al. Gastropexy with an automatic stapling instrument for the treatment of gastric dilatation and volvulus in 20 dogs. Can Vet J 2009;50(7):733–40.

64. Ullmann B, Seehaus N, Hungerbühler S, et al. Gastric dilatation volvulus: a retrospective study of 203 dogs with ventral midline gastropexy. J Small Anim Pract 2016;57(1):18–22.

65. Arbaugh M, Case JB, Monnet E. Biomechanical comparison of glycomer 631 and glycomer 631 knotless for use in canine incisional gastropexy. Vet Surg 2013;42:205–9.

66. Belch A, Rubinos C, Barnes DC, et al. Modified tube gastropexy using a mushroom-tipped silicone catheter for management of gastric dilatation-volvulus in dogs. J Small Anim Pract 2017;58(2):79–88.

67. Waschak MJ, Payne JT, Pope ER, et al. Evaluation of percutaneous gastrostomy as a technique for permanent gastropexy. Vet Surg 1997;26(3):235–41.

68. Eggertsdóttir AV, Stigen Ø, Lønaas L, et al. Comparison of the recurrence rate of gastric dilatation with or without volvulus in dogs after circumcostal gastropexy versus gastrocolopexy. Vet Surg 2001;30(6):546–51.

69. Benitez ME, Schmiedt CW, Radlinsky MG, et al. Efficacy of incisional gastropexy for prevention of GDV in dogs. J Am Anim Hosp Assoc 2013;49(3):185–9.

70. Przywara JF, Abel SB, Peacock JT, et al. Occurrence and recurrence of gastric dilatation with or without volvulus after incisional gastropexy. Can Vet J 2014; 55(10):981–4.

71. Hammel SP, Novo RE. Recurrence of gastric dilatation-volvulus after incisional gastropexy in a rottweiler. J Am Anim Hosp Assoc 2006;42(2):147–50.

72. Wacker CA, Weber UT, Tanno F, et al. Ultrasonographic evaluation of adhesions induced by incisional gastropexy in 16 dogs. J Small Anim Pract 1998;39(8): 379–84.

73. Leib MS, Konde LJ, Wingfield WE, et al. Circumcostal gastropexy for preventing recurrence of gastric dilatation-volvulus in the dog: an evaluation of 30 cases. J Am Vet Med Assoc 1985;187(3):245–8.

74. Stampley AR, Burrows CF, Ellison GW. The use of retrievable electrodes for recording gastric myoelectric activity after spontaneous gastric dilatation volvulus in dogs. Cornell Vet 1992;82(4):423–34.

75. Hall JA, Willer RL, Seim HB 3rd, et al. Gastric emptying of nondigestible radiopaque markers after circumcostal gastropexy in clinically normal dogs and dogs with gastric dilatation-volvulus. Am J Vet Res 1992;53(10):1961–5.

76. Ward MP, Patronek GJ, Glickman LT. Benefits of prophylactic gastropexy for dogs at risk of gastric dilatation volvulus. Prev Vet Med 2003;60:319–29.

77. Steelman-Szymeczek SM, Stebbins ME, Hardie EM. Clinical evaluation of a right-sided prophylactic gastropexy via a grid approach. J Am Anim Hosp Assoc 2003;39(4):397–402.

78. Dujowich M, Keller ME, Reimer SB. Evaluation of short- and long-term complications after endoscopically assisted gastropexy in dogs. J Am Vet Med Assoc 2010;236(2):177–82.

79. Tavakoli A, Mahmoodifard M, Razavifard AH. The superiority of paracostal endoscopic-assisted gastropexy over open incisional and belt loop gastropexy in dogs: a comparison of three prophylactic techniques. Iran J Vet Res 2016; 17(2):118–23.

80. Balsa IM, Culp WT, Johnson EG, et al. Efficacy of Two Radiologic-Assisted Prophylactic Gastropexy Techniques. Vet Surg 2016;45(4):464–70.

81. Haraguchi T, Kimura S, Itoh H, et al. Comparison of postoperative pain and inflammation reaction in dogs undergoing preventive laparoscopic-assisted and incisional gastropexy. J Vet Med Sci 2017;79(9):1524–31.

82. Imhoff DJ, Cohen A, Monnet E. Biomechanical Analysis of Laparoscopic Incisional Gastropexy With Intracorporeal Suturing Using Knotless Polyglyconate. Vet Surg 2015;44(Suppl 1):39–43.

83. Rivier P, Furneaux R, Viguier E. Combined laparoscopic ovariectomy and laparoscopic-assisted gastropexy in dogs susceptible to gastric dilatation-volvulus. Can Vet J 2011;52(1):62–6.

84. Balsa IM, Culp WTN, Drobatz KJ, et al. Effect of Laparoscopic-assisted Gastropexy on Gastrointestinal Transit Time in Dogs. J Vet Intern Med 2017;31(6):1680–5.

85. Gazzola KM, Nelson LL, Fritz MC, et al. Effects of prophylactic incisional gastropexy on markers of gastric motility in dogs as determined by use of a novel wireless motility device. Am J Vet Res 2017;78(1):100–6.

86. Coleman KA, Boscan P, Ferguson L, et al. Evaluation of gastric motility in nine dogs before and after prophylactic laparoscopic gastropexy: a pilot study. Aust Vet J 2019;97(7):225–30.

87. Rawlings CA, Foutz TL, Mahaffey MB, et al. A rapid and strong laparoscopic-assisted gastropexy in dogs. Am J Vet Res 2001;62(6):871–5.

88. Loy Son NK, Singh A, Amsellem P, et al. Long-Term Outcome and Complications Following Prophylactic Laparoscopic-Assisted Gastropexy in Dogs. Vet Surg 2016;45(S1):O77–83.

89. Stiles M, Case JB, Coisman J. Elective gastropexy with a reusable single-incision laparoscopic surgery port in dogs: 14 cases (2012-2013). J Am Vet Med Assoc 2016;249(3):299–303.

90. Baron JK, Casale SA, Monnet E, et al. Paramedian incisional complications after prophylactic laparoscopy-assisted gastropexy in 411 dogs. Vet Surg 2020;49(Suppl 1):O148–55.

91. Rawlings CA, Mahaffey MB, Bement S, et al. Prospective evaluation of laparoscopic-assisted gastropexy in dogs susceptible to gastric dilatation. J Am Vet Med Assoc 2002;221(11):1576–81.

92. Mayhew PD, Brown DC. Prospective evaluation of two intracorporeally sutured prophylactic laparoscopic gastropexy techniques compared with laparoscopic-assisted gastropexy in dogs. Vet Surg 2009;38:738–46.

93. Coleman KA, Monnet E. Comparison of laparoscopic gastropexy performed via intracorporeal suturing with knotless unidirectional barbed suture using a needle driver versus a roticulated endoscopic suturing device: 30 cases. Vet Surg 2017;46(7):1002–7.

94. Takacs JD, Singh A, Case JB, et al. Total laparoscopic gastropexy using 1 simple continuous barbed suture line in 63 dogs. Vet Surg 2017;46(2):233–41.

95. Spah CE, Elkins AD, Wehrenberg A, et al. Evaluation of two novel self-anchoring barbed sutures in a prophylactic laparoscopic gastropexy compared with intracorporeal tied knots. Vet Surg 2013;42(8):932–42.

96. Deroy C, Hahn H, Bismuth C, et al. Simplified Minimally Invasive Surgical Approach for Prophylactic Laparoscopic Gastropexy in 21 Cases. J Am Anim Hosp Assoc 2019;55(3):152–9.

97. Fracassi L, Crovace AM, Staffieri F, et al. Biomechanical evaluation of an absorbable fixation strap for use in total laparoscopic gastropexy in dogs. Am J Vet Res 2020;81(7):594–9.
98. Lacitignola L, Fracassi L, Di Bella C, Zizzo N, Passantino G, Tinelli A, Crovace AM, Staffieri F. Absorbable fixation straps for laparoscopic gastropexy in dogs. Vet Surg 2021 Jul;(50 Suppl 1):O78–88.
99. Hardie RJ, Flanders JA, Schmidt P, et al. Biomechanical and histological evaluation of a laparoscopic stapled gastropexy technique in dogs. Vet Surg 1996; 25(2):127–33.
100. Balsa IM, Giuffrida MA, Mayhew PD. A randomized controlled trial of three-dimensional versus two-dimensional imaging system on duration of surgery and mental workload for laparoscopic gastropexies in dogs. Vet Surg 2021; 50(5):944–53.
101. Sharp CR, Rozanski EA, Finn E, et al. The pattern of mortality in dogs with gastric dilatation and volvulus. J Vet Emerg Crit Care (San Antonio) 2020; 30(2):232–8.
102. Boller M, Nemanic TS, Anthonisz JD, et al. The Effect of Pet Insurance on Presurgical Euthanasia of Dogs With Gastric Dilatation-Volvulus: A Novel Approach to Quantifying Economic Euthanasia in Veterinary Emergency Medicine. Front Vet Sci 2020;7:590615.

Updates in Upper Respiratory Surgery

Heidi Phillips, VMD

KEYWORDS

- Brachycephalic • Airway syndrome • Nasal turbinates • Soft palate
- Laryngeal saccules • Laryngeal collapse • Tonsillectomy • Epiglottis

KEY POINTS

- Primary components of brachycephalic obstructive airway syndrome (BOAS) include stenosis of the alar wings and folds; aberrant, obstructive nasal turbinates; overlong and thickened soft palate; everted mucosa of the laryngeal ventricles; and everted and enlarged tonsils, macroglossia, and hypoplastic trachea
- Several clinical scoring systems have been developed in efforts to increase the sensitivity of physical examination for determination of the severity of BOAS and to provide indications for particular treatments. Use of a 3-minute exercise test is most useful in conjunction with careful auscultation.
- Stenotic nares appear to be the predominant primary abnormality causing clinical signs of brachycephalic cats. Ala-vestibuloplasty and ventral skin fold resection have been described as successful treatments.
- Norwich terrier upper airway syndrome is an emerging condition of some Norwich terrier dogs that warrants anatomic, diagnostic imaging and therapeutic investigation independent of BOAS.

INTRODUCTION

There are at least 24 recognized dog breeds with brachycephalic conformation, including the affenpinscher, Boston terrier, Fila Brasileiro, Brussels griffon, bulldog, French bulldog, Boxer, Cavalier King Charles Spaniel, Dogue de Bordeaux, Japanese chin, Lhasa apso, bullmastiff, Pekingese, pug, and shih tzu breeds.[1,2] Despite knowledge of the encumbrances imposed upon these pets, demand for severe brachycephalic conformation in small animals persists.[3,4] French and English bulldogs have remained among the top 10 breeds registered with the American Kennel Club since 2014 and are among the top 5 breeds registered since 2017.[5] Even more concerning, registration of brachycephalic breeds has skyrocketed in the United Kingdom in recent years, with registration of French bulldogs increasing 15-fold, from 2200 in 2010 to more than 33,000 in 2020.[6] In Australia, a study evaluating characteristics

Small Animal Surgery, Department of Veterinary Clinical Medicine, University of Illinois College of Veterinary Medicine, 1008 West Hazelwood Drive, Urbana, IL 61802, USA
E-mail address: philli@illinois.edu

Vet Clin Small Anim 52 (2022) 339–368
https://doi.org/10.1016/j.cvsm.2021.12.002
0195-5616/22/© 2021 Elsevier Inc. All rights reserved.
vetsmall.theclinics.com

of kennel club–registered breeds found that the cephalic index, a ratio of skull width to height, increased substantially among registered breeds from 1986 to 2013, indicating an escalating preference for dogs with shorter, wider heads.[7] Although ownership of purebred cats is less common than ownership of purebred dogs, brachycephalic feline breeds also remain a popular choice of pet. Exotic shorthair and Persian cats have been among the top 4 most popular cat breeds registered with the Cat Fanciers' Association since 2012.[8]

Although many abnormalities comprise the clinical brachycephalic syndrome, chronic, debilitating, and potentially fatal upper airway obstruction is most threatening to both quality of life and survival.[1,9–12] Brachycephalic obstructive airway syndrome (BOAS) affects both brachycephalic canine and feline breeds and results predominantly from a severely shortened craniofacial conformation without concomitant reduction in the volume of nasal, nasopharyngeal, and/or oropharyngeal soft tissues.[11,13–22] Stenotic nares, elongated soft palate, and hypoplastic trachea have long been considered the primary components of BOAS that cause increased airway resistance and more negative intraluminal pressure on inspiration.[9,11,19] Clinical signs commonly associated with the respiratory tract in dogs include snoring or stertor, stridor, other inspiratory dyspnea, coughing, choking, difficulty eating, exercise intolerance, cyanosis, syncope, and death.[3,11,14,17–20,22–29]

Secondary airway abnormalities result from chronically increased resistance to airflow, and include enlarged and everted tonsils and laryngeal saccules, laryngeal and pharyngeal mucosal edema, and laryngeal collapse.[11,22,23,28–30] Pharyngeal collapse is also thought to be associated with brachycephaly, and concurrent laryngeal collapse has been shown to worsen the clinical respiratory signs of brachycephalic syndrome.[31,32] Bronchial collapse also has been documented in brachycephalic dogs and may be due entirely to chronically increased negative airway pressures or to chondromalacia of the lower airways.[33,34]

Canine brachycephaly also causes life-threatening cardiopulmonary disorders, including hypoxemia, hypercapnea, hiatal hernia, aspiration pneumonia, polycythemia, heat stroke, and hypertension.[3,21] Neoplastic disorders of the cardiopulmonary system, such as chemodectomas, also are associated with brachycephaly.[3,21,22,25,35] Sleep apnea may cause systemic hypertension in brachycephalic dogs and has been purported to occur in cats.[3,25,36] In severe cases, brachycephalic dogs may require ventilation for respiratory fatigue secondary to aspiration pneumonia,[24] and acquired myocardial damage and systemic inflammation may occur in brachycephalic dogs and cats. Cardiac troponin 1 levels were elevated in a majority of brachycephalic dogs in 2 reports.[37,38]

Given the grave implications of chronic upper airway obstruction, surgery is indicated to correct primary abnormalities early in life to improve quality of life and prevent development of secondary changes.[11,13,22] Traditional surgical intervention of BOAS has focused on widening the external nares, shortening the soft palate, and excising everted mucosa of the laryngeal ventricles.[3,9,13,19,20] Despite variability in the frequency of reported complications, an emerging and consistent problem with the use of traditional surgical techniques has proved the persistence of clinical signs.[39–41] Clinical signs reported to persist after traditional brachycephalic airway surgery include snoring during sleep in 73.9% of dogs, stertor and/or stridor while conscious in 50% of dogs, excessive panting in 28.3%, and other dyspnea in 21.7% of dogs.[41] Failure of response to surgery may be more common in dogs affected by secondary effects of brachycephaly, such as laryngeal collapse, and such dogs may require permanent tracheostomy.[24,39,40,42] Recent advances in diagnostic imaging and assessment have revealed components of brachycephaly and anatomic details regarding airway obstruction that may allow for more complete treatment of upper airway obstruction in brachycephalic dogs and cats and improved responses to multilevel upper airways surgeries that combine traditional and novel procedures.[3,14,17–20,27,31,32,34,43–62]

With growing concern for the plight of brachycephalic pets, investigators of brachycephalic dogs have reported dogs exhibit a constellation of abnormalities not only manifested by respiratory noise and difficulty but also by problems with exercise and heat tolerance, eating, drinking, and sleeping as well as numerous concerns related to general welfare and quality of life.[3,4,12,21,22,35,55,58,59,63–71] Although Trostel and Frankel[73] demonstrated positive outcomes in brachycephalic dogs treated by resection alaplasty, and other studies have shown both subjective as well as objective measurable reductions in clinical signs following routine upper airway surgery,[9,11,27,35,38,41,72,73] clinical signs of respiratory distress have persisted or worsened in many patients; gastrointestinal problems, such as regurgitation, vomiting, gastritis, duodenitis, hiatal hernia, and aspiration pneumonia, have plagued some pets,[35,63,64,68,69,74–76] and sleep disturbances, such as obstructive sleep apnea, have become more prevalent or more recognized.[3,15,16,19,20,25,36,47] Reportedly, traditional upper airway surgery, including vertical or horizontal wedge or punch resection alaplasty, cut-and-suture staphylectomy, and resection of everted mucosa of the laryngeal ventricles, is effective in diminishing clinical signs in as few as 45% of cases.[15,16,65,77]

To more fully characterize and understand the primary anatomic abnormalities and secondary effects that contribute to fixed or dynamic and recalcitrant upper airway obstructions in dogs with persistent BOAS, several researchers have conducted imaging-based anatomic studies of brachycephalic dogs using computed tomography (CT), endoscopy, and magnetic resonance imaging (MRI). Advanced imaging in brachycephalic dogs also has led to greater understanding of the anatomic abnormalities contributing to BOAS in dogs and development of novel surgical options to address them.[19,20,48,51,78]

This article discusses updates in brachycephalic and other upper respiratory surgery, including schemata for classifying brachycephalic dogs in terms of severity of disease and indications for monitoring and treatment, new characterizations of the primary and secondary components of brachycephaly, and updates to traditional brachycephalic surgical procedures as well as novel surgeries to treat BOAS, the effects of brachycephaly on some feline breeds, mechanical or functional disorders of the epiglottis, and upper airway syndrome in Norwich terriers.

VALIDATION SCORE FOR BRACHYCEPHALIC OBSTRUCTIVE AIRWAY SYNDROME

With the dramatic rise in popularity of brachycephalic breeds in the United States and Europe, the potential for unintended suffering for brachycephalic pets is great, as is the need for education of owners, breeders, and veterinary professionals.[5,8,12,79] Although many brachycephalic dogs and cats suffer from a clinical brachycephalic syndrome, some do not, and a predetermination of pets at greatest risk of physiologic compromise would aid in breeding, or cessation of breeding efforts, and application of the highest standard of care.[12,59,62] Although many veterinarians rely on careful anamnesis, detailed physical examination, visual airway inspection, and advanced diagnostic imaging studies, including radiographic, CT, MRI, and fluoroscopic studies to diagnose BOAS in animals presented for care, an effective clinical grading system that clearly differentiates dogs at risk for BOAS or affected by BOAS from dogs not at risk or unaffected would increase the sensitivity of physical examination for determination of BOAS, facilitate timely treatment of affected dogs and cats, and permit minimally invasive assessment of response to surgical interventions.[3,4,21,22,58,59,65,66,79–82]

An exercise test was developed to more accurately diagnose laryngeal collapse in brachycephalic dogs. Investigators found that the sensitivity of the clinical examination for diagnosis of laryngeal collapse in brachycephalic dogs was improved from approximately 57% to more than 93% following a 3-minute trot test.[59] Although auscultation of laryngeal stridor was highly specific for a diagnosis of laryngeal collapse in this cohort, it was not terribly sensitive.[59] To improve sensitivity of detection of laryngeal collapse, careful auscultation of the larynx and a 3-minute trot test should be included as part of a more comprehensive clinical scoring assessment of dogs presented for evaluation for BOAS.[59,79]

A Brachycephalic Syndrome Functional score was developed based on a 6-minute walking test, upper airway noise recordings, and airway auscultation; the score was used to evaluate the association of morphometric and phenotypic characteristics of French bulldogs with signs of brachycephalic syndrome.[4] Nasal stenosis accounted for 32% of the variation in the Brachycephalic Syndrome Functional score, indicating this morphometric parameter had a serious impact on the respiratory health of dogs in the study, and the nares should be evaluated carefully and treated as completely as possible in brachycephalic dogs.[4]

A brachycephalic risk score was developed to objectively and accurately predict the risk of major complications or death in dogs undergoing corrective surgery for BOAS (**Table 1**).[62] Although the score was performed as part of a retrospective study using clinical data available at the time of presentation and admission to assess for correlations to outcome, scoring was able to discriminate between dogs likely to have a positive or negative outcome following surgical intervention for BOAS.[62] The scoring system assigned 0.5 to 2 points per variable, including temperature at admission, breed, prior airway surgery, plan for concurrent procedures unrelated to the airway, body condition score (BCS), presence and character of upper respiratory noise, need for oxygen or sedation, and need for intubation. The investigators concluded dogs with scores less than 3 were at low risk for major complications or death, and dogs with scores 3 or greater were at high risk for morbidity or mortality related to BOAS. Preoperative variables associated with increased risk for major complications from airway surgery, including death, were French or English bulldog breed; increasing age; admission during warmer months; BCS greater than or equal to 4/5; exercise intolerance; prior airway surgery; emergent admission; concurrent procedures performed unrelated to the airway; heart rate at admission greater than 120 beats per minute; respiratory rate at admission greater than 30 breaths per minute; rectal temperature at admission greater than 102°F; any requirement for sedation, oxygen, or intubation at admission; radiologic evidence of aspiration pneumonia at admission; and increasing anesthetic American Society of Anesthesiologists score. Operative or perianesthetic variables associated with negative outcome included diagnosis of stage 2 or greater laryngeal collapse and increased surgical time. A brachycephalic risk score of 4 or greater was 70% sensitive and greater than 80% specific for negative outcome.[62]

The University of Cambridge in partnership with The Kennel Club of the United Kingdom developed a respiratory function grading scheme and protocol for assessment of brachycephalic dogs for characterization of BOAS signs.[14,79] Within the scheme are prompts for evaluators, and recommendations include a thorough physical examination prior to and immediately following a 3-minute trot test, during which dogs are meant to trot at 4 to 5 miles per hour. Functional grading is performed while evaluating for respiratory noise, including stertor or stridor; inspiratory effort; and other dyspnea, cyanosis, or syncope. Grades are assigned for variables based on presence or absence, frequency, and severity of signs before and after the exercise test

Table 1
Brachycephalic risk score[62]

Score Category				
Breed	Brachycephalic breed, NOT English or French bulldog 0 points	English or French bulldog 0.5 point		
Surgical history	No history of prior airway surgery 0 points	History of prior airway surgery 1.5 points		
Procedures planned	No additional procedures planned 0 points	Additional procedures planned 1.5 points		
BCS	BCS ≤2.5 1 point	2.5<BCS≤3.5 0 points	BCS >3.5 1 point	
Level of compromise at admission	No stertor or stertor only at exercise 0 points	Stertor at rest 1.5 points	Oxygen and sedation needed at admission 2 points	Intubation needed; unable to extubate without surgery 4 points
Admission rectal temperature	Admission rectal temperature ≤100°F 1.5 points	100°F (37.8°C) less than rectal temperature ≤101°F (38.3°C) 1 point	101°F (38.3°C) less than rectal temperature ≤ 103°F (39.4°C) 0.5 points	Admission rectal temperature >103°F (39.4°C) 0 points

(**Table 2**).[79] In addition to providing a means of objective initial comparison for respiratory performance among dogs, the functional grading system for BOAS also was compared with whole-body barometric plethysmography (WBBP) data.[14] Using physical examination, an exercise tolerance test, and computational WBBP data, a classifier was developed with quadratic discriminant analysis of respiratory parameters to distinguish French bulldogs with and without BOAS, and a BOAS index was calculated for each dog. Sensitivity, specificity, positive predictive value, and negative predictive value of the classifier were 0.97, 0.93, 0.95, and 0.97, respectively, for a training group. The classifier then was validated using a test group of 20 French bulldogs, with an accuracy of 0.95. The investigators concluded WBBP offers objective screening for the diagnosis of BOAS in French bulldogs.[14] Unfortunately, WBBP is not readily available to most general practice or tertiary referral clinics. If widely available, the classifier could provide objective disease probabilities for dogs at the time of testing and monitor disease progression. This classification scheme could also assist in improving welfare of French bulldog and other brachycephalic breeds.[14]

ASSESSMENT OF THE BRACHYCEPHALIC DOG

The author recommends primary veterinarians or specialists presented symptomatic brachycephalic dogs for upper airway evaluation or surgery conduct a detailed and

Table 2
University of Cambridge functional grading system[79]

		Respiratory Noise	Inspiratory Effort	Dyspnea/Cyanosis/Syncope
Grade 0	Pre-ET[a]	Not audible	Not present	Not present
	Post-ET	Not audible	Not present	Not present
Grade I	Pre-ET	Not audible to mild stertor, and/or moderate intermittent nasal stertor when sniffing	Not present	Not present
	Post-ET	Mild stertor, and/or moderate intermittent nasal stertor when sniffing, and/or intermittent gentle stertor when panting	Not present to mild	Not present
Grade II	Pre-ET	Mild to moderate stertor	Not present to moderate	Not present
	Post-ET	Moderate to severe stertor	Moderate to severe and/or regurgitation of foam/saliva	Dyspnea, cyanosis, or syncope not present
Grade III	Pre-ET	Moderate to severe stertor or any stridor	Moderate to severe	Dyspnea; may or may not be presented with cyanosis. Inability to exercise
	Post-ET	Severe stertor or any stridor	Severe and/or regurgitation of foam/saliva	Dyspnea; may or may not be presented with cyanosis

[a] ET, exercise test.

thorough anamnesis. Veterinarians should aim to discuss the following topics with owners. For the highest quality anamnesis, these topics must be addressed by veterinarians directly, because owners often fail to mention clinically relevant symptoms.

- Character of respiratory noise
- Timing, frequency, and duration of respiratory noise and dyspnea
- Association of respiratory noise and dyspnea to exercise, eating, drinking, or sleeping
- Quality of sleep and evidence of sleep apnea, especially periods of hypopnea or apnea followed by sudden arousal and increased respiratory effort
- Presence of daytime somnolence, for example, sleeping while sitting
- Efforts by the pet to manipulate the head and neck during wakefulness or sleep into an elongated or arched position. Pets often hang the head over an owner's limb, arm of a chair, or edge of a bed or position a toy or bone within the mouth, presumably to facilitate passage of airflow.

For initial examination of a symptomatic brachycephalic dog, the dog should be examined as soon as possible on arrival to the clinic. The dog should be kept calm, and only gentle restraint should be used. If the dog is agitated from travel or presentation to the clinic, supervised time should be provided to allow to dog to calm.[79] The dog should be observed for inspiratory or respiratory effort and timing, frequency, character, and duration of respiratory noise. With the head held in a neutral position by the mandibles to avoid compression of the soft tissues of the cervical region, the author begins auscultation at the nares, listening for airflow by manually obstructing each naris alternately as the dog permits. The skin around the nares and the thoracic inlet should be observed for evidence of collapse on inspiration, an indicator of the increased inspiratory effort required to overcome significant upper airway obstruction. Auscultation should proceed to the larynx, avoiding pressure on the larynx, while observing thoracic wall and abdominal wall excursions and use of the diaphragm and accessory muscles of respiration on inspiration and expiration.[79] Finally, auscultation should proceed to the thorax. Auscultation of stridor should prompt concern for laryngeal collapse, although the absence of stridor is not indicative of a functional larynx. If the dog is stable without a history of cyanosis or syncope, an exercise test can be performed with the goal to trot the dog or walk at a fast pace for 3 minutes. Thorough auscultation should be repeated after the exercise test.[14,79]

At the author's institution, a prolonged fast greater than 12 hours to 24 hours is performed prior to sedated oral examination, diagnostic imaging, and surgery to minimize the risk of regurgitation and aspiration, and intravenous (IV) gastrointestinal protectant drugs are initiated at admission, including cisapride, 0.5 mg/kg IV every 8 hours; maropitant, 1 mg/kg IV every 24 hours; pantoprazole, 1 mg/kg IV every 12 hours; and metoclopramide, 2 mg/kg/d constant rate infusion. In the author's experience, sedated oral examination and diagnostic imaging should be performed the day of surgery in a single session along with surgery, if indicated.

UNDERSTANDING NEW PRIMARY COMPONENTS AND SECONDARY EFFECTS OF BRACHYCEPHALY
Aberrant Turbinates

Although aberrant turbinate growth was reported as an additional feature of brachycephaly in both dogs and cats as early as 2007, the problem only recently has become more universally accepted as a primary anatomic abnormality contributing to clinical signs.[19,20,28,29,48,56] Using CT and rigid anterior and posterior rhinoscopy of French bulldogs, English bulldogs, and pugs, investigators noted the common presence and variable manifestation of aberrant and malformed conchal tissue causing obstruction of the intranasal meatuses by inappropriate contact of the intranasal mucosal surfaces. Rostral aberrant turbinates were defined as conchal lamellae from the ventral or medial nasal conchae spreading rostral to the first branch of the plica alaris (**Fig. 1**).[19,65] Caudal aberrant turbinates (CATs) were defined as turbinates visible in the ventral nasal meatus possibly extending into the nasopharyngeal meatus or beyond the vomer into the nasopharynx (**Fig. 2**).[19,65] Rostral aberrant turbinates (RATs) and nasopharyngeal or CATs as well as intranasal mucosal contact points **Fig. 3** were identified in 66% to 72% (RATs and CATs) and 87% (intranasal mucosal contact points) of brachycephalic dogs examined, respectively.[19,28,29] Deviations of the nasal septum also were reported in approximately one-half of all dogs and approximately 100% of pugs.[20] In another study, nasopharyngeal turbinates were identified in 21% of brachycephalic small animals, including 21% of dogs and 20% of cats examined. Pugs accounted for 32% of all dogs in the study population and 82% of dogs with nasopharyngeal turbinates.[48] The effect of turbinate abnormalities, although not directly established, also has been implied in computational fluid dynamics studies, where significant resistance to airflow can be predicted within nasal passages affected by aberrant turbinates.[83,84] Investigators also have provided information on the proposed pathophysiologic mechanism whereby aberrant turbinates develop in some breeds.[19] Although the craniofacial skull of brachycephalic dogs is marked by inhibition of postnatal growth, by contrast, the turbinates show tremendous postnatal growth as well as differentiation, resulting in development of crowded and malformed nasal turbinates in some severely affected brachycephalic dogs.[19,85,86]

A novel endosurgical procedure, laser-assisted turbinectomy (LATE) (**Figs. 4** and **5**), recently was introduced and shown to yield promising findings, resulting in decreased mucosal contact points in the nasal passages and improved nasal patency (see **Fig. 5**).[20,28,29] Endoscopic-assisted laser turbinectomy was performed to safely and

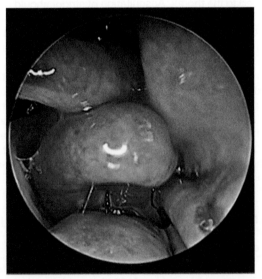

Fig. 1. Rostral aberrant turbinate, right nasal passage. A rostral aberrant turbinate is seen arising from the plica alaris and causing obstruction of the right nasal passage. Image obtained with a 2.7-mm 0° rigid endoscope.

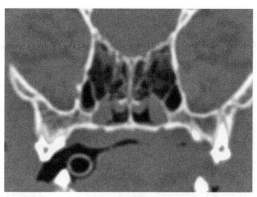

Fig. 2. Caudal aberrant turbinate, axial CT image, right nasal passage. A caudal aberrant turbinate is seen extending into the right nasopharyngeal meatus.

efficiently remove the ventral nasal concha and aberrant turbinates growing rostrally and caudally in 158 dogs of 1 report, and a clear passage for nasal airflow was crafted in all dogs.[20] Complications included minor, transient, intraoperative hemorrhage in 32% of dogs and regrowth of obstructive turbinates requiring additional resection in only 16% of dogs 6 months following the initial LATE procedure (**Fig. 6**).[20] A separate study was performed to evaluate the efficacy of LATE in treating BOAS and to investigate potential indications.[65] Investigators of this study found that dogs that did not show satisfactory clinical improvement from traditional brachycephalic airway surgery, including conventional resection alaplasty and staphylectomy, did benefit from LATE, and the proportion of soft tissue at the rostral entrance of the choana as measured on CT was a reliable predictor of candidacy for LATE in French bulldogs and pugs.[65] Investigators also found that LATE largely reduced the incidence of regurgitation and sleep disturbances, and WBBP documented improvement to satisfactory respiratory function in 80% of operated dogs.[65] WBBP provides noninvasive measurement of respiratory function by placement of dogs in barometric chambers equipped with pneumotachographs. Respiration is sensed by pressure transducers, and signals are amplified and assessed by commercial software to yield information on

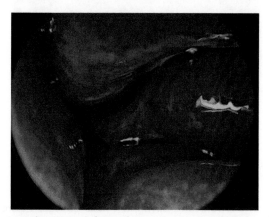

Fig. 3. Increased mucosal contact, left nasal passage. Increased points of mucosal contact among turbinates. Image obtained with a 2.7-mm 0° rigid endoscope.

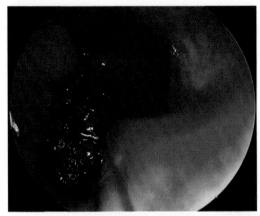

Fig. 4. An example of LATE, right nasal passage. A diode laser is used to resect a rostral aberrant turbinate at its base. A red rubber catheter is positioned ventrally in the nasal passage to aid in removal of smoke and blood. Image obtained with a 2.7-mm 0° rigid endoscope.

respiratory rate, inspiratory and expiratory times, tidal and minute volumes, and peak inspiratory and expiratory flow rates. Protocols for the assessment of these data have been described and validated.[14]

The LATE procedure was pioneered by Professor Gerhard Oechtering at the University of Leipzig, Germany, and has generated interest among veterinary surgeons and owners of brachycephalic dogs. The procedure also is offered by Dr Jane Ladlow and colleagues at the University of Cambridge and Hamilton Specialist Referrals, Buckinghamshire, England, and by the author (HP) at the University of Illinois, Urbana. Along with French bulldogs, English bulldogs, and pugs, the author has performed this procedure for Boston terrier and Cavalier King Charles spaniel breeds. The author recommends owners of brachycephalic dogs suspected to potentially benefit from LATE pursue traditional treatment of nares, palate, laryngeal saccule, and tonsillar abnormalities with a regional specialist before considering travel to a select institution for

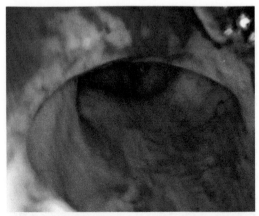

Fig. 5. An example of a LATE-treated airway, left nasal passage. View of the open nasopharynx achieved by rigid anterior rhinoscopy following LATE. Image obtained with a 2.7-mm 0° rigid endoscope.

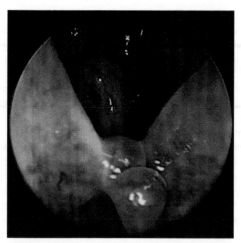

Fig. 6. An example of regrowth of nasal turbinates with synechia. Two months following initial LATE, regrowth of turbinates to the point of obstruction has occurred with the presence of synechia. Image obtained with a 2.7-mm 0° rigid endoscope.

evaluation for LATE, because some dogs show satisfactory improvement in respiration after accurate performance of traditional brachycephalic surgery. The author also asks all owners of potential LATE candidates to submit videos of the pet breathing during wakefulness and sleep, including the head, neck, thorax, and abdomen in the videos. At the author's institution, evaluation for LATE includes this video assessment of behaviors at home; detailed and thorough anamnesis; thorough physical examination; complete blood cell count, serum biochemical profile, and urinalysis; sedated oral examination; CT examination of the head, cervical, and thoracic airways; anterior and posterior rigid rhinoscopy using 0° and 120° rigid rhinoscopy, respectively; and laryngoscopy with the aid of doxapram, 1 mg/kg IV.

Elongated and Thickened Soft Palate

The overlong palate has long been accepted as a primary anatomic component of brachycephalic syndrome, and numerous methods have been described, including the cut-and-sew method, partial resection by CO_2 laser, and partial resection by vessel sealing device.[1,9–11,13,45,47,55,64,76,82,87–92] If the CO_2 laser is used, the author recommends the oral and nasal mucosa of the cut soft palate be apposed with a continuous suture pattern of 4-0 poliglecaprone 25 to prevent disruption to the site and exposure of palatine muscle and soft tissues, which may lead to granulation tissue formation. The author has found the addition of suture apposition is not a requirement with the use of vessel sealing devices and prefers the cut-and-sew method of staphylectomy or use of a vessel sealing device.

The contribution of the soft palate to brachycephalic syndrome initially was accepted to be only excessive palatal length but has been expanded more recently to also include pathologic thickening.[1,9,53,91,93–95] Pathologic changes associated with gross palatal thickening have been documented microscopically. Several studies have reported histologic changes to the brachycephalic canine soft palate, including myofiber atrophy, diminished palatine peripheral nerve branches, and increased stroma and salivary tissue compared with palates from mesaticephalic dogs.[87,88,91] One study demonstrated that dogs severely affected by brachycephalic syndrome had significantly thicker soft palates on CT compared with dogs that were minimally affected by brachycephalic syndrome.[78] Another study found the smallest dimensions of the nasopharynx in both pugs and French bulldogs were dorsal to the caudal soft palate.[51]

To newly characterize the palate's role in BOAS, some investigators have used CT or MRI.[14,16,17,51,53,61,78,83,84,96] Since the publication of Findji and Dupre's folded flap palatoplasty,[47] several investigators have confirmed that thickness of the soft palate, independent of excessive length, contributes substantially to airway narrowing and obstruction in some brachycephalic dogs.[1,9,47,51,78,93–95,97] In 1 CT study, brachycephalic dogs, and French bulldogs, in particular, were found to have significantly thicker palates than normocephalic dogs, and thickness increased with severity of the brachycephalic conformation.[78] The investigators hypothesized that muscular hypertrophy, mucosal edema, or both contributed to the relative increase in thickness caused by airflow resistance at the nares, the vestibulum nasi, and the cavum nasi.[78] This hypothesis was supported by histologic evidence showing hyperplasia of the superficial epithelium and mucus glands in the brachycephalic palate along with myofiber atrophy, extensive swelling of the interfibrillar matrix, and edema of the lamina propria.[87,91,93] Other investigators have focused on measurement of the nasopharyngeal airway using CT and confirmed that soft palate thickness contributes to nasopharyngeal airway obstruction and likely to sleep-disordered breathing in brachycephalic dogs.[51,98,99] The author also has found that soft palate thickness is greater in brachycephalic dogs than mesaticephalic dogs when normalized to body weight, most significantly at the rostral aspect of the soft palate, nearest the posterior nasal spine61 (**Fig. 7**), and routinely employs CT to evaluate soft palate thickness in any brachycephalic dog presented with signs of sleep apnea.

Although routine staphylectomy addresses BOAS-associated laryngeal obstruction due to excessive soft palate length,[1,9–11,13,45,47,55,64,76,82,87–92] the nasopharyngeal and oropharyngeal obstructions caused by a thickened soft palate can be mitigated by either more rostral excision for staphylectomy or folded flap palatoplasty.[47,97,98] In a prospective study of dogs with BOAS, maximal nasopharyngeal occlusion was always located 1 cm to 2 cm directly caudal to the hamular pterygoids.[97] The investigators proposed that an incision at this site for staphylectomy would result in resection of the most offensive portion of the soft palate, accounting for excessive length and thickness.[97] The author prefers folded flap palatoplasty performed with dogs placed in sternal recumbency and the maxilla suspended.[47,65] With the tongue pulled rostrally, traction can be placed on the caudal edge of the oral mucosa of the soft palate. Electrocautery is used to mark the most rostral aspect of the proposed excision, usually approximately 2 cm caudal to the posterior nasal spine. The oral mucosa is marked and incised in a trapezoidal shape from the rostral incision to the free edge of the caudal palate using bipolar cautery and Metzenbaum scissors (**Fig. 8**). Beginning rostrally and continuing caudally, the palatine muscles and other soft tissues are excised along with the oral mucosa using a combination of blunt and sharp dissection leaving the nasal mucosa and submucosa intact (**Fig. 9**). Hemostasis is achieved with continued use of fine-tipped bipolar cautery. Closure is performed by folding the remaining palatal tissue rostrally to appose the free caudal edge of the nasal mucosa to the rostral incised edge of the oral mucosa (**Fig. 10**).[47,65,98]

Stenotic Nares

Stenotic nares have been cited as a common primary component of BOAS and a significant contributor to clinical signs, and approximately half of French bulldogs studied had severely stenotic nares based on a published scale.[4,15,16,65] Airflow through the nares and nasal vestibule accounts for 76.5% of total airflow resistance in the

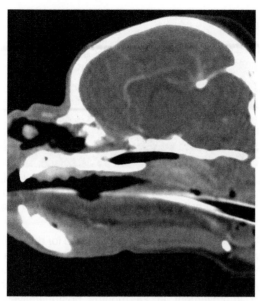

Fig. 7. Increased thickness of the soft palate. Sagittal CT image of a brachycephalic dog showing a thickened soft palate causing obstruction of the nasopharynx.

respiratory tract of normal dogs,[11,28,29] and the Poiseuille law states that a 50% reduction in radius results in a 16-fold increase in resistance to flow.[27,83,84] Therefore, any decrease in the dimension of the nares, nasal passages, or laryngeal airways increases upper airway resistance in brachycephalic breeds significantly compared with nonbrachycephalic breeds. Early reported techniques for management of stenotic nares included Trader's[100] technique of alar amputation and vertical, horizontal, or lateral wedge resection alaplasty.[66,72,100,101] Up to 25% of juvenile dogs were found to "breathe normally" following application of Trader's technique.[66,72,73,100,101] A more recent study found that French bulldogs showed increased saturation of the arterial blood with oxygen 4 weeks following vertical wedge resection alaplasty.[60] Alapexy is a technique in which the ala nasi are permanently abducted by apposition of 2

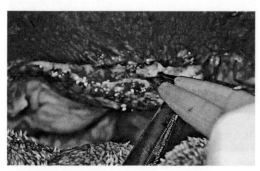

Fig. 8. Initial incision, folded flap palatoplasty. An initial incision is made rostrally in the oral mucosa and soft tissues of the soft palate during folded flap palatoplasty, using fine-tipped bipolar cautery and sharp dissection. Image obtained with a 10-mm 0° rigid endoscope.

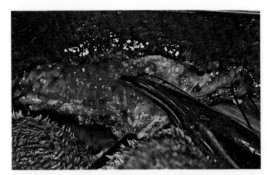

Fig. 9. Dissection during folded flap palatoplasty continues carefully through the soft tissues of the soft palate using a combination of blunt and sharp dissection. Care is taken not to penetrate the nasal mucosa. Image obtained with a 10-mm 0° rigid endoscope.

incisions lateral to the alar wing and has been advocated for dogs failing resection alaplasty or in dogs with very flaccid nasal cartilages.[73,102] Success rates for these procedures have been thought to be generally good, with 83% of dogs undergoing punch resection alaplasty having "excellent" outcomes and all dogs undergoing alapexy showing significant improvement at 24 months postoperatively.[73,102] Increased breeding and ownership of dogs suffering from ever more severe brachycephalic conformation, however, thankfully has been met with increased advocacy for brachycephalic pets and greater awareness of the physiologic effects of the brachycephalic conformation. Awareness and education as to the clinical implications of some respiratory symptoms, gastrointestinal problems, and sleep-disordered breathing have prompted some surgeons and owners to express dissatisfaction with results achieved by traditional nares-altering surgeries and to pursue alternative therapies.[9,15,17,18,21,27,35,39–41,49,50,54,64,68,76,83,84,95,96,98,103]

Ala-vestibuloplasty is a novel procedure whereby relief of stenosis of the external nares and internal nasal vestibule (**Fig. 11**) is achieved by removal of both the ala nasi, or alar wings, and the vestibula nasi, or alar folds.[58,65] This technique has

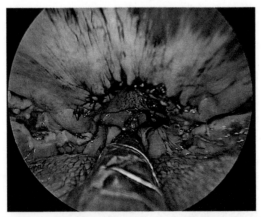

Fig. 10. Completed folded flap palatoplasty. Closure is achieved by folding the remaining palatal tissue rostrally to appose the free caudal edge of the nasal mucosa and submucosa to the rostral incised edge of the oral mucosa. Image obtained with a 10-mm 0° rigid endoscope.

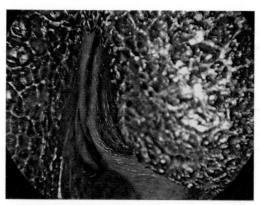

Fig. 11. Stenotic nares. Obstruction of the external naris and internal nasal vestibule is evident in this ventromedial image of the left naris. The alar wing and alar fold cause obstruction externally and internally, respectively. Both obstructions are addressed by treatment with ala-vestibuloplasty. Image obtained with a 2.7-mm 0° rigid endoscope.

been reported to contribute to very good success rates following multilevel upper airway surgery, but descriptions of this technique are limited.[15,16,19,20,58,65,92,98] Ala-vestibuloplasty reportedly is performed by grasping the dorsal part of the alar fold with curved hemostats.[15,16] An initial incision is made by a #11 blade horizontally to dissect the ventral connection of the alar fold to the vestibule. The dorsal part of the alar fold then is rotated gently with the hemostats laterally, enabling the blade to be positioned to resect the dorsomedial and caudal portions of the alar fold, widening the nasal vestibule and alleviating both external and internal stenoses of the nares **(Fig. 12)**.[15,16,57] The author has performed this procedure in more than 50 dogs and 20 cats, with excellent results and no significant complications.

Dorsal offset rhinoplasty was reported as an alternate technique to treat stenotic nares in 34 dogs and was defined as removal of a dorsal wedge of nasal planum from each naris with apposition of the rostral abaxial tissue to the caudal axial tissue,

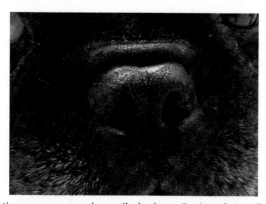

Fig. 12. Postoperative appearance, ala-vestibuloplasty. During ala-vestibuloplasty, the dorsomedial and caudal portion of the alar fold is resected along with the axial portion of the alar wing, widening the nasal vestibule and alleviating both external and internal stenosis of the nares. Image obtained with a 2.7-mm 0° rigid endoscope.

resulting in translocation of the alar cartilage in both median and dorsal planes (**Fig. 13**).[46] Only 50% of dogs had long-term follow-up, but 94% of owners able to be contacted reported high satisfaction with the procedure. Collapse of the naris was reported as a rare complication.[46] It is not clear if the presence or absence of concurrent abnormalities affected outcome in this cohort of patients.

Macroglossia

Although macroglossia anecdotally has been accepted as a prominent feature of brachycephaly, the tongue's contribution to BOAS only recently has been investigated.[52,61,99] Jones and colleagues[52] compared the dimensions and CT density of the soft palate and tongue in brachycephalic and mesaticephalic dogs by evaluating area of the soft palate and tongue at 2 points aligning in a sagittal plane with the caudal nasal spine and pterygoid hamulae. Tongues of brachycephalic dogs were found to be larger and denser than tongues of mesaticephalic dogs, and the investigators concluded that brachycephalic dogs have a relative macroglossia that can be considered a primary anatomic anomaly contributing to BOAS.[52] Other investigators have documented differences in tongue size among brachycephalic breeds; French and English bulldogs showed relative macroglossia compared with mesaticephalic breeds whereas pugs showed no evidence of macroglossia in 1 study.[99] The author's own data show that brachycephalic dogs not only have greater tongue volume than mesaticephalic dogs when normalized to body weight but also greater fat volume and tendencies toward sleep-disordered breathing.[61] Although targeted volume reduction of the tongue and soft palate may offer promise for more complete treatment of severe BOAS and sleep-disordered breathing, there are no studies describing experimental or clinically substantiated techniques for surgical correction of macroglossia in affected brachycephalic dogs.[61,99]

Enlarged and Everted Tonsils

Partial removal of the palatine tonsils, if they are enlarged or everted, is accomplished using a harmonic scalpel, bipolar electrothermal vessel sealing device or using bipolar forceps and Metzenbaum scissors (**Fig. 14**).[43,45] Although it is difficult to assess the impact of excision of enlarged or everted tonsils on outcome and prognosis, because this procedure is rarely performed in isolation for dogs treated surgically for BOAS, the author advocates tonsillectomy as part of a modified multilevel upper airway surgical treatment of dogs with BOAS, and tonsillectomy facilitates folded flap palatoplasty.[15,16,47,98] Tonsillectomy is included as part of multimodal treatment of snoring and obstructive sleep apnea in people to reduce obstruction at the level of the caudal palate and to stiffen the palate by fibrosis.[104–106]

BRACHYCEPHALIC SYNDROME IN CATS

Considering the significant literature dedicated to the anatomic abnormalities, clinical syndrome, and surgical interventions of brachycephalic dogs, it is clear brachycephalic cats are poorly studied as a similarly at-risk population.[107–109] The prevalence of primary abnormalities attributable to brachycephaly in cats is not known nor are the full-spectrum of effects brachycephalic conformation has on cats.[72,80,82,90,110–112] Stenotic nares have been reported as a cause for upper airway disease in cats, yet few data have been published on nares-altering procedures in cats.[44,72,73,100] Pulmonary edema secondary to elongated soft palate and pulmonary hypertension both have been reported in a young, Persian cat.[90] Nasopharyngeal or caudal aberrant turbinates have been described in both dogs and cats.[28,48] Yet, despite these reports

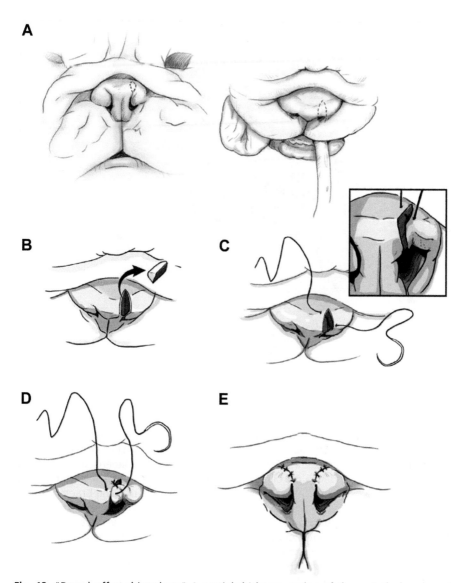

Fig. 13. "Dorsal offset rhinoplasty" A partial thickness wedge of the rostral, dorsal most aspect of the nasal planum and nasal cartilages is planned (*A*) and removed (*B*). The first suture placed apposes the rostral most aspect of the abaxial edge with the caudal most aspect of the axial edge (*C*). This results in a caudal and dorsal translocation of the alar cartilage (*C*, inset). The closure is completed in a simple interrupted pattern (*D*). The procedure is repeated on the opposite side (*E*). (*From* Dickerson VM, Dillard CMB, Grimes JA, Wallace ML, McAnulty JF, Schmiedt CW. Dorsal offset rhinoplasty for treatment of stenotic nares in 34 brachycephalic dogs. Vet Surg. 2020 Dec;49(8):1497-1502. doi: 10.1111/vsu.13504. Epub 2020 Aug 27. PMID: 32853422)

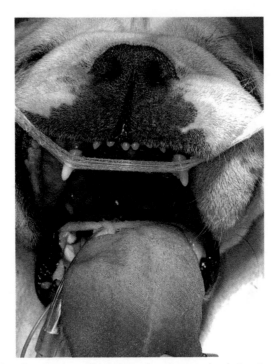

Fig. 14. Enlarged and everted tonsils. Enlarged and everted palatine tonsils in a brachyce-phalic dog.

and a published scale of feline brachycephaly, data describing clinical signs of illness or documenting quality of life issues in brachycephalic cats are severely lacking.[112] Because cats often exhibit subtle manifestations of disease while harboring serious clinical problems,[113] the author finds it incumbent on veterinarians to thoroughly investigate and clearly define the clinical signs and disorders associated with a feline brachycephalic syndrome.[107–109] The authors' investigations of feline brachycephaly described here weree funded by the Winn Feline Foundation Miller Trust and consider the airway and cardiopulmonary consequences of upper airway obstruction. This effortrepresents a major advancement in the care of brachycephalic cats and advo-cacy of responsible breeding and pet ownership.[36]

In a prospective, survey-based study, owners of nearly 1200 cats identified their cats' breed and volunteered to complete a survey of questions about their cats' res-piratory, gastrointestinal, sleep, and activity-related parameters. Brachycephalic cats were reported by their owners to have more frequent respiratory symptoms, such as snoring, sneezing, coughing, and nasal discharge; more activity-related symptoms, such as dyspnea during activity, shorter duration of activity, slower recovery from ac-tivity, and lower activity levels; more gastrointestinal signs, such as hypersalivation, halitosis, and difficulty chewing; and more ocular and aural problems, such as ocular and otic discharge, periocular staining, and more frequent need for ear cleaning, compared with nonbrachycephalic cats. Because brachycephalic cats exhibited clin-ically relevant symptoms, the investigators concluded medical or surgical interven-tions may improve these symptoms and warranted further investigation.[49]

A follow-up surgical study was performed. Brachycephalic cats were assessed pre-operatively by CT of the oronasal, cervical, and thoracic airways; rigid anterior and posterior rhinoscopy and laryngoscopy; contrast echocardiography and assessment of cardiac troponin 1 and N-terminal prohormone of brain natriuretic peptide; and a similar structured owner questionnaire, as in the aforementioned study. Ala-vestibuloplasty was performed bilaterally (**Fig. 15**), and cats and owner questionnaire responses were re-evaluated at least 8 weeks postoperatively. All cats had stenotic nares, prolonged normalized pulmonary artery transit time, and a hyperattenuating pulmonary pattern preoperatively. Postoperatively, cats demonstrated improved normalized pulmonary artery transit time on contrast echocardiography and decreased frequency and severity of abnormal respiratory symptoms and behaviors, as reported by owners. The investigators concluded that anatomic, echocardio-graphic, and CT changes were common in 1 cohort of clinically affected brachyce-phalic cats. Ala-vestibuloplasty was adapted from dogs to cats and was performed with only minor complications. Based on this research, stenotic nares appear to be the predominant airway abnormality of brachycephalic cats. Ala-vestibuloplasty also appears to be a safe procedure in brachycephalic cats that improves cardiac and CT abnormalities and respiratory symptoms.[50]

Finally, investigators of a recent study of 5 brachycephalic cats proposed the ventral skin fold may be a significant contributor to stenotic nares in cats, unlike in dogs.[44] Resection of the skin fold, followed by bilateral single pedicle advancement flaps, was reported as a novel technique and appeared to be successful in treating stenotic nares in the 5 cats studied.[44]

EPIGLOTTIC RETROVERSION

Although not a disease exclusive to brachycephalic dogs, epiglottic retroversion has been reported in the affenpinscher, Boston terrier, Brussels griffon, Cavalier King Charles spaniel, French bulldog, Japanese chin, pug, boxer, and shih tzu breeds in addition to other small breed dogs, including Yorkshire, Norwich, and Jack Russell terriers and Maltese and Chihuahua dogs.[114] Epiglottic retroversion occurs when the epiglottis becomes caudally displaced and possibly entrapped dorsal to the caudal edge of the soft palate, causing intermittent or persistent

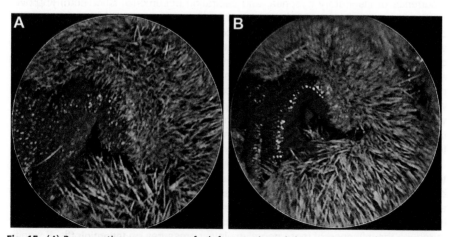

Fig. 15. (*A*) Preoperative appearance of a left stenotic naris in a cat. Image obtained with a 1.9-mm 0° rigid endoscope. (*B*) Postoperative appearance of the left naris and nasal vesti-bule following ala-vestibuloplasty. Image obtained with a 1.9-mm 0° rigid endoscope.

obstruction of the rima glottidis.[114,115] Although it is not clear if epiglottic retroversion and entrapment have shared etiology, failure of the hyoepiglottic muscles to draw the epiglottis ventrally and rostrally occurs during periods of inspiratory dyspnea and more negative airway pressures.[115] Other hypotheses for pathogenesis include epiglottic malacia or fracture and denervation of the hypoglossal or glossopharyngeal nerves associated with peripheral neuropathy or trauma.[116] Stertor, stridor, sneezing, coughing, gagging, reverse sneezing, and cyanosis are common clinical signs, and dogs that are female or obese may be predisposed.[114–116] Concurrent respiratory disorders are noted in 34% to 79% of dogs and include components of BOAS, such as stenotic nares, elongated soft palate, aberrant turbinates, relative macroglossia, enlarged or everted palatine tonsils or mucosa of the laryngeal ventricles, and laryngeal collapse, in addition to other respiratory issues, including nasal septum deviation, tracheal or bronchial collapse, pharyngeal collapse, and laryngeal paralysis.[114,116]

Epiglottic retroversion is diagnosed on sedated airway examination, with laryngoscopy or fluoroscopy, and the condition is classified as low grade or high grade.[114–116] In low-grade patients, the epiglottis is elevated from the tongue base throughout the respiratory cycle and does not move ventrally on inspiration, causing partial obstruction of the rima glottidis. In high-grade patients, the epiglottis is displaced caudally by retroflexion on inspiration or pulled into the rima glottidis, causing complete obstruction of the rima glottidis.[116,117] Temporary epiglottopexy can be achieved by placement of a single mattress suture of 2-0 to 5-0 polypropylene between the epiglottis and tongue, engaging the full thickness of the cartilage of the epiglottis and the glossopharyngeal mucosa of the tongue.[117,118] To achieve fibrosis between the epiglottis and tongue for permanent epiglottopexy, a wedge of mucosa must be removed from each tissue and the wounds apposed with a continuous suture of 3-0 to 5-0 poliglecaprone 25 or polydioxanone.[117,118] In cases of failure of epiglottopexy, partial amputation of one-third to two-thirds of the distal epiglottis may be performed and titrated as needed to permit patency of the rima glottidis.[114] The dorsal and ventral mucosa of the cut surface of the epiglottis should be apposed with suture following amputation to prevent retraction of the mucosa.[114]

Complications associated with epiglottopexy include failure of the pexy suture, recurrence of inspiratory dyspnea, and aspiration pneumonia. Short-term improvement was seen in 54% to 83% of cases, but a recurrence of clinical signs occurred commonly, suggesting failure in epiglottopexy by suture breakage or pull-through in some cases or progression of concurrent airway diseases.[114,116,117] Only 33% of dogs were free of clinical signs at long-term follow-up in 1 study.[117] Partial or subtotal epiglottectomy has resulted in more consistent and permanent relief of clinical respiratory signs with long-term successful outcomes in up to 85% of dogs, but dysphagia was reported in 67% of dogs undergoing epiglottectomy in 1 study.[117] Another disadvantage of partial or subtotal epiglottectomy is the potential for aspiration of aerosolized food and water particles. Aspiration pneumonia has not been reported, however, following partial or subtotal epiglottectomy in studies performed to date.[114,116–118]

Epiglottic retroversion is thought to rarely be a primary cause of respiratory symptoms and occurs more commonly secondary to other underlying primary disorders, causing more negative airway pressures and abnormal forces on the epiglottis.[114,116–118] It is the author's preference to perform temporary epiglottopexy in cases of significant concurrent airway issues that can be managed aggressively to reduce the influence of more negative airway pressures on the epiglottis. If significant concurrent airway obstruction is not present or cannot be satisfactorily managed, then permanent epiglottopexy or partial or subtotal epiglottectomy may be preferred.

NORWICH TERRIER–SPECIFIC DISEASE

Dogs with a skull width-to-length ratio greater than 0.8 are categorized as brachyce-phalic, whereas mesaticephalic dogs have a smaller width-to-length ratio.[119,120] Quanti-tative linkage of proportional brachycephaly with BOAS was confirmed in a prospective study of 754 dogs that showed risk of BOAS increased sharply in a nonlinear manner as relative muzzle length shortened.[3] Although the same study concluded that BOAS only occurred in dogs whose muzzles contributed less than half the craniofacial length, the Norwich terrier breed standard mandates a wide skull with the facial skull one-third shorter than the cephalic skull.[121] Most commonly classified as having mesaticephalic conformation, the Norwich terrier had been found to suffer many respiratory afflictions normally attributed to brachycephaly, inspiring additional study.[121–123]

Investigators examined 23 Norwich terriers by clinical physical examination, sedated oral examination, endoscopic examination of the respiratory tract, and radio-graphic measurement of the skull.[121] Two indices were measured, the skull index and the length-width index. Although measurement and calculation of length-width indices and craniofacial angles yielded results consistent with mesaticephaly in this cohort of Norwich terriers, measurement and calculation of skull indices denoted brachy-cephaly.[121] To classify dogs according to facial and cephalic skull conformation, and to account for different sizes between breeds in studies, indices, such as the skull index, length-width index, and many others, have been used.[70,99,119,120,124] Because no craniofacial index has been validated for use in accurately comparing dogs, how-ever, results of research using any craniofacial index to draw comparisons or conclu-sions of dogs with varying size or conformation should be interpreted with caution until any craniofacial index is validated as a means of standardization among dogs.[3,15,16,124]

Clinically, Norwich terriers have been found to show clinical signs, such as increased respiratory noise, including stertor, frequent cough, excessive panting, and difficulty sleeping.[121–123,125] Some investigators have concluded Norwich terriers suffer from a variant upper airway obstructive syndrome, Norwich terrier upper airway syndrome, with pathologic features distinct from and overlapping with BOAS.[121,122,125] In 1 study of 16 dogs, airway obstruction in Norwich terriers appeared due mostly to laryngeal narrowing caudal to the vocal fold causing decreased luminal diameter,[122] a keyhole or V-shaped lumen, and severe redundancy of supraglottic mu-cosa (**Fig. 16**).[122,126]

Subsequently, an Norwich terrier upper airway syndrome scoring system was pro-spectively constructed to classify anatomic abnormalities affecting the breed based on number and severity of obstructive lesions detected on laryngoscopy.[123] To utilize the system, veterinarians should perform a complete upper airway examination of the nares, hard palate, soft palate, palatine tonsils, lateral and dorsal pharyngeal walls, epiglottis, hyoepiglottis and valleculae, cuneiform and corniculate processes of the larynx, piriform recesses, laryngeal mucosa, vestibular and vocal folds, laryngeal ven-tricles, and the immediate infraglottic lumen.[122,123,126] The 5 variables found to distin-guish clinical Norwich terriers from nonclinical terriers most readily include characteristics of the dorsal pharyngeal wall, supraglottic laryngeal mucosa, cunei-form processes of the arytenoid cartilages, laryngeal ventricles, and the infraglottic lumen.[122,123,126] The nasal vestibule, nasal passages, choanae, nasopharynx, and soft palate thickness also should be evaluated with CT and a slung maxilla, especially in dogs with sleep-disordered breathing.[122,123,126]

Although nares-altering procedures, palatoplasty, and resection of enlarged and everted tonsils and everted mucosa of the laryngeal ventricles can be performed

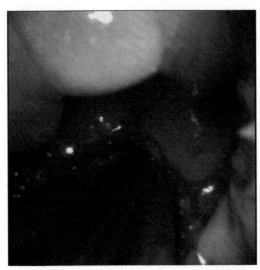

Fig. 16. Redundant supraglottic mucosa. Redundant and edematous supraglottic mucosa and lateral and dorsal pharyngeal walls in a Norwich terrier.

readily, as for brachycephalic dogs, resection or minimization of redundant supraglottic mucosa and lateral or dorsal pharyngeal walls in Norwich terriers is more challenging and not well described or studied.[123] Narrowing of the infraglottic lumen and medial displacement of the cuneiform processes may be amenable to permanent tracheostomy or partial laryngectomy,[15,16,42,123] but further study is required.

Whole-genome sequencing and genome-wide association analyses have found a genetic variant of a canine chromosome common to Norwich terriers and BOAS-susceptible French and English bulldogs. Loss of function of a metallopeptidase may cause airway edema and contribute to BOAS.[125] Such compelling findings may partially dissociate respiratory disease from head conformation and point researchers toward other genetic and morphologic variables. It is possible Norwich terriers are becoming more short-faced, that breeding is propagating genetic variants that code for morphology and physiology that increase risk for BOAS, or that Norwich terriers have an upper airway syndrome with etiology entirely distinct from BOAS.[121–123,125,126] Because owners and breeders of Norwich terriers have expressed concern regarding signs of an upper airway syndrome in the breed, the Norwich and Norfolk Terrier Club has formed a committee advocating for health and for genetics research on upper airway syndrome in Norwich terriers.[63] Any transition toward brachycephaly within the breed should be met by reproductive measures to prevent further digression to phenotypically and physiologically affected animals.[121,122,127]

CLINICS CARE POINTS

- Best practice coordination of care for brachycephalic dogs includes thorough anamnesis and detailed physical assessment. Care should be taken to discern the timing, frequency, and severity of respiratory noise and difficulty, especially concerning association with exercise, eating, drinking, and sleeping.

- CT allows assessment of thickness as well as length of the soft palate in brachycephalic dogs. Folded flap palatoplasty successfully addresses both the pathologic length and thickness of the soft palate in some dogs.
- Prolonged fast and use of multimodal gastrointestinal protectant therapy should be considered in brachycephalic dogs undergoing anesthesia and surgery to minimize risk of regurgitation and aspiration.
- Brachycephalic cats presented for respiratory, gastrointestinal, activity-related, or sleep-related symptoms should be evaluated for stenotic nares, and treatments, including ala-vestibuloplasty and ventral skin fold resection, should be considered.

DISCLOSURE

The author has no commercial or financial conflicts of interest.

REFERENCES

1. Dupre G, Heidenreich D. Brachycephalic syndrome. Vet Clin Small Anim 2016; 46:691–707.
2. Einspruch B. Norwich terrier upper airway syndrome. District of Columbia (USA): The Norwich Terrier Club of America; 2016. Available at: https://norwichterrierclub.org/ntuas/.
3. Packer RM, Hendricks A, Tivers MS, et al. Impact of facial conformation on canine health: brachycephalic obstructive airway syndrome. Plos One 2015; 10:e0137496.
4. Ravn-Mølby E-M, Sindahl L, Nielsen SS, et al. Breeding French bulldogs so that they breathe well-A long way to go. PLoS One 2019;14:e0226280.
5. AKC Most Popular Breeds. 2019. Available at: https://www.akc.org/most-popular-breeds/. Accessed October 5, 2021.
6. Breed Registration Statistics. 2020. Available at: https://www.thekennelclub.org.uk/registration/breed-registration-statistics/. Accessed October 5, 2021.
7. Teng KT, McGreevy PD, Toribio J-ALML, et al. Trends in popularity of some morphological traits of purebred dogs in Australia. Canine Genet Epidemiol 2016;3:2–9.
8. CFA Most Popular Breeds. 2019. Available at: https://cfa.org/cfa-news-releases/top-breeds-2019/. Accessed January 5, 2020.
9. Fasanella FJ, Shivley JM, Wardlaw JL, et al. Brachycephalic airway obstructive Syndrome in dogs: 90 cases (1991-2008). J Am Vet Med Assoc 2010;237: 1048–51.
10. Lodato DL, Hedlund CS. Brachycephalic airway syndrome: pathophysiology and diagnosis. Compend Contin Educ Vet 2012;34:E3.
11. Meola SD. Brachycephalic airway syndrome. Top Companion Anim Med 2013; 28(3):91–6.
12. Pohl S, Roedler FS, Oechtering GU. How does multilevel upper airway surgery influence the lives of dogs with severe brachycephaly? Results of a structured pre- and postoperative owner questionnaire. Vet J 2016;210:39–45.
13. Hendricks JC. Brachycephalic airway syndrome. Vet Clin North Am Small Anim Pract 1992;22:1145–53.
14. Liu NC, Sargan DR, Adams VJ, et al. Characterization of brachycephalic obstructive airway syndrome in French bulldogs using whole-body barometric plethysmography. Plos One 2015;10:e0130741.

15. Liu N-C, Oechtering GU, Adams VJ, et al. Outcomes and prognostic factors of surgical treatments for brachycephalic obstructive airway syndrome in 3 breeds. Vet Surg 2017;46:271–80.

16. Liu NC, Troconis EL, Kalmar L, et al. Conformational risk factors of brachycephalic obstructive airway syndrome (BOAS) in pugs, French bulldogs, and bulldogs. Plos One 2017;12(8):e0181928.

17. Noller C, Oechtering GU, Budras KD. Anatomical aspects of the brachycephalic airway syndrome in cats and dogs. Paper presented at: 24th Symposium of the Veterinary Comparative Respiratory Society; 2006 October 8-10; Jena, Germany.

18. Oechtering GU, Hueber J, Noller C. Medicine Forum 2008 June.

19. Oechtering GU, Pohl S, Schlueter C, et al. A novel approach to brachycephalic syndrome 1 Evaluation of anatomical intranasal airway obstruction. Vet Surg 2016;45:165-172.

20. Oechtering GU, Pohl S, Schlueter C, et al. A novel approach to brachycephalic syndrome. 2. Laser-assisted turbinectomy (LATE). Vet Surg 2016;45:173–81.

21. Pratschke K. Current thinking about brachycephalic syndrome: more than just airways. Comp Anim 2014;19:70–8.

22. Roedler FS, Pohl S, Oechtering GU. How does severe brachycephaly affect dog's lives? Results of a structured preoperative owner questionnaire. Vet J 2013;198:606–10.

23. Bernaerts F, Talavera J, Leemans J, et al. Description of original endoscopic findings and respiratory functional assessment using barometric whole-body plethysmography in dogs suffering from brachycephalic airway obstruction syndrome. Vet J 2010;183:95–102.

24. Hoareau GL, Mellema MS, Silverstein DC. Indication, management, and outcome of brachycephalic dogs requiring mechanical ventilation. J Vet Emerg Crit Care 2011;21:226–35.

25. Hoareau GL, Jourdan G, Mellema M, et al. Evaluation of arterial blood gases and arterial blood pressures in brachycephalic dogs. J Vet Intern Med 2012; 26:897–904.

26. Hoareau G, Mellema M. Pro-coagulant thromboelastographic features in the bulldog. J Small Anim Pract 2015;56:103–7.

27. Hueber JP, Smith HJ, Reinhold P, et al. Brachycephalic airway syndrome: effects of partial turbinectomy on intranasal airway resistance. Paper presented at: 25th Veterinary Comparative Respiratory Society; 2007 October 10-13; West Lafayette, Indiana.

28. Schuenemann R, Oechtering GU. Inside the brachycephalic nose: intranasal mucosal contact points. J Am Anim Hosp Assoc 2014;50:149–58.

29. Schuenemann R, Oechtering GU. Inside the brachycephalic nose: conchal regrowth and mucosal contact points after laser-assisted turbinectomy. J Am Anim Hosp Assoc 2014;50:237–46.

30. Harvey CE, Venker-von Haagan A. Surgical management of pharyngeal and laryngeal airway obstruction in the dog. Vet Clin North Am 1975;5:515–35.

31. Hara Y, Teshima K, Seki M, et al. Pharyngeal contraction secondary to its collapse in dogs with brachycephalic airway syndrome. J Vet Med Sci 2020; 82(1):64–7.

32. Rubin JA, Holt DE, Reetz JA, et al. Signalment, clinical presentation, concurrent diseases, and diagnostic findings in 28 dogs with dynamic pharyngeal collapse (2008-2013). J Vet Intern Med 2015;29:815–21.

33. De Lorenzi D, Bertoncello D, Drigo M. Bronchial abnormalities found in a consecutive series of 40 brachycephalic dogs. J Am Vet Med Assoc 2009; 235:835–40.

34. Yoon H, Yu J, An G, et al. CT and radiographic evaluation of bronchial collapsibility at forced expiration in asymptomatic brachycephalic dogs. Vet Radiol Ultrasound 2020;61:167–80.

35. Poncet CM, Dupre GP, Freiche VG, et al. Long-term results of upper respiratory syndrome surgery and gastrointestinal tract medical treatment in 51 brachycephalic dogs. J Small Anim Pract 2006;47:137–42.

36. Malik R, Sparkes A, Bessant C. Brachycephalia–a bastardisation of what makes cats special. J Feline Med Surg 2009;11:889–90.

37. Planellas M, Cuenca R, Tabar M-D, et al. Evaluation of C-reactive protein, haptoglobin and cardiac troponin 1 levels in brachycephalic dogs with upper airway obstructive syndrome. BMC Vet Res 2012;8:152–7.

38. Planellas M, Cuenca R, Tabar M-D, et al. Clinical assessment and C-reactive protein (CRP), haptoglobin (Hp), and cardiac troponin I (ctni) values of brachycephalic dogs with upper airway obstruction before and after surgery. Can J Vet Res 2015;79:58–63.

39. Mercurio A. Complications of upper airway surgery in companion animals. Vet Clin North Am Small Anim Pract 2011;41:969–80, vi–vii.

40. Ree JJ, Milovancev M, Malintyre LA, et al. Factors associated with major complications in the short-term postoperative period in dogs undergoing surgery for brachycephalic airway syndrome. Can Vet J 2016;57:976–80.

41. Torrez CV, Hunt GB. Results of surgical correction of abnormalities associated with brachycephalic airway obstruction syndrome in dogs in Australia. J Small Anim Pract 2006;47:150–4.

42. Gobbetti M, Romussi S, Buracco P, et al. Long-term outcome of permanent tracheostomy in 15 dogs with severe laryngeal collapse secondary to brachycephalic airway obstructive syndrome. Vet Surg 2018;47:648–53.

43. Belch A, Matiasovic M, Rasotto R, et al. Comparison of the use of Ligasure versus a standard technique for tonsillectomy in dogs. Vet Rec 2017;180: 186–96.

44. Berns CN, Schmiedt CW, Dickerson VM, et al. Single pedicle advancement flap for treatment of feline stenotic nares: technique and results in five cases. J Feline Med Surg 2020;22:1238–42.

45. Cook DA, Moses PA, Mackie JT. Clinical effects of the use of a bipolar vessel sealing device for soft palate resection and tonsillectomy in dogs, with histological assessment of resected tonsillar tissue. Aust Vet J 2015;93:445–51.

46. Dickerson VM, Dillard CMB, Grimes JA, et al. Dorsal offset rhinoplasty for treatment of stenotic nares in 34 brachycephalic dogs. Vet Surg 2020;49:1497–502.

47. Findji L, Dupre G. Folded flap palatoplasty for treatment of elongated soft palates in 55 dogs. Vet Med Austria/Wien Tierärztl Mschr 2008;95:56–63.

48. Ginn JA, Kumar MSA, McKiernan BC, et al. Nasopharyngeal turbinates in brachycephalic dogs and cats. J Am Anim Hosp Assoc 2008;44:243–9.

49. Gleason HE, McCoy AM, Phillips H. Feline brachycephaly is associated with respiratory, gastrointestinal, and activity abnormalities as reported by owners. Paper presented at: American College of Veterinary Surgeons Surgical Summit; 2020 October 21-24; Germantown (MD).

50. Gleason HE, Phillips H, Keating S, Hamel PES, McCoy AM, Fries R. Ala vestibuloplasty improves cardiopulmonary and lifestyle parameters in brachycephalic

cats. Paper presented at: American College of Veterinary Surgeons Surgical Summit; 2020 October 21-24; Germantown MD, USA.

51. Heidenreich D, Gradner G, Kneissl S, et al. Nasopharyngeal dimensions from computed tomography of pugs and French bulldogs with brachycephalic airway syndrome. Vet Surg 2016;45:83-90.

52. Jones BA, Stanley BJ, Nelson NC. The impact of tongue dimension on air volume in brachycephalic dogs. Vet Surg 2020;49:512–20.

53. Kim YJ, Lee N, Yu J, et al. Three-dimensional volumetric magnetic resonance imaging (MRI) Analysis of the soft palate and nasopharynx in brachycephalic and non-brachycephalic dog breeds. J Vet Med Sci 2019;81:113–9.

54. Ladlow J, Liu N-C, Kalmar L, et al. Brachycephalic obstructive airway syndrome. Vet Rec 2018;182:375–8.

55. Lilja-Maula L, Lappalainen AK, Hyytiäinen HK, et al. Comparison of submaximal exercise test results and severity of brachycephalic obstructive airway syndrome in English bulldogs. Vet J 2017;219:22–6.

56. Oechtering GU, Hueber JP, Kiefer I. Laser assisted turbinectomy (LATE)- a novel approach to brachycephalic syndrome. Vet Surg 2007;36:E11.

57. Oechtering G. Brachycephalic syndrome – new information on an old congenital 501 disease. Vet Focus 2010;20:2–9.

58. Oechtering GU, Schuenemann R. Brachycephalics-trapped in man-made misery. Paper presented at: Association of Veterinary Soft Tissue Surgeons Meeting; 2010 January 2-3; Cambridge, UK. http://www.avsts.org.uk/sites/avsts.org.uk/files/event-proceedings/avsts_autumn_2010.pdf.

59. Riggs J, Liu NC, Sutton DR, et al. Validation of exercise testing and laryngeal auscultation for grading brachycephalic obstructive airway syndrome in pugs, French bulldogs, and English bulldogs by using whole-body barometric plethysmography. Vet Surg 2019;48:488–96.

60. Sławuta P, Nicpoń J, Domańska S. Influence of the wing-of-the-nostrils correction procedure on the change of the acid-base balance parameters and oxygen concentration in the arterial blood in French bulldogs. Pol J Vet Sci 2011;14:77–80.

61. Song A, Phillips H, McCoy A, Oliveira C. Volumetric study of the soft palate and tongue: how tissue composition and dimension contribute to brachycephalic obstructive airway syndrome. Paper presented at: American College of Veterinary Surgeons Surgical Summit; 2020 October 21-24; Germantown, MD, USA.

62. Tarricone J, Hayes GM, Singh A, et al. Development and validation of a brachycephalic risk (BRisk) score to predict the risk of complications in dogs presenting for surgical treatment of brachycephalic obstructive airway syndrome. Vet Surg 2019;48:1253–61.

63. Eivers C, Chicon Rueda R, Liuti T, et al. Retrospective analysis of esophageal imaging features in brachycephalic versus non-brachycephalic dogs based on videofluoroscopic swallowing studies. J Vet Intern Med 2019;33:1740–6.

64. Fenner JVH, Quinn RJ, Demetriou JL. Postoperative regurgitation in dogs after upper airway surgery to treat brachycephalic obstructive airway syndrome: 258 cases (2013-2017). Vet Surg 2020;49:53–60.

65. Liu N-C, Genain M-A, Kalmar L, et al. Objective effectiveness of and indications for laser- assisted turbinectomy in brachycephalic obstructive airway syndrome. Vet Surg 2019;48:79–87.

66. Packer R, Hendricks A, Burn CC. Do dog owners perceive the clinical signs related to conformational inherited disorders as "normal" for the breed? A potential constraint to improving canine welfare. Anim Welf 2012;21:81–93.

67. Phillips H, Corrie J, Engel DM, et al. Clinical findings, diagnostic test results, and treatment outcome in cats with hiatal hernia: 31 cases (1995-2018). J Vet Intern Med 2019;33:1970–6.

68. Poncet CM, Dupre GP, Freiche VG, et al. Prevalence of gastrointestinal tract lesions in 73 brachycephalic dogs with upper respiratory syndrome. J Small Anim Pract 2005;46:273–9.

69. Reeve EJ, Sutton D, Friend EJ, et al. Documenting the prevalence of hiatal hernia and oesophageal abnormalities in brachycephalic dogs using fluoroscopy. J Small Anim Pract 2017;58:703–8.

70. Selba MC, Oechtering GU, Heng HG, et al. The impact of selection for facial reduction in dogs: geometric morphometric analysis of canine cranial shape. Anat Rec 2020;303(2):330–46.

71. Shaw TE, Harkin KR, Nietfeld J, et al. Aortic body tumor in full-sibling English bulldogs. J Am Anim Hosp Assoc 2010;46:366–70.

72. Harvey CE. Surgical correction of stenotic nares in a cat. J Am Anim Hosp Assoc 1986;22:31–2.

73. Trostel CT, Frankel DJ. Punch resection alaplasty technique in dogs and cats with stenotic nares: 14 cases. J Am Anim Hosp Assoc 2010;46:5–11.

74. Broux O, Clercx C, Etienne A-L, et al. Effects of manipulations to detect sliding hiatal hernia in dogs with brachycephalic airway obstructive syndrome. Vet Surg 2018;47:243–51.

75. Gianella P, Caccamo R, Bellino C, et al. Evaluation of metabolic profile and C-reactive protein concentrations in brachycephalic dogs with upper airway obstructive syndrome. J Vet Intern Med 2019;33:2183–92.

76. Kaye BM, Rutherford L, Perridge DJ, et al. Relationship between brachycephalic airway syndrome and gastrointestinal signs in three breeds of dog. J Small Anim Pract 2018;59:670–3.

77. Monnet E. Brachycephalic airway syndrome. In: Slatter D, editor. Textbook of small animal surgery, Vol 1, 3rd edition. Philadelphia (PA): Saunders; 2002. p. 808–13.

78. Grand JG, Bureau S. Structural characteristics of the soft palate and meatus nasopharyngeus in brachycephalic and non-brachycephalic dogs analyzed by CT. J Small Anim Pract 2011;52:232–9.

79. University of Cambridge. Brachycephalic obstructive airway syndrome (BOAS). Cambridge, UK: Department of Veterinary Medicine University of Cambridge; 2021. Available at: https://www.vet.cam.ac.uk/boas.

80. Farnworth MJ, Chen R, Packer RMA, et al. Flat feline faces: Is brachycephaly associated with respiratory abnormalities in the domestic cat (Felis catus)?. In: Staffieri F, editor. Plos ONE 2016;11(8)::e0161777.

81. Feng T, McConnell C, O'Hara K, et al. Nationwide Brachycephalic Breed Disease Prevalence Study - March 2017. 2017. Available at: http://nationwidedvm.com/wp-Content/uploads/2017/03/nwbrachycelphalicstudy0317.pdf. Accessed J October 6, 2021.

82. Künzel W, Breit S, Oppel M. Morphometric investigations of breed-specific features in feline skulls and considerations on their functional implications. Anat Histol Embryol 2003;32:218–23.

83. Fernández-Parra R, Pey P, Zilberstein L, et al. Use of computational fluid dynamics to compare upper airway pressures and airflow resistance in brachycephalic, mesocephalic, and dolichocephalic dogs. Vet J 2019;253:105392.

84. Hostnik ET, Scansen BA, Zielinski R, et al. Quantification of nasal airflow resistance in English bulldogs using computed tomography and computational fluid dynamics. Vet Radiol Ultrasound 2017;58:542–51.

85. Harris HA. Congenital absence of the middle turbinate bone associated with precocious ossification of the limb bones in a stillborn female. J Anat 1926;20: 148–51.

86. Thilander B. Basic mechanisms in craniofacial growth. Acta Odontol Scand 1995;53:144–51.

87. Arai K, Kobayashi M, Harada Y, et al. Histopathologic and immunohistochemical features of soft palate muscles and nerves in dogs with an elongated soft palate. Am J Vet Res 2016;77(1):77–83.

88. Arrighi S, Pichetto M, Roccabianca P, et al. The anatomy of the dog soft palate. I. Histological evaluation of the caudal soft palate in mesaticephalic breeds. Anat Rec 2011;294(7):1261–6.

89. Asher L, Diesel G, Summers JF, et al. Inherited defects in pedigree dogs. part 1: Disorders related to breed standards. Vet J 2009;182(3):402–11.

90. Corgozinho KB, Pereira AN, Cunha SCDS, et al. Recurrent pulmonary edema secondary to elongated soft palate in a cat. J Feline Med Surg 2012;14:417–9.

91. Crosse KR, Bray JP, Orbell G, et al. Histological evaluation of the soft palate in dogs affected by brachycephalic obstructive airway syndrome. N Z Vet J 2015; 63:319–25.

92. Dupré G, Findji L, Oechtering G. Brachycephalic airway syndrome. In: Monnet E, editor. Small animal soft tissue surgery. 1st edition. Chichester (UK): Wiley Blackwell; 2013. p. 167–80.

93. Pichetto M, Arrighi S, Roccabianca P, et al. The anatomy of the dog soft palate. II. Histological evaluation of the caudal soft palate in brachycephalic breeds with grade I brachycephalic airway obstructive syndrome. Anat Rec 2011; 294:1267–72.

94. Pichetto M, Arrighi S, Gobbetti M, et al. The anatomy of the dog soft palate. III. Histological evaluation of the caudal soft palate in brachycephalic neonates. Anat Rec 2015;298:618–23.

95. Riecks TW, Birchard SJ, Stephens JA. Surgical correction of brachycephalic syndrome in dogs: 62 cases (1991-2004). J Am Vet Med Assoc 2007;230: 1324–8.

96. Haimel G, Dupré G. Brachycephalic airway syndrome: a comparative study between pugs and French bulldogs. J Small Anim Pract 2015;56:714–9.

97. Sarran D, Caron A, Testault I, et al. Position of maximal nasopharyngeal maximal occlusion in relation to hamuli pterygoidei: use of hamuli pterygoidei as landmarks for palatoplasty in brachycephalic airway obstruction syndrome surgical treatment. J Small Anim Pract 2018. https://doi.org/10.1111/jsap.12909.

98. Hinchliffe TA, Liu NC, Ladlow J. Sleep-disordered breathing in the Cavalier King Charles spaniel: a case series. Vet Surg 2019;48:497–504.

99. Seidenburg JS, Dupré G. Tongue and upper airway dimensions: A comparative study between three popular brachycephalic breeds. Animals 2021;11:662–75.

100. Trader RL. Nose operation. J Am Vet Med Assoc 1949;114:210–1.

101. Harvey CE. Upper airway obstruction surgery. 1. Stenotic nares surgery in brachycephalic dogs. J Am Anim Hosp Assoc 1982;18:535–7.

102. Ellison GW. Alapexy: an alternative technique for repair of stenotic nares in dogs. J Am Anim Hosp Assoc 2004;40:484–9.

103. Fawcett A, Barrs V, Awad M, et al. Consequences and management of canine brachycephaly in veterinary practice: perspectives from Australian veterinarians and veterinary specialists. Animals 2018;9:3.
104. Adzrell B, Wong EHC, Saraiz A, et al. The effectiveness of combined tonsillectomy and anterior palatoplasty in the treatment of snoring and obstructive sleep apnoea (OSA). Eur Arch Otorhinolaryngol 2017;274:2005–11.
105. Ellis PD. Laser palatoplasty for snoring due to palatal flutter: a further report. Clin Otolaryngol Allied Sci 1994;19:350–1.
106. Mair EA, Day RH. Cautery-assisted palatal stiffening operation. Otolaryngol Head Neck Surg 2000;122:547–56.
107. Häußler TC, Pückler von KH, Thiel C, et al. Measurement of the normal feline pituitary gland in brachycephalic and mesocephalic cats. J Feline Med Surg 2018;20:578–86.
108. Keyes M. Brachycephalic cats - is it too late for the Persian? J Feline Med Surg 2010;12:55.
109. Schmidt MJ, Kampschulte M, Enderlein S, et al. The relationship between brachycephalic head features in modern Persian cats and dysmorphologies of the skull and internal 2017 hydrocephalus. J Vet Intern Med 2017;31:1487–501.
110. Farnworth MJ, Packer RMA, Sordo L, et al. In the eye of the beholder: owner preferences for variations in cats' appearances with specific focus on skull morphology. Animals 2018;8(2):30.
111. Mestrinho LA, Louro JM, Gordo IS, et al. Oral and dental anomalies in purebred, brachycephalic Persian and Exotic cats. J Am Vet Med Assoc 2018;253:66–72.
112. Schlueter C, Budras KD, Ludewig E, et al. Brachycephalic feline noses: CT and anatomical study of the relationship between head conformation and the nasolacrimal drainage system. J Feline Med Surg 2009;11:891–900.
113. Little SE. Preface. In: Little SE, editor. The cat clinical medicine and management. St. Louis (MO): Elsevier Saunders; 2012. p. xiii.
114. Mullins RA, Stanley BJ, Flanders JA, et al. Intraoperative and major postoperative complications and survival of dogs undergoing surgical management of epiglottic retroversion: 50 dogs (2003-2017). Vet Surg 2019;48:803–19.
115. Leonard HC. Collapse of the larynx and adjacent structures in the dog. J Am Vet Med Assoc 1960;137:360–3.
116. Skerrett SC, McClaran JK, Fox PR, et al. Clinical features and outcome of dogs with epiglottic retroversion with or without surgical treatment: 24 cases. J Vet Intern Med 2015;29:1611–8.
117. Van Ginneken K, Van Goethem B, Devriendt N, et al. Epiglottic retroversion in 9 dogs. Vlaams Diergeneeskundig Tijdschrift 2020;89:152–8.
118. Flanders JA, Thompson MS. Dyspnea caused by epiglottic retroversion in two dogs. J Am Vet Med Assoc 2009;235:1330–5.
119. Evans HE, de Lahunta A. The skeleton. In: Evans HE, de Lahunta A, editors. Miller's anatomy of the dog. 4th edition. St Louis (MO): Elsevier Saunders; 2013. p. 80–157.
120. Koch D, Wiestner T, Balli A, et al. Proposal for a new radiological index to determine skull conformation in the dog. Schweiz Arch Tierheilkd 2012;154:217–20.
121. Koch DA, Rosaspina M, Montavon PM, et al. Comparative investigations on the upper respiratory tract in Norwich terriers, brachycephalic, and mesaticephalic dogs. Schweizer Archiv fur Tierheilkunde 2014;156:119–24.
122. Johnson L, Mayhew P, Steffey M, et al. Upper airway obstruction in Norwich terriers: 16 cases. J Vet Intern Med 2013;27:1409–15.

123. Johnson LR, Mayhew PD, Culp WTN, et al. Results of owner questionnaire describing long-term outcome in Norwich terriers with upper airway syndrome. J Vet Intern Med 2021;35:1950–6.
124. Caccamo R, Buracco P, La Rosa G, et al. Glottic and skull indices in canine brachycephalic airway obstructive syndrome. BMC Vet Res 2014;10:12.
125. Marchant TW, Dietschi E, Rytz U, et al. An ADAMTS3 missense variant is associated with Norwich Terrier upper airway syndrome. PLoS Genet 2019;15: e1008102.
126. Lai GP, Stanley BJ, Nelson NC, et al. Clinical and laryngoscopic characterization of Norwich terrier upper airway syndrome (NTUAS): preliminary results. Paper presented at: European College of Veterinary Surgeons Annual Meeting; 2018 July 5-7; Athens, Greece.
127. Pink JJ, Doyle RS, Hughes JM, et al. Laryngeal collapse in seven brachycephalic puppies. J Sm Anim Pract 2006;47:131 5.

Updates in Hepatobiliary Surgery
New Data on Portosystemic Shunts and Cholecystectomy in Dogs and Cats

Mandy L. Wallace, DVM, MS; Diplomate, American College of Veterinary Surgeons (Small Animal)

KEYWORDS

- Portosystemic shunt • Cholecystectomy • Hepatobiliary surgery
- Extrahepatic portosystemic shunt • Gallbladder

KEY POINTS

- Gradual occlusion devices for extrahepatic portosystemic shunts result in good to excellent outcomes in most patients, with no major differences in outcome despite device used.
- Surgical attenuation of extrahepatic portosystemic shunts results in improved survival and quality of life when compared with medical management in dogs of all ages.
- In cats, thin film banding of an extrahepatic portosystemic shunt can result in inconsistent shunt closure, leading to variable clinical improvement in this species.
- Although the postoperative mortality rate for cholecystectomy is still relatively high, this can be lowered by early surgical intervention for gallbladder mucoceles when patients do not yet have clinical signs of hepatobiliary disease.
- Catheterization of the common bile duct is not necessary in every dog undergoing a cholecystectomy and should be reserved for cases where common bile duct obstruction is present. Normograde catheterization is recommended, when possible, to prevent potential complications.

INTRODUCTION

Portosystemic shunts (PSS) are vascular anomalies connecting blood from the portal system directly to the systemic circulation without passage through the liver for clearance of toxins, leading to neurologic, gastrointestinal, and urinary tract signs. These anomalous vessels may be either within the liver parenchyma (intrahepatic PSS [IHPSS]) or outside of the liver parenchyma (extrahepatic PSS [EHPSS]).[1] Recent studies have focused on comparing long-term outcome between surgical options,

Small Animal Surgery, Department of Small Animal Medicine and Surgery, University of Georgia, 2200 College Station Road, Athens, GA 30605, USA
E-mail address: mandywl@uga.edu

Vet Clin Small Anim 52 (2022) 369–385
https://doi.org/10.1016/j.cvsm.2021.11.001
0195-5616/22/© 2021 Elsevier Inc. All rights reserved.
vetsmall.theclinics.com

new methods of evaluating postoperative shunt occlusion, and best practices in pre-operative management.

DIAGNOSIS OF PORTOSYSTEMIC SHUNTS

Initial suspicion for presence of a PSS is either due to suggestive clinical signs noted by the owner or through changes on standard bloodwork (**Table 1**). Tests for hepatic dysfunction such as preprandial and postprandial serum bile acid levels or blood ammonia levels are often performed when PSS is suspected. In symptomatic patients, fasting serum bile acid levels have a very high sensitivity (98%) for PSS, and a combination of both fasting serum bile acid levels and fasting ammonia levels had the highest specificity (97%) for PSS in one study.[2] Measurement of protein C activity is another test that can be performed to differentiate between dogs with PSS and dogs with microvascular dysplasia-portal vein hypoplasia (MVD-PVH). One study found that 88% of dogs with PSS had abnormal protein C levels (less than 70%), whereas more than 90% of dogs with MVD-PVH had normal protein C levels (greater than 70%).[3]

Diagnostic imaging provides both a definitive diagnosis of PSS and may also aid in surgical planning. The most used imaging modalities include abdominal ultrasonography, nuclear scintigraphy, and computed tomography angiography (CTA). CTA has gained favor recently for use in surgical planning (both open surgery and interventional techniques) due to improved sensitivity and specificity for PSS diagnosis compared with abdominal ultrasonography.[1] In addition, CTA does not use radioactive material, as is used in nuclear scintigraphy requiring isolation of the animal for up to 24 hours.[1] One disadvantage of CTA is that the patient must be either heavily sedated or under general anesthesia. However, a study evaluating CTA performed under general anesthesia before surgery did not find a negative impact of preoperative CTA on complication rate or patient outcome.[4]

PREOPERATIVE MEDICAL MANAGEMENT

Medical management before surgical attenuation of PSS is often recommended to decrease signs of hepatic encephalopathy prior to the patient undergoing general anesthesia. The mainstays of medical management include lactulose, antibiotics (metronidazole, neomycin, amoxicillin), hepatic support diet, and omeprazole (for IHPSS cases to prevent gastric ulceration).[1] Although these medications are often given in combination, not all dogs or cats require all components to show improvement in clinical signs. A recent study in dogs undergoing nonsurgical PSS management found that a hepatic support diet alone resulted in similar quality of life and survival time when compared with patients receiving both a hepatic support diet

Table 1	
Bloodwork abnormalities commonly seen in dogs and cats with a portosystemic shunt	
Complete Blood Count	**Biochemistry Panel**
Normochromic, microcytic nonregenerative anemia	Decreased blood urea nitrogen
Leukocytosis	Hypoalbuminemia
Neutrophilia	Hypoglycemia
	Hypocholesterolemia
	Mild increase in ALT and/or ALP

and lactulose, highlighting the importance of diet change as a component of medical management.[5] Therapeutic plasma exchange was also recently reported to decrease signs of hepatic encephalopathy in a patient refractory to medical management before surgical attenuation.[6]

Levetiracetam as a component of preoperative medical management for EHPSS patients has been the subject of recent scrutiny. An initial study evaluating the utility of levetiracetam for the reduction of postattenuation seizures (PAS) found that dogs receiving levetiracetam were significantly less likely to experience PAS.[7] Recently, several studies have evaluated this, including one study of 940 dogs, and found no difference in PAS occurrence with and without preoperative levetiracetam administration.[4,8–10] Based on the results of these studies, it seems that preoperative levetiracetam is likely not beneficial for prevention of PAS.

MEDICAL MANAGEMENT VERSUS SURGICAL ATTENUATION

Because of the potential for perioperative mortality with PSS attenuation, it is worth investigating if surgical attenuation results in enough improvement to be worth undertaking the risk of perioperative death. Surgical attenuation of PSS is known to decrease clinical signs, increase postoperative liver volume, improve portal vasculature, and decrease C-reactive protein levels.[9,11–14] When evaluating the long-term outcome in dogs with EHPSS, 89% of dogs treated with medical management only died or were euthanized during the study period (Median Survival Time [MST] 836 days) compared with only 21% of dogs having surgery (MST not reached).[13] Similarly, when evaluating 351 dogs that were diagnosed with EHPSS at 5 years of age or older, survival was improved in dogs undergoing surgical attenuation, with survival estimates of 10.9 years with surgery and 3.4 years with medical management.[9] These studies show the importance of surgical attenuation of EHPSS in dogs.

SURGICAL OPTIONS

Surgical EHPSS attenuation options have evolved over the past 15 years, with an increase in popularity of gradual occlusion devices, such as the ameroid constrictor (AC) and thin film bands (TFB). Advantages of these devices include gradual closure of the anomalous vessel allowing the portal system time to adapt to increased blood flow, decreased need to measure portal pressures intraoperatively, and in theory, decreased risk of portal hypertension and acute postoperative complications.[1]

ACs (**Fig. 1**) close the vessel via 2 methods. The casein inner ring swells by taking up abdominal fluid to partially close the vessel, with the remainder of the closure coming from a foreign body reaction to the casein. When evaluated in vivo, the inner diameter of the AC closed an average of 31%, with the remainder of EHPSS closure coming from soft tissue filling within the ring secondary to an inflammatory response.[15] The most rapid closure of the shunt occurs within 3 to 14 days after AC placement, with some animals developing a thrombus within the vessel, resulting in complete obstruction of the shunt within days of surgery.[1]

TFB is another surgical option for gradual occlusion of PSS. This material closes the shunt vessel by creating a foreign body reaction, leading to closure via inflammation. Initially called cellophane banding, studies evaluating the materials used found that the majority were not actually cellophane material, leading to the change in nomenclature to TFB.[16,17] This lack of consistency in materials leads to significant variation in closure times, with closure times ranging from less than 10 weeks to more than 6 months after surgery between individual patients and makes comparison of studies evaluating outcome with TFB challenging.[18–20]

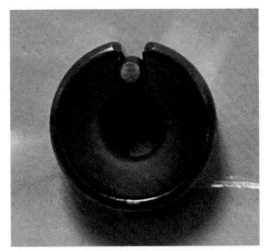

Fig. 1. Ameroid constrictor. The inner gray ring is composed of casein, a milk protein, which partially swells within the body after placement and then leads to a foreign body reaction, which results in vessel attenuation.

TFB are typically secured with hemoclips after being placed around the shunt vessel. The standard configuration is 4 hemoclips placed in an alternating fashion on a 3-layer band (**Fig. 2**); however, a study to determine the most secure configuration found that a single medium-sizes hemoclip withstood the physiologic forces needed to secure the band around the vessel and that a 4-layer band was less likely to fail when compared with a 3-layer band.[21]

In cats, TFB has been somewhat controversial with anecdotal reports that TFB would be less likely to cause PSS closure due to a decreased inflammatory reaction. A study evaluating the attenuation caused by TFB placed around an intraabdominal vessel in cats found that vessel occlusion was inconsistent and often incomplete

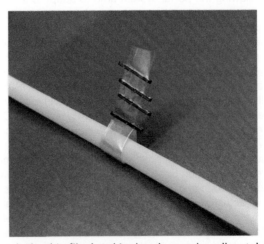

Fig. 2. Thin film band. The thin film band is placed around a yellow tube representative of an EHPSS. Four alternating hemoclips are used to secure the band around the vessel.

8 weeks after TFB placement.[22] In addition, recanalization of an EHPSS at 6 months after TFB surgery has been reported in one cat that initially had complete shunt attenuation.[23] However, in a retrospective case series of 34 cats undergoing TFB of an EHPSS, bile acids normalized in 25/28 cats that survived the initial postoperative period, with only one cat with abnormal bile acids having a patent shunt at the time of a second exploratory surgery. Overall, 3 cats had evidence of some residual shunting.[24] These inconsistent results may be due to variation in thin film materials used or variations between cats.

Another option for EHPSS attenuation is a self-retaining polyacrylic acid-silicone device (**Fig. 3**). This device closes the vessel via gradual physical occlusion over a 6- to 8-week time period without relying on an inflammatory reaction. The advantages of this device are the consistency in closure times and the ease of application. In a small clinical trial, this device led to complete occlusion by 8 weeks in 4/6 of dogs, with the remaining 2/6 having only mild residual flow.[25] This device is not yet commercially available but shows promise for being a new option in EHPSS attenuation.

Minimally invasive attenuation of EHPSS has been reported in 2 cases performed laparoscopically, as well as in a cadaveric study evaluating thoracoscopic placement of AC and TFB for portoazygous shunts[26,27]; however, for IHPSS, minimally invasive attenuation has become more common. Percutaneous transvenous coil embolization (PTCE) of IHPSS involves placement of a vascular stent into the caudal vena cava with thrombogenic coils inserted into the IHPSS, allowing for gradual occlusion through clot formation (**Fig. 4**). This procedure has been shown to be safe and effective, while limiting morbidity and mortality; however, it does require training in interventional radiology, as well as specialized equipment.[1] PTCE of EHPSS has been reported in a limited number of cases, with some cases having complete resolution of clinical signs; however, complications including migration of coils to the main pulmonary artery leading to death have occurred in other dogs with EHPSS.[28–30]

SURGICAL COMPLICATIONS

Complications of PSS surgery include PAS, portal hypertension, hemorrhage, hypoglycemia, gastric ulceration (with IHPSS), central blindness (cats), failure of shunt

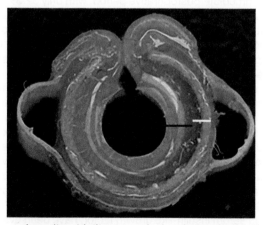

Fig. 3. Self-retaining polyacrylic acid silicone gradual occlusion device. The inner ring (black bar) is a silicone tubing filled with a proprietary polyacrylic acid and inorganic salt mixture, whereas the outer ring (white bar) is a second silicone tubing containing a plastic polymer ring to maintain the shape of the device.[25]

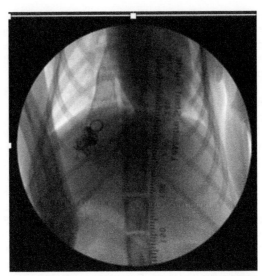

Fig. 4. Fluoroscopic image of percutaneous transvenous coil embolization of an intrahepatic portosystemic shunt. Note the vascular stent present within the caudal vena cava with thrombogenic coils placed within the shunt vessel.

closure, and sudden death, among others.[1] PAS occur in approximately 5% to 8% of dogs and 8% to 24% of cats.[1,24,31–33] A recent study revealed that 11% of dogs and 62% of cats developed postattenuation neurologic signs, with 5% of dogs and 22% of cats having PAS.[8,33] Risk factors for development of these conditions included preoperative hepatic encephalopathy and increasing age in dogs and lower postoperative osmolality in cats.[8,33] In addition, pugs may be at an increased risk of postattenuation neurologic signs when compared with other breeds, with 28.6% of pugs in a recent study experiencing these signs, leading to death or euthanasia within 30 days of surgery, compared with 3.3% of other dog breeds.[34] Most of the dogs experiencing PAS do not survive the immediate postoperative period, with only 32.3% of dogs surviving to 30 days after surgery in one study.[31] Factors that have been positively associated with survival in patients experiencing PAS include having a history of seizures preoperatively and development of only focal seizures postoperatively.[31] Unfortunately, no preventative preoperative or intraoperative measure has been consistently shown to result in a decrease in PAS.

Failure of shunt closure with gradual occlusion devices has recently been reported in 18% of dogs with AC placement and 35% of TFB cases.[15,35] In cats, failure of shunt closure has been reported in up to 57% after AC placement and 3% to 20% after TFB placement.[24,36,37] Despite this failure of complete attenuation, most cases were free of clinical signs, which calls into question the clinical impact of mild residual flow. Determination of residual flow postoperatively currently requires either advanced diagnostic imaging or nuclear scintigraphy for definitive diagnosis, as paired serum bile acid levels and fasting ammonia levels are not reliable to determine if complete occlusion has occurred or not.[38] Several blood tests, including the lidocaine/MEGX test, serum hyaluronic acid, and serum insulin-like growth factor, have been evaluated recently to determine usefulness in evaluation of postoperative shunt attenuation.[39–41] Although these show promise, they are often still inferior to advanced imaging, are not easily accessible in most practices, and require further evaluation to determine clinical usefulness. As most dogs and cats do not undergo postoperative imaging to confirm EHPSS closure unless there are continued clinical signs related to liver dysfunction, failure of shunt closure is likely underdiagnosed in clinical patients.

OUTCOME WITH SURGICAL ATTENUATION

Outcomes with surgical attenuation for PSS are good to excellent overall, with most patients having long survival times and minimal need for medical management long term. Several recent studies have compared outcomes between dogs undergoing AC versus TFB attenuation. Overall, no differences were found in postoperative complications, postoperative mortality, or long-term outcome between the 2 procedures.[42–44] Postoperative mortality ranged from 2% to 8%, with long-term clinical outcome regarded as excellent in 39% to 45% or good in 55% to 61%.[42–44] One study found that dogs undergoing TFB were more likely to need revision surgery due to persistent shunting.[44] These studies indicate that the placement of AC or TFB likely results in similar patient outcomes.

In cats, both AC and TFB have been evaluated separately, but they have not been compared in a single study. With the AC, development of postoperative complications occurred in 33% to 77% of cats, with a 0% to 4% postoperative mortality rate. Long-term outcome was considered excellent in 33% to 77%, despite a persistent shunting rate of 42% to 57%.[45,46] With TFB, postoperative complications occurred in 22% to 32% of cats, with 12% to 22% mortality in the postoperative period. At long-term follow-up, 44% to 89% of cats were free of clinical signs.[24,47] These results indicate that both devices can result in excellent long-term outcomes in cats.

For IHPSS, treatment with PTCE resulted in excellent outcomes in 66% of dogs in one study, with a median survival time of 2204 days.[32] In another study, 92% of dogs were free of clinical signs 3 months after the procedure, with liver volume increasing in 15/25 dogs available for imaging. However, liver volume was still lower than normal in 11/15 dogs.[11] PTCE has also been reported in 4 cats with excellent outcomes in 3/4, with one cat developing an acquired EHPSS, resulting in lower urinary tract signs.[48] In addition, one study evaluated PTCE compared with TFB for IHPSS and found that dogs treated with TFB had more minor postoperative complications and were hospitalized longer than dogs undergoing PTCE. Five-year survival rates were 75% for dogs undergoing TFB and 80% for dogs undergoing PTCE.[49] These studies indicate that excellent short and long-term results can be achieved in a minimally invasive procedure with PTCE, and this procedure should be considered for all dogs with IHPSS.

UPDATES IN CHOLECYSTECTOMY
Introduction

Cholecystectomy, removal of the gallbladder, is performed for various types of gallbladder pathology including gallbladder mucoceles (GBM), bacterial cholangiohepatitis, cholecystolithiasis, and biliary neoplasia. Although this procedure is commonly performed, concern for postoperative complications and reportedly high postoperative mortality rates can deter early surgical intervention for benign diseases; however, new data may shift this paradigm. In addition, laparoscopic cholecystectomy is the standard of care in people and has become a frequently used option in veterinary surgical practice over the past few years.

Breed Predispositions for Gallbladder Mucoceles

The most common reason for cholecystectomy in dogs is presence of a GBM, with other causes, such as cholecystolithiasis, being rare in this species.[50] Certain dog breeds are predisposed to development of GBM, including the Shetland Sheepdog, American Cocker Spaniel, Chihuahua, Pomeranian, and Miniature Schnauzer.[51] Recently, Border terriers have been added to this list, with this predisposition possibly being secondary to impaired cholecystokinin release.[51,52]

Diagnosis of Gallbladder Disease

Suspicion for presence of gallbladder disease is usually based on a combination of clinical signs and bloodwork abnormalities, with definitive diagnosis usually occurring via diagnostic imaging. Clinical signs related to gallbladder disease typically are nonspecific and may include vomiting, anorexia, lethargy, and abdominal pain. In cases where extrahepatic biliary obstruction (EHBO) is present, the patient may also have icterus due to elevated total bilirubin levels.[50] Other common bloodwork abnormalities include elevated serum alkaline phosphatase, elevated alanine aminotransferase, and neutrophilia.[50] Proteinuria has recently been demonstrated in dogs with GBM and was found to worsen with the severity of illness.[53]

Diagnostic imaging for gallbladder disease has traditionally focused on abdominal ultrasonography. Ultrasonography can be used to identify presence of a GBM (via typical stellate or "kiwi" appearance of material within the gallbladder; **Fig. 5**) and other abnormalities, such as common bile duct dilation, cholecystolithiasis, and evidence of gallbladder wall rupture.[50] Distinction between a GBM and biliary sludge via ultrasonography is important, as biliary sludge may be present in animals without gallbladder disease. In a study of 200 sequential abdominal ultrasonographic examinations in dogs, 66.5% had hyperechoic gallbladder material, whereas only 2% of cases had a GBM. A larger amount of sludge was seen in older dogs, in dogs with hypothyroidism, and in dogs with hyperadrenocorticism.[54] Interestingly, in another study, animals with gallbladder sludge did not develop symptoms of gallbladder disease or develop GBM, nor did the sludge resolve over a period of 1 year in most healthy animals.[55]

Accurate diagnosis of biliary rupture via ultrasonography is important, as this information is often used to determine if emergency surgical intervention is recommended. The sensitivity of ultrasonography for detection of biliary rupture is reportedly between 56% and 88%.[56] A recent study showed ultrasonography to be a better predictor of biliary rupture than serum total bilirubin concentrations. Ultrasonography correctly identified biliary rupture in 85.7% of dogs, whereas 40% of dogs with biliary rupture had normal total serum bilirubin values.[57] Comparison of abdominal effusion total

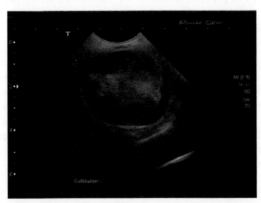

Fig. 5. Ultrasonographic image of a gallbladder mucocele. Note the stellate or "kiwi" appearance of the non–gravity-dependent material within the gallbladder.

bilirubin to serum total bilirubin remains vital to confirm bile peritonitis when samples can be obtained via abdominocentesis. If the total bilirubin level in the abdominal fluid is greater than or equal to 2 times higher than the peripheral blood bilirubin level, bile peritonitis is likely.[60]

Decision-Making in Management of Gallbladder Mucoceles and Timing of Cholecystectomy

Although making the decision to move forward with cholecystectomy can be straight-forward in cases of EHBO and/or gallbladder rupture, it can be a more difficult deci-sion in patients in whom a GBM is incidentally found. Initial treatment of GBM that is not causing EHBO often focuses on medical management and evaluation for any concurrent diseases, which may predispose the patient to having a GBM. Medical management typically includes use of ursodeoxycholic acid (Ursodiol), which is a nontoxic bile acid and choleretic. Concerns exist over increased risk of gallbladder rupture with use of Ursodiol; however, this concern has not been substantiated. It should be used with caution, or not used at all, in dogs with partial or complete EHBO.[50]

Dogs with GBM should also be evaluated for presence of hypothyroidism and hyperadrenocorticism, as these endocrine diseases have been shown to increase odds of GBM development by 3 and 29 times, respectively.[58] Treatment of the under-lying disease in these cases may improve the GBM or lead to complete resolution, although very few cases evaluating this are reported in the literature. In one case series that evaluated GBM in dogs treated for hyperadrenocorticism, improvement was seen in the GBM via ultrasound in 4/15 cases; however, complete resolution was not seen in any case.[59] A case report of 2 dogs with hypothyroidism had complete resolution of their GBM after treatment with only levothyroxine and Ursodiol; however, this is a very small number of patients and likely does not reflect the population overall.[60]

Medical management alone for GBM when compared with cholecystectomy has been evaluated to determine the effect of treatment choice on long-term outcome. Medical management alone was found to have significantly decreased long-term sur-vival with a median survival time of 1340 days compared with 1802 days for dogs un-dergoing cholecystectomy. Interestingly, dogs that failed medical management and then underwent cholecystectomy had a survival time of only 203 days (**Fig. 6**).[61] The results of this study indicate that surgical management of GBM is preferable for long-term survival, despite an initially higher risk of mortality postoperatively.

Several studies have sought to evaluate the impact of the presence of clinical signs at the time of surgery on surgical outcome in dogs with GBM. Dogs that were not exhibiting clinical signs related to their GBM at the time of cholecystectomy had a lower mortality rate across studies, with mortality rates ranging from 2% to 6% in nonclinical dogs compared with 17% to 23% in clinically affected dogs.[62–64] These findings support early surgical intervention in patients with confirmed GBM to decrease risk of postoperative mortality; however, it is important to note that some nonclinical cases did not survive the postoperative period, highlighting that cholecys-tectomy is not a benign procedure.

Open Cholecystectomy Surgery

Open cholecystectomy is performed via a ventral midline approach, with the gall-bladder dissected from the hepatic parenchyma via a combination of blunt and sharp dissection with the instruments used varying between surgeons.[50] In cases where common bile duct obstruction is present, normograde or retrograde catheterization of the common bile duct is performed to ensure patency and to flush any obstructive

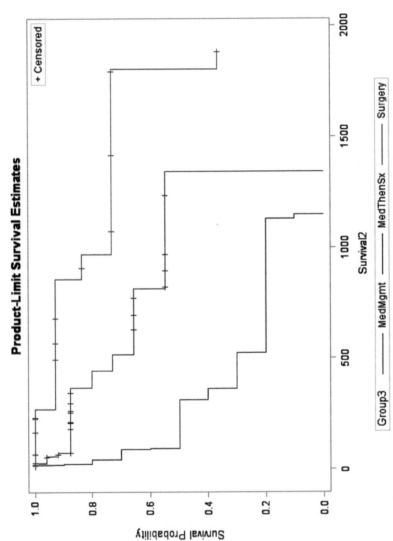

Fig. 6. Survival probability (starting 14 days postdiagnosis) of dogs with gallbladder mucocele undergoing medical management only, failed medical management followed by cholecystectomy, or cholecystectomy only. Note that the cholecystectomy group has a significantly longer survival time than the other 2 groups.[61]

material out of the duct. Retrograde catheterization requires a duodenotomy to allow visualization of the major duodenal papilla and passage of a red rubber catheter. Normograde catherization can be performed after transection of the cystic duct before suture ligation or hemoclip application; however, catheterization in this direction can be challenging in patients with a friable cystic duct or highly tortuous common bile duct.

Recent studies have evaluated the influence of catheterization and method of catheterization on various surgical variables, complications, and outcome. One study found that although postoperative complications overall were not different between those with and without intraoperative catheterization of the common bile duct, postoperative pancreatitis occurred more commonly, and surgical times were longer in those patients where catherization was performed.[65] Another study compared normograde with retrograde catheterization of the common bile duct. Dogs were more likely to experience complications after retrograde catheterization and were more likely to have persistence of gastrointestinal signs postoperatively. In addition, total bilirubin levels only decreased by 39% after retrograde catheterization compared with a 70% decrease after normograde catheterization.[66] This can likely be attributed to inflammation at the major duodenal papilla secondary to catheterization insertion attempts during retrograde catheterization. Based on these data, it is recommended to strongly consider whether catheterization is necessary in an individual patient and if needed, to perform normograde catheterization when possible.

Postoperative complications with cholecystectomy include bile peritonitis, pancreatitis, nonresolution of clinical signs, and reobstruction of the common bile duct.[50] These complications may result in the need for a second surgical procedure or in the worst cases, death. Overall mortality in recent studies has ranged from 9% to 20%, which is lower than the previously reported mortality of up to 40%.[61–64,67–69] Factors that have recently been associated with mortality in dogs with GBM undergoing cholecystectomy include presence of clinical signs, increasing age, presence of jaundice, azotemia, hypoalbuminemia, concurrent hyperadrenocorticism, postoperative ileus, postoperative pancreatitis, and Pomeranian breed, among others.[63,64,67] In addition, presence of gallbladder rupture and bile peritonitis increased risk of death by 2.7 times when compared with those with an intact gallbladder.[56] Intraoperative hypotension and presence of cholecystitis were not found to affect survival.[67,68] Although the mortality rate is still higher than would be expected, the improvement seen recently in mortality rates is likely due to a combination of early surgical intervention and advances in the fields of veterinary anesthesia and critical care.

Laparoscopic Cholecystectomy

Laparoscopic cholecystectomy is reserved for dogs without EHBO, choledocholithiasis, or evidence of a gallbladder wall rupture.[50] Case selection for laparoscopic cholecystectomy is variable and depends on a variety of factors, including clinician comfort with laparoscopic procedures. Any patient with common bile duct dilation, suspicion of sludge within the common bile duct, or possible common bile duct obstruction may not be a good candidate for a laparoscopic approach due to the inability to flush the duct to remove obstruction or ensure obstruction is not present. A 4-port technique is used with the camera port placed on midline just caudal to the umbilicus and 3 instrument ports placed in paramedian positions, one on the left and 2 on the right. A technique using a single port access system has been described in a case series of 15 dogs. With this technique, the single port is placed subumbilically, with a second port placed as needed to complete the procedure either to the right or left side of the umbilicus in a paramedian position.[70] A second port was placed in addition to the single access port in 13/15 cases in one case series, and 1 or 2 additional ports were placed in 7/7 cases in another series.[70,71]

Outcome with laparoscopic cholecystectomy has been reported in 3 case series, with a total of 111 cases reported. Conversion to open laparotomy was reported in 4% to 30% of cases, with conversions occurring due to the presence of adhesions, preoperative or intraoperative biliary leakage, hemorrhage, inability to safely ligate the cystic duct, acute respiratory compromise, and cardiac arrest.[70–72] According to one case series, the need to convert to laparotomy decreased when using the single port access system if an additional port was placed at the beginning of the surgical procedure.[70] Another case series found no difference in conversion rate when a single port access system was compared with a multiport approach.[71]

Across the available data, 3/111 (3%) required reoperation for postoperative bile peritonitis, with 2 leaking from the cystic duct and one leaking from a hepatic duct. Intraoperative death occurred in 2/111 (2%) due to acute circulatory failure and diaphragmatic injury from an electric scalpel. Four out of one hundred eleven (4%) died within 2 weeks of surgery secondary to acute heart failure, liver dysfunction, systemic sepsis, and septic peritonitis from leakage around a gastrostomy tube.[70–72] None died secondary to postoperative biliary leakage. Follow-up at greater than 30 days after surgery was available for 19/20 dogs in one case series, with 74% of dogs still alive at the time of follow-up. Of the 5 dogs that were not alive at the time of follow-up, all had died of causes unrelated to hepatobiliary disease.[71]

The results of these studies indicate that with appropriate training and case selection, laparoscopic cholecystectomy is a safe and effective surgical option with minimal risk for postoperative complications. However, owners must be prepared that conversion to open laparotomy may occur in up to 30% of cases. Further research is needed comparing open with laparoscopic cholecystectomy to evaluate for any differences in outcome between the 2 procedures. In addition, further research is needed to understand which patients are the best candidates for a laparoscopic procedure as compared with an open procedure.

SUMMARY

In conclusion, there have been many advancements recently in the treatment of PSS and GBM. Surgery remains the mainstay of treatment in both conditions, with recent studies reaffirming the benefits of surgery regarding long-term survival and quality of life. Although risks are still present in both procedures, more information is available to help surgeons mitigate those risks, resulting in improved surgical outcomes.

CLINICS CARE POINTS

- Surgical attenuation of EHPSS, even in dogs diagnosed later in life, results in improved survival times and quality of life compared with medical management only.
- Use of levetiracetam before EHPSS surgery likely does not decrease risk for development of postattenuation seizures.
- Recent studies indicate that early surgical intervention via cholecystectomy in dogs with GBM decreases postoperative mortality.
- With appropriate training, laparoscopic cholecystectomy is a safe option for dogs with nonobstructive gallbladder disease.

DISCLOSURE

The author has nothing to disclose.

REFERENCES

1. Berent AC, Tobias KM. Hepatic vascular anomalies. In: Johnston SA, Tobias KM, editors. Veterinary surgery: small animal. 2nd edition. St. Louis: Elsevier; 2018. p. 1852–85.
2. van Straten G, Spee B, Rothuizen J, et al. Diagnostic value of the rectal ammonia tolerance test, fasting plasma ammonia and fasting plasma bile acids for canine portosystemic shunting. Vet J 2015;204:282–6.
3. Toulza O, Center SA, Brooks MB, et al. Evaluation of plasma protein C activity for detection of hepatobiliary disease and portosystemic shunting in dogs. J Am Vet Med Assoc 2006;229:1761–71.
4. Brunson BW, Case JB, Ellison GW, et al. Evaluation of surgical outcome, complications, and mortality in dogs undergoing preoperative computed tomography angiography for diagnosis of an extrahepatic portosystemic shunt: 124 cases (2005-2014). Can Vet J 2016;57:59–64.
5. Favier RP, de Graaf E, Corbee RJ, et al. Outcome of non-surgical dietary management with or without lactulose in dogs with congenital portosystemic shunts. Vet Q 2020;40:108–14.
6. Culler CA, Reinhardt A, Vigani A. Successful management of clinical signs associated with hepatic encephalopathy with manual therapeutic plasma exchange in a dog. J Vet Emerg Crit Care 2020;30:312–7.
7. Fryer KJ, Levine JM, Peycke LE, et al. Incidence of postoperative seizures with and without levetiracetam pretreatment in dogs undergoing portosystemic shunt attenuation. J Vet Intern Med 2011;25:1379–84.
8. Strickland R, Tivers MS, Adamantos SE, et al. Incidence and risk factors for neurological signs after attenuation of single congenital portosystemic shunts in 253 dogs. Vet Surg 2018;47:745–55.
9. Wallace ML, Grimes JA, Edwards L, et al. Outcome of medical versus surgical management of a congenital extrahepatic portosystemic shunt in older dogs: a multi-institutional retrospective study. Vet Surg 2021;54–5. ACVS 2021 surgery summit abstracts.
10. Mullins RA, Villamil CS, de Rooster H, et al. Effect of prophylactic treatment with levetiracetam on the incidence of postattenuation seizures in dogs undergoing surgical management of single congenital extrahepatic portosystemic shunts. Vet Surg 2019;48:164–72.
11. Culp WTN, Zwingenberger AL, Giuffrida MA, et al. Prospective evaluation of outcome of dogs with intrahepatic portosystemic shunts treated via percutaneous transvenous coil embolization. Vet Surg 2018;47:74–85.
12. Zwingenberger AL, Daniel L, Steffey MA, et al. Correlation between liver volume, portal vascular anatomy, and hepatic perfusion in dogs with congenital portosystemic shunt before and after placement of ameroid constrictors. Vet Surg 2014; 43:926–34.
13. Greenhalgh SN, Reeve JA, Johnston T, et al. Long-term survival and quality of life in dogs with clinical signs associated with a congenital portosystemic shunt after surgical or medical treatment. J Am Vet Med Assoc 2014;245:527–33.
14. Tivers MS, Handel I, Gow AG, et al. Attenuation of congenital portosystemic shunt reduces inflammation in dogs. PLoS One 2015;10:e0117557.

15. Hunt GB, Culp WTN, Mayhew KN, et al. Evaluation of in vivo behavior of ameroid ring constrictors in dogs with congenital extrahepatic portosystemic shunts using computed tomography. Vet Surg 2014;43:834–42.
16. Smith RR, Hunt GB, Garcia-Nolen TC, et al. Spectroscopic and mechanical evaluation of thin film commonly used for banding congenital portosystemic shunts in dogs. Vet Surg 2013;42:478–87.
17. Field EJ, Scurr DJ, Piggott MJ, et al. The chemical and ultra-structural analysis of thin plastic films used for surgical attenuation of portosystemic shunts in dogs and cats. Res Vet Sci 2019;126:192–8.
18. Landon BP, Abraham LA, Charles JA. Use of transcolonic portal scintigraphy to evaluate efficacy of cellophane banding of congenital extrahepatic portosystemic shunts in 16 dogs. Aust Vet J 2008;86:169–79.
19. Youmans KR, Hunt GB. Cellophane banding for the gradual attenuation of single extrahepatic portosystemic shunts in eleven dogs. Aust Vet J 1990;70:531 7.
20. Frankel D, Seim H, MacPhail C, et al. Evaluation of cellophane banding with and without intraoperative attenuation for treatment of congenital extrahepatic portosystemic shunts in dogs. J Am Vet Med Assoc 2006;228:1355–60.
21. Joffe MR, Hall E, Tan C, et al. Evaluation of different methods of securing cellophane bands for portosystemic shunt attenuation. Vet Surg 2019;48:42–9.
22. Freund KA, Wallace ML, Secrest SA, et al. Thin film occlusion of an intra-abdominal vein in cats. Vet Surg 2020;49:354–62.
23. Crowley J, Foo T, Boland L, et al. Recanalization of a congenital extrahepatic portosystemic shunt previously attenuated with cellophane banding in a cat. JFMS Open Rep 2018;4. 2055116918795717.
24. Valiente P, Trehy M, White R, et al. Complications and outcome of cats with congenital extrahepatic portosystemic shunts treated with thin film: thirty-four cases (2008-2017). J Vet Intern Med 2020;34:117–24.
25. Wallace ML, Ellison GW, Giglio RF, et al. Gradual attenuation of a congenital extrahepatic portosystemic shunt with a self-retaining polyacrylic acid-silicone device in 6 dogs. Vet Surg 2018;47:722–8.
26. Miller JM, Fowler JD. Laparoscopic portosystemic sunt attenuation in two dogs. J Am Anim Hosp Assoc 2006;42:160–4.
27. Carroll KA, Dickson RE, Scharf VF. Feasibility of thoracoscopic attenuation of the azygos vein as a model for portoazygos shunts: a canine cadaveric study. Vet Surg 2021;50:345–52.
28. Léveillé R, Johnston SE, Birchard SJ. Transvenous coil embolization of portosystemic shunt in dogs. Vet Radiol Ultrasound 2003;44:32–6.
29. Léveillé R, Pibarot P, Soulez G, et al. Transvenous coil embolization of an extrahepatic portosystemic shunt in a dog: a naturally occurring model of portosystemic malformations in humans. Pediatr Radiol 2000;30:607–9.
30. Bussadori R, Bussadori C, Millán L, et al. Transvenous coil embolization for the treatment of single congenital portosystemic shunts in six dogs. Vet J 2008;176:221–6.
31. Mullins RA, Villamil CS, Selmic LE, et al. Prognostic factors for short-term survival of dogs that experience postattenuation seizures after surgical correction of single congenital extrahepatic portosystemic shunts: 93 cases (2005-2018). Vet Surg 2020;49:958–70.
32. Weisse C, Berent AC, Todd K, et al. Endovascular evaluation and treatment of intrahepatic portosystemic shunts in dogs: 100 cases (2001-2011). J Am Vet Med Assoc 2014;244:78–94.

33. Strickland R, Tivers MS, Fowkes RC, et al. Incidence and risk factors for neurological signs after attenuation of a single congenital portosystemic shunt in 50 cats. Vet Surg 2021;50:303–11.

34. Wallace ML, MacPhail CM, Monnet E. Incidence of postoperative neurologic complications in pugs following portosystemic shunt attenuation surgery. J Am Anim Hosp Assoc 2018;54:46–9.

35. Nelson NC, Nelson LL. Imaging and clinical outcomes in 20 dogs treated with thin film banding for extrahepatic portosystemic shunts. Vet Surg 2016;45:736–45.

36. Hunt GB, Kummeling A, Tisdall PL, et al. Outcomes of cellophane banding for congenital portosystemic shunts in 106 dogs and 6 cats. Vet Surg 2004;33: 25–31.

37. Havig M, Tobias KM. Outcome of ameroid constrictor occlusion of single extrahepatic portosystemic shunts in cats: 12 cases (1993-2000). J Am Vet Med Assoc 2002;220:337–41.

38. Vallarino N, Pil S, Devriendt N, et al. Diagnostic value of blood variables following attenuation of congenital extrahepatic portosystemic shunt in dogs. Vet Rec 2020;187:e48.

39. Devriendt N, Serrano G, Croubels S, et al. Evaluation of serum lidocaine/monoethylglycylxylidide concentration to assess shunt closure in dogs with extrahepatic portosystemic shunts. J Vet Intern Med 2021;35:261–8.

40. Devriendt N, Serrano G, Meyer E, et al. Serum hyaluronic acid, a marker for improved liver perfusion after gradual surgical attenuation of extrahepatic portosystemic shunt closure in dogs. Vet J 2021;268:105064.

41. Serrano G, Devriendt N, Paepe D, et al. Serum insulin-like growth factor-1 as a marker of improved liver function and surgical outcome in dogs with congenital extrahepatic portosystemic shunts. Vet J 2021;274:105716.

42. Otomo A, Singh A, Jeong J, et al. Long-term clinical outcomes of dogs with single congenital extrahepatic portosystemic shunts attenuated with thin film banding or ameroid ring constrictors. Vet Surg 2020;49:436–44.

43. Traverson M, Lussier B, Huneault L, et al. Comparative outcomes between ameroid ring constrictor and cellophane banding for treatment of single congenital extrahepatic portosystemic shunts in 49 dogs (1998-2012). Vet Surg 2018;46: 179–87.

44. Matiasovic M, Chanoit GPA, Meakin LB, et al. Outcomes of dogs treated for extrahepatic congenital portosystemic shunts with thin film banding or ameroid constrictor. Vet Surg 2020;49:160–71.

45. Havig M, Tobias KM. Outcome of ameroid constrictor occlusion of single congenital extrahepatic portosystemic shunts in cats: 12 cases (1993-2000). J Am Vet Med Assoc 2002;220:337–41.

46. Kyles AE, Hardie EM, Mehl M, et al. Evaluation of ameroid ring constrictors for the management of single extrahepatic portosystemic shunts in cats: 23 cases (1996-2001). J Am Vet Med Assoc 2002;220:1341–7.

47. Cabassu J, Seim HB, MacPhail CM, et al. Outcomes of cats undergoing surgical attenuation of congenital extrahepatic portosystemic shunts through cellophane banding: 9 cases (2000-2007). J Am Vet Med Assoc 2011;238:89–93.

48. Culp WTN, Griffin MA, Case JB, et al. Use of percutaneous transvenous coil embolization in the treatment of intrahepatic portosystemic shunts in four cats. J Am Vet Med Assoc 2020;257:70–9.

49. Case JB, Marvel SJ, Stiles MC, et al. Outcomes of cellophane banding or percutaneous transvenous coil embolization of canine intrahepatic portosystemic shunts. Vet Surg 2018;47:O59–66.

50. Mayhew PD, Weisse C. Liver and biliary system. In: Johnston SA, Tobias KM, editors. Veterinary surgery: small animal. 2nd edition. St. Louis: Elsevier; 2018. p. 1829–52.
51. Allerton F, Swinbourne F, Barker L, et al. Gall bladder mucoceles in Border terriers. J Vet Intern Med 2018;32:1618–28.
52. Barker L, Tivers MS, Kathrani A, et al. Serological markers of gluten sensitivity in Border terriers with gall bladder mucoceles. J Sm Anim Pract 2020;61:630–6.
53. Lindaberry C, Vaden S, Aicher KM, et al. Proteinuria in dogs with gallbladder mucocele formation: a retrospective case control study. J Vet Intern Med 2021;35:878–86.
54. Cook AK, Jambhekar AV, Dylewski AM. Gallbladder sludge in dogs: ultrasonographic and clinical findings in 200 patients. J Am Anim Hosp Assoc 2016;52:125–31.
55. DeMonaco SM, Grant DC, Larson MM, et al. Spontaneous course of biliary sludge over 12 months in dogs with ultrasonographically identified biliary sludge. J Vet Intern Med 2016;30:771–8.
56. Jaffey JA, Graham A, VanEerde E, et al. Gallbladder mucocele: variables associated with outcome and the utility of ultrasonography to identify gallbladder rupture in 219 dogs. J Vet Intern Med 2018;32:195–200.
57. Wilson K, Powers D, Grasperge B, et al. Dogs with biliary rupture based on ultrasound findings may have normal total serum bilirubin values. Vet Radiol Ultrasound 2021;62:236–45.
58. Mesich MLL, Mayhew PD, Paek M, et al. Gall bladder mucoceles and their association with endocrinopathies in dogs: a retrospective case-control study. J Small Anim Pract 2009;50:630–5.
59. Kim KH, Han SM, Jeon KO, et al. Clinical relationship between cholestatic disease and pituitary-dependent hyperadrenocorticism in dogs: a retrospective case series. J Vet Intern Med 2017;31:335–42.
60. Walter R, Dunn ME, d'Anjou MA, et al. Nonsurgical resolution of gallbladder mucocele in two dogs. J Am Vet Med Assoc 2008;232:1688–93.
61. Parkanzky M, Grimes J, Schmiedt C, et al. Long-term survival of dogs treated for gallbladder mucocele by cholecystectomy, medical management, or both. J Vet Intern Med 2019;33:2057–66.
62. Friesen SL, Upchurch DA, Hollenbeck DL, et al. Clinical findings for dogs undergoing elective and nonelective cholecystectomies for gall bladder mucoceles. J Sm Anim Pract 2021;62:547–53.
63. Jaffey JA, Pavlick M, Webster CR, et al. Effect of clinical signs, endocrinopathies, timing of surgery, hyperlipidemia, and hyperbilirubinemia on outcome in dogs with gallbladder mucocele. Vet J 2019;251:105350.
64. Youn G, Waschak MJ, Kunkel KAR, et al. Outcome of elective cholecystectomy for the treatment of gallbladder disease in dogs. J Am Vet Med Assoc 2018;252:970–5.
65. Piegols HJ, Hayes GM, Lin S, et al. Association between biliary tree manipulation and outcome in dogs undergoing cholecystectomy for gallbladder mucocele: a multi-institutional retrospective study. Vet Surg 2021;50:767–74.
66. Putterman AB, Selmic LE, Kindra C, et al. Influence of normograde versus retrograde catheterization of bile ducts in dogs treated for gallbladder mucocele. Vet Surg 2021;50:784–93.
67. Hattersley R, Downing F, Gibson S, et al. Impact of intra-operative hypotension on mortality rates and post-operative complications in dogs undergoing cholecystectomy. J Sm Anim Pract 2020;61:624–9.

68. Rogers E, Jaffey JA, Graham A, et al. Prevalence and impact of cholecystitis on outcome in dogs with gallbladder mucocele. J Vet Emerg Crit Care 2020;30: 97–101.
69. Besso JG, Wrigley RH, Gliatto JM, et al. Ultrasonographic appearance and clinical findings in 14 dogs with gallbladder mucocele. Vet Radiol Ultrasound 2000; 41:261–71.
70. Simon A, Monnet E. Laparoscopic cholecystectomy with single port access system in 15 dogs. Vet Surg 2020;49:O156–62.
71. Scott J, Singh A, Mayhew PD, et al. Perioperative complications and outcome of laparoscopic cholecystectomy in 20 dogs. Vet Surg 2016;45:O49–59.
72. Kanai H, Hagiwara K, Nukaya A, et al. Short-term outcome of laparoscopic cholecystectomy for benign gall bladder diseases in 76 dogs. J Vet Med Sci 2018;80: 1747–53.

Current Concepts in Urinary Surgery

Pamela Schwartz, DVM, DACVS, CCRP

KEYWORDS

- Ureteral obstruction • Ureteral stent • Subcutaneous ureteral bypass (SUB)
- Ureterotomy • Urinary incontinence • Transurethral bulking agent
- Hydraulic occluder

KEY POINTS

- Minimally invasive treatment options for ureteral obstructions and ectopic ureters are becoming more readily available in veterinary medicine.
- Ureteral stents have become the first choice for treatment of canine ureteral obstruction caused by ureteroliths due to the propensity for the mineralization of the subcutaneous ureteral bypass system.
- The subcutaneous ureteral bypass system has become the first choice for many clinicians for the treatment of feline ureteral obstruction that does not respond to medical management regardless of cause.
- For animals that have refractory urinary incontinence after appropriate surgical treatment of all anatomic abnormalities and failure of medical management, additional treatments, such as cystoscopic transurethral bulking agents and hydraulic occluders can be considered.

 Video content accompanies this article at http://www.vetsmall.theclinics.com.

INTRODUCTION

The incidence of urinary disease in cats and dogs requiring surgical intervention has been increasing steadily over the past few years.[1-3] Several challenges have been encountered historically when treating the urinary system in veterinary patients. These include delicate and diminutive anatomy, difficultly obtaining a diagnosis (need for advanced imaging), lack of improvement with medical management, and high

Disclosure: The authors have nothing to disclose.
Surgeon and Department Chair, The Animal Medical Center, 510 East 62 Street, New York, NY 10065, USA
[a] Vet Stent-Ureter feline, 2.5 F, multifenestrated, Infiniti Medical LLC, Menlo Park, Calif.
[b] SUB device, Norfolk Vet Products, Skokie, Ill.
[c] AUSTM, Norfolk Vet Products, Skokie, Ill.
E-mail address: Pamela.Schwartz@amcny.org

Vet Clin Small Anim 52 (2022) 387–417
https://doi.org/10.1016/j.cvsm.2021.12.003
0195-5616/22/© 2021 Elsevier Inc. All rights reserved.

morbidity and mortality rates associated with several surgical techniques.[4–7] Minimally invasive treatment options are becoming more readily available in veterinary medicine, which may help circumvent many of these challenges.

Endourology refers to the use of minimally invasive techniques to both inspect and perform definitive treatment on the urinary tract.[5] There are several advantages to using interventional radiology (IR) and interventional endoscopic (IE) techniques in comparison to traditional surgical procedures, including shorter hospital stays, decreased pain, fewer complications, reduced morbidity and mortality rates.[2,5] This chapter focuses on the advancements in urologic surgery in both dogs and cats with primary focus on the treatment of ureteral obstruction and urinary incontinence.

URETERAL OBSTRUCTION

With the increased availability of various imaging modalities, including point of care ultrasound, the diagnosis of ureteral obstruction has become more commonplace (**Fig. 1**). It is well documented, that the longer a ureter is obstructed, the more irreversible damage to the kidney parenchyma may occur, which is clinically important as animals with ureteral obstruction often have some degree of underlying renal disease.[1,5,6,8–10] In one study, only 13.4% of cats had a significant decrease in serum creatinine in response to medical management and 32.7% of cats did not respond and died or were euthanized within 1 month of diagnosis of ureteral calculi.[7] These factors and the low success rate of medical management, warrant other interventions, if medical management alone does not show improvement after a 24 to 48 hour period.[7,8]

The most common cause of feline ureteral obstruction is calcium oxalate ureterolithiasis.[2,11,12] Additional etiologies of ureteral obstruction in dogs and cats may include ureteral stricture, dried solidified blood stones, neoplasia, ureteritis, iatrogenic ligation, and circumcaval ureters.[2,12,13] Traditional open surgical procedures reported to relieve ureteral obstruction include ureterotomy, neoureterocystostomy, ureteral resection and end-to-end anastomosis, ureteronephrectomy, and renal transplantation.[5,7,8,14,15] Previous studies in both cats and dogs have shown high morbidity and mortality rates, in addition to a high rate of recurrence of obstruction. In a large study of cats undergoing ureterotomy or ureteroneocystostomy for the management of ureteral calculi, the postoperative complication rate and perioperative mortality rate were 31% and 18%, respectively (**Table 1**).[7] Urine leakage and persistent ureteral obstruction after surgery were the most common complications.[7] In contrast, one study comparing cats following open ureteral surgery with and without stents had much lower mortality rates of 9% and

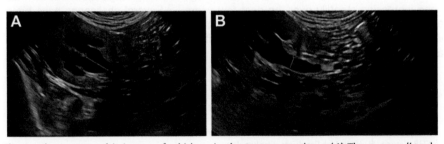

Fig. 1. Ultrasonographic image of a kidney in the transverse plane. (*A*) The *orange line* denotes renal pelvic dilation. (*B*) The *orange line* denotes the proximal ureter diameter. (Adapted from, McEntee, E. P., et al Evaluation of preoperative ultrasonographic parameters to predict renal recovery in long-term survivors after the treatment of feline ureteral obstructions: 2012–2019. J Feline Med Surg 2021 https://doi.org/10.1177/1098612X211023645 with permission of SAGE Publications.)

Table 1
Comparison of various ureteral interventions in cats

Procedure	Morality Rate	Anesthesia Time (Median)	Procedure Time (Median)	Intra-op Complications	Postoperative	Short Term	Long Term
Medical Management (Kyles et al,[7] 2005)	33% died or euthanized with 1 mo					Only 13.5% responded to medical management (improved azotemia)	
Traditional Surgical Techniques: Ureterotomy, ureteroneo-cystostomy, ureterone-phrectomy, ureteral resection and anastomosis (Kyles et al,[7] 2005)/ Ureterotomy, reimplantation (Roberts et al,[6] 2011)	18%; Mortality rate of cats that underwent a 2nd surgery because of uroabdomen was 27%/21% died postop at a median of 3 d after surgery		160 minutes[6]		31%[7]	Uroabdomen 16%[7]; persistent ureteral obstruction 11% of cats with ureteroneo-cystostomy[7]; 2.9% after ureterotomy[7]; 6% uroabdomen post-op[6]	Second episode of ureterolithiasis in 40% occurred a median of 12.5 mo after initial diagnosis[7]; no long-term follow-up [6]

(continued on next page)

Table 1
(continued)

Procedure	Morality Rate	Anesthesia Time (Median)	Procedure Time (Median)	Intra-op Complications	Postoperative	Short Term	Long Term
Stent: (Berent et al,[9] 2014) 95% successful stent placement	7.5% periop		110 min	8.9% major procedure related complications: 2 urine leakage from ureteral tear during stent placement (spontaneously resolved), 2 urine leakage from ureterotomy incision (resolved with closed suction drain), 1 urine leakage from urinary bladder stay suture site requiring reoperation, 1 stent malposition; 2 (2.8%) needed to return to surgery for fixation of a complication (bladder leak and stent malposition)	23% UTI before discharge	31.7% UTI within 1 mo; pollakiuria or stranguria in 4.5% <1 wk; pollakiuria or stranguria in 9.8% from 1 wk – <1 mo; 1 stent migration 3 wk post-op; 1 cat with progressive azotemia	13% UTI >1 mo; reobstruction 19%; stent migration 5.9%; stent exhange required in 27% a median of 67.5 d after surgery; dysuria 1.7%; hematuria 18%

| Ureteral surgery vs stent placement (Wormser et al,[16] 2016) | Perioperative mortality rates were 9% with and 8% without stents | Not noted | Not noted | Not noted | Uroabdomen in 7% of cats that had ureteral surgery: 4 had ureterotomy (3 with stents placed, 1 without), 3 had stent only, 1 ureteral reimplantation with stent - led to additional surgery for 1 cat and euthanasia for 1 | 5% stent migration within 5 d requiring additional surgery | 20% chronic lower urinary tract disease (hematuria, dysuria, stranguria); proportion of cats with lower urinary tract signs significantly higher for cats that had stents. 7 required stent modification, removal, or replacement; 11% chronic UTIs; UTIs were significantly greater in cats that had stents placed; 22% had recurrent ureteral obstruction (no difference between stent vs no stent) |
| Stent surgery combined or not with traditional surgery (Manassero et al,[15] 2014) | 8.0% Periop mortality rate; 1 y mortality rate of 25% | Not noted | Not noted | 40% of cases required incising the urothelium of the ureterovesical papilla to allow dilator/stent placement; | 6.7% (1 case) had uroabdomen postop that had a second surgery | 6.7% (1 case) had stent migration requiring replacement; UTI in 1 case; 3 cases with self limiting stranguria; 3 cases with |

(continued on next page)

Table 1
(continued)

Procedure	Morality Rate	Anesthesia Time (Median)	Procedure Time (Median)	Intra-op Complications	Postoperative	Short Term	Long Term
				Failure to direct stent placement in 26% due to stricture or ureteral tear requiring ureteral resection and anastomosis			stent obstruction requiring surgical removal resulting in death in 1 cat; migration of ureteroliths along the stent in 50% of stents
Stent: (Kulendra et al,[17] 2014)	15%	315 min	182 min	19 ureters required a traditional surgical technique to place the stent	19.2% uroabdomen - 4/5 had an additional surgery		stent replacement in 19.2%; mild dysuria 27%, moderate dysuria 9%, severe dysuria 27%
Stent vs SUB (Deroy et al,[18] 2017)	Perioperative mortality rate 18% for stents and 13% for SUBs	Not noted	77 min stent group; 47 min SUB group		18.5% uroabdomen in the stent group only		44% of stent group required additional procedures because of stent occlusion (7), uroabdomen (3), and severe and refractory signs of cystitis (2); 2 cats with severe cystitis had replacement of stent with a SUB, and dysuria resolved.

| SUB (Berent et al,[19] 2018) | 6% | Not noted | 70 min | 7%: leak at catheter-port junction (2%) requiring reattachment of the catheter, blood clot within the device (2%) requiring flushing, kinking of a catheter (2%) requiring repositioning before closure, renal bleeding during nephrostomy tube placement (1%) that was self-limiting, and self-limiting subcapsular bleeding (1%) | blood clot in the SUB device 5%, leak in the SUB device 3%, dysuria 3%, urethral obstruction 2%, worsening azotemia 1.4%, kinking of the device 1%; surgical revision was needed in 7% | blood clot blocking one of the catheters 2%, a stone blocking the system 1%, urethral obstruction 1% | Device blockage due to mineralization 25%, kinking 3%, blood clot 1%, exchange of device due to mineralization 13%, urethral obstruction 1.7% | Two (9%) in SUB group required additional surgical procedures because of SUB occlusion and lower urinary tract obstruction; Only cats with stents had flank pain 23% |

(continued on next page)

Table 1
(continued)

Procedure	Morality Rate	Anesthesia Time (Median)	Procedure Time (Median)	Intra-op Complications	Postoperative	Short Term	Long Term
SUB (Kulendra et al,[12] 2021)	10.5%	185 min	115 min	Urine leakage at kidney and nephrostomy catheter 5.2%, profuse hemorrhage 3.2%, nephrostomy catheter coiled through dorsal surface of kidney 2.1%, pigtail of nephrostomy catheter difficult to coil in the renal pelvis and folded back on itself 2.1%, leakage from pyelogram site 1%, subcapsular leakage of contrast around nephrostomy tube 1%		Catheter kinks - a change in technique to have minimal tubing in the subcutaneous space meant the rate reduced from 13% to 2%	Minor complication rate of 19% and major complication rate of 48% most of which occurred after hospital discharge; post-op UTI in cats surviving to discharge 31%; revision surgery required in 27.3%

SUB, 54% also had a ureterotomy (Butty et al,[20] 2021)	4%	Not noted	125 min (SUB only) 180 (with ureterotomy)	7% (kink of nephrostomy catheter at body wall; connection of pelvis and subcapsular space)	38%: transient worsening of kidney values 15.4%, severe postobstructive diuresis 7.7%, severe hematuria 3.8%, severe anemia 11.5%, coagulopathy and neurologic signs 3.8%, seroma 3.8%	30%: UTI (9.5%), pollakiuria/dysuria without UTI (9.5%), difficulty flushing SUB device (4.3%), subcapsular effusion (4.3%), persistent seroma around subcutaneous port (4.3%)	52%: chronic UTI 19%, pollakiuria/dysuria without evidence of UTI 19%, kink of tubing at abdominal wall 7.7%, nonpatent tubing without kink 7.7%, perirenal effusion 3.8%, subcapsular hematoma 3.8%, displacement of the subcutaneous port 3.8%
SUB (Vrijsen et al,[21] 2020)	20.80%	137.8 min	100 min	16.7% (ischemic encephalopathy, fluid overload, persistent hyperkalemia)	43.5% developed perioperative complications, most commonly device obstruction and UTI	50% (most frequently SUB obstruction, UTI, sterile cystitis and pyelonephritis)	87.5% (most frequently SUB obstruction, UTI, sterile cystitis and pyelonephritis); 79.2% overall complication rate - SUB obstruction 33.3%, lower UTI 20.8%, pyelonephritis 20.8%, sterile cystitis 12.5%; 25% underwent a revision surgery

8%, respectively.[16] The most common complication was uroabdomen in cats both with and without stents, but there was no difference in the reobstruction rate between the 2 groups.[16] It should be said that the authors of this paper had extensive training in ureteral surgery most likely leading to their lower complications rates. An additional study in cats evaluating ureterotomy for calculi removal reported a mortality rate of 21% and postoperative uroabdomen in 6% of cases.[6] A study investigating the surgical management of ureteral calculi in dogs reported a 12.5% mortality rate within 2 weeks of surgery.[10] Due to the lack of follow-up imaging in most of the cases, the incidence of complications such as stricture formation or recurrence of ureterolithiasis is not truly known from this study. However, 25% of dogs ultimately died or were euthanized due to clinical signs related to the urinary tract (azotemia, hematuria, stranguria).[10] Because of these reasons, placement of ureteral stents for both dogs and cats has been investigated as an alternative to traditional surgical techniques.

URETERAL STENTS IN CATS

Ureteral stents are small gauge polyurethane devices spanning the ureter from the renal pelvis of the kidney to the urinary bladder (**Fig. 2**). Ureteral dilation allows urine to flow past an obstruction or stricture around the stent.[9] Because of the presence of this passive dilation, stent obstruction with progressive calculi or sediment does not always lead to the reobstruction of the kidney. Initial cases of stent placement in cats proved problematic as either human pediatric or early veterinary prototype stents were used and were too large in diameter.[9] This led to ureteral damage during placement and lengthy procedures. Although a commercially available double-pigtail feline ureteral stent[a] was developed, challenges with stent placement in cats persist. While mortality rates in some studies seem to be lower than traditional open surgical techniques, complications including, ureteral damage during the placement of the guidewire or dilator make ureteral stenting less attractive in feline patients. If the ureteral obstruction is located more proximally, stent placement can be even more challenging due to the small diameter of the more distal ureter.[9] Endoscopic placement of stents in cats can be attempted; however, most cases require an open surgical approach to assist in the placement of the guidewire, dilator, and stent.[9,17] In a large study of stents placed in cats for benign ureteral obstruction, the need for stent exchange was seen in 19% of patients because of stent occlusion, migration, or stent irritation.[9] Cats with a ureteral stricture were more likely to obstruct poststent placement, as fibrous tissue may not allow for the passive dilation of the ureter.[9] One study in 15 cats, looked at the use of stents placed alone or in conjunction with traditional surgical techniques.[15] This study reported a postoperative mortality rate of 8% and no postoperative leakage of urine from the ureter in any case.[15] Periodic and long-term complications were encountered, including dysuria, urinary tract infection (UTI), sent migration requiring replacement, and stent obstruction requiring removal.[15] The ureterovesical junction (UVJ) location is a proposed mechanism for irritation and a high rate of lower urinary tract signs noted long term in cats, in particular dysuria.[9,16–18] One study comparing cats that had ureteral surgery with and without stents noted that the proportion of cats with lower urinary tract signs during the follow-up period was significantly higher among cats that received stents compared with those that did not (37% vs 2%).[16] The feline UVJs are located in the proximal urethra, in contrast to dogs, whereby they enter the bladder at the trigone.[9] Pigtailed stents exiting the UVJ will curl in the proximal urethral leading to continual irritation and stimulation of the trigone. Because the placement of stents in cats can be technically challenging,

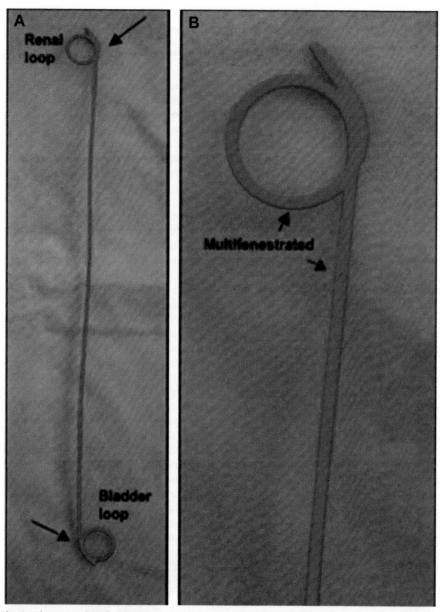

Fig. 2. Photographs of a double pigtail ureteral stent. (*A*) The stent has 2 loops (*arrows*); after placement, 1 loop is contained within the renal pelvis, and the other loop is contained within the urinary bladder. The stent shaft extends through the entire length of the ureteral lumen. (*B*) Multiple fenestration of the ureteral stent allows for urine drainage. (Adapted from Lam, N.K., et al., Endoscopic placement of ureteral stents for the treatment of congenital bilateral ureteral stenosis in a dog. J Am Vet Med Assoc, 2012. 240(8): p. 985; with permission (see Figure 5 in original).)

and morbidity rates were still high, stent placement in cats with ureteral obstruction has largely been replaced with subcutaneous ureteral bypass (SUB) devices.[16–18]

URETERAL STENTS IN DOGS

In contrast to cats, because of their anatomic and size differences, ureteral stents in dogs can be placed minimally invasively in most cases with low postoperative morbidity (**Fig. 3**). Benign ureteral obstruction secondary to ureterolithiasis is the most common cause leading to ureteral obstruction in dogs, as it is in cats.[22] Iatrogenic ureteral trauma (spay ligation), pyonephrosis, and congenital ureteral stenosis are additional causes of benign ureteral obstruction.[23–25] Ureteral stents are also preferred in dogs compared with SUBs because they can be removed or replaced easily and because mineralization of stents occurs less frequently than with the SUB device.[13,25]

In female dogs of almost any size, stent placement for benign ureteral obstruction is performed through a rigid cystoscope and fluoroscopic guidance.[22,25] In male dogs weighing >7 kgs, a flexible cystoscope can be attempted to gain access into the bladder.[22] Because the working channel of the flexible cystoscope is not large enough to accommodate the ureteral catheter, a stiffened guidewire is placed through the working channel to gain access to the ureter and kidney, the cystoscope is then removed off the wire, and the remaining stent placement is performed with fluoroscopic guidance.[22] However, some dogs are too small to accommodate the flexible cystoscope. In those cases, percutaneous perineal access into the ischial urethra followed by serial dilation and rigid cystoscopy is performed.[22,25] If minimally invasive stent placement is unsuccessful, an open surgical procedure can be performed with stent placement accomplished via cystotomy and retrograde catheterization of the ureters or in conjunction with traditional surgical techniques.[22]

In the first study to publish short- and long-term outcomes of stent placement for benign ureteral obstruction in dogs, all stents were able to be placed with the majority placed endoscopically.[22] The mortality rate was low (2%) with the one dog's death being attributed to progressive sepsis which was present before stent placement and therefore considered unrelated the stent. Short- and long-term complications were considered minor; however, the need for stent exchange or an alternative procedure such as the placement of a SUB device was warranted in 16% of dogs because of stent occlusion, stent migration, or recurrent UTI (**Table 2**). In contrast to cats, none of the dogs experienced dysuria following stent placement, most likely due to the more cranial placement of the UVJ.[22] In a study evaluating ureteral stent placement

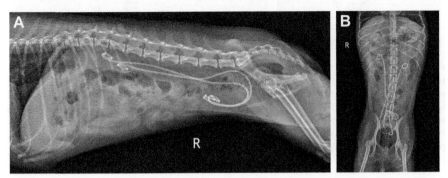

Fig. 3. Lateral (A) and V/D (B) radiographs of a dog after the placement of bilateral ureteral stents.

Table 2
Comparison of traditional surgical techniques versus stent placement for ureteral interventions in dogs

Procedure	Morality Rate	Anesthesia Time (Median)	Procedure Time (Median)	Intra-op Complications	Short Term	Long Term
Traditional Surgical Techniques: Ureterotomy, Ureterotomy with pyelotomy, ureteronephrectomy nephroureterectomy (Synder et al,[10] 2005)	12.5% within 2 wk; 31.3% within 3 mo	Not noted	Not Noted	None	2 (12.5%) required additional surgery 1 and 4 mo post-op for nephrolithiasis and recurrent ureterolithiasis. One dog was subsequently euthanized due to post-op complications. The second dog recovered but developed a stricture at the surgical site 1-mo post-op requiring nephroureterectomy; 3 dogs with pre-op azotemia remained azotemic post-op; worsening azotemia in 2 dogs at 8 and 90 d post-op	2 (12.5%) required additional surgery 1 and 4 mo post-op for nephrolithiasis and recurrent ureterolithiasis. One dog was subsequently euthanized due to post-op complications. The second dog recovered but developed a stricture at the surgical site 1-mo post-op requiring nephroureterectomy; 3 dogs with pre-op azotemia remained azotemic post-op; worsening azotemia in 2 dogs at 8 and 90 d post-op

(continued on next page)

Table 2
(continued)

Procedure	Morality Rate	Anesthesia Time (Median)	Procedure Time (Median)	Intra-op Complications	Short Term	Long Term
Stent placement for pyonephrosis (Kuntz et al,[25] 2015)	7.69%	Not noted	Not noted	Guide wire could not be placed past the obstruction in 1 dog and ureteral wall penetration occured - converted to open surgery with ureterotomy and then stent placed - this dog's azotemia and sepsis progressed and the dog was euthanized; stent occlusion from coating of the guide wire shearing off during placement not recognized until 48 h later and required stent exchange	Of 8 dogs that had blood work within 14 d, 3 remained azotemic	1 dog had encrustation of the stent 5 mo post-op requiring exchange; 5 dogs remained azotemic; recurrent UTI in 7/12 dogs; transient dysuria in 3 dogs; recurrence of urolithiasis in 1 dog 14 mo after stent placement; euthanasia due to the progression of renal disease in 2 dogs
Stents for benign ureteral obstruction (Pavia et al,[22] 2018)	2.3%		Endoscopic placement 60 min; surgical approach 113 min	5% major (3 dogs) - shearing of the outer coating of the guide wire within the stent requiring stent replacement; ureteral perforation with the ureteral catheter requiring conversion to an open surgery for stent placement; ureteral avulsion requiring ureteral R&A over a ureteral stent	Hematuria 20% self-limiting	UTI 26%; stent exchange 12%; replacement with a SUB 5%

in dogs for pyonephrosis, stents were able to be placed in all dogs with the majority placed endoscopically. The perioperative morality rate was 7.8% (1/13) as one dog was euthanized due to worsening azotemia and sepsis after surgery. This dog required conversion to laparotomy and a ureterotomy in addition to stent placement. Two major intraoperative complications were noted, one requiring surgical conversion and the second requiring stent exchange. Stent encrustation causing reobstruction of the ureter occurred in 1 dog 5 months after initial placement and required stent exchange, which was performed endoscopically as an outpatient. No dogs experienced dysuria long term.[25]

Ureteral stents can also be placed for the treatment of malignant ureteral obstruction in dogs.[26] Transitional cell carcinoma (TCC) is most commonly seen due to its frequent location at the trigone and local extension to the ureters.[8,26] When ureteral stents are placed in a minimally invasive manner due to malignancy, they are typically placed in antegrade fashion, due to the lack of visibility of the UVJ during cystoscopy, with the patient in lateral recumbency and the affected kidney up.[26] In a study of 12 dogs with malignant ureteral obstruction, stents were placed percutaneously in all but 1 dog, which was placed surgically. The median survival time from stent placement in this study was 57 days. It is important to note that there was no treatment standardization in the dogs within this study. The authors of this study recommend dogs with TCC have frequent monitoring so that a stent can be placed preemptively via cystoscopy before the obstruction of the UVJ.[26] If diagnosed late in the course of the disease, these tumors can be firm and very difficult to traverse with guidewires endoscopically. A small caudal abdominal approach with an outside-in (Seldinger) needle/catheter approach is commonly used in these cases. Briefly, this technique uses an 18 or 20-gauge long needle/catheter to pierce the ureter near the entrance into the urinary bladder. The needle is passed from the ureter into the urinary bladder and then out of the ventral surface of the urinary bladder. A guidewire is placed into the needle and then the needle is gently removed placing the guidewire into the ureter. A guidewire is then passed cranially under fluoroscopic guidance into the renal pelvis. The stent is placed over the guidewire into the renal pelvis. The distal pigtail is placed within the urinary bladder with a combination of fluoroscopic guidance and gentle manipulation. This technique decreases the contamination of the abdomen with neoplastic cells as a cystotomy incision is not performed. If necessary, a single suture can be placed at the ventral bladder needle/guidewire and ureteral exit site.

As mortality rates and complications associated with the placement of ureteral stents in dogs are similar or less than traditional open techniques, it should be considered as a first choice for the treatment of ureteral obstruction due to the possibility of minimally invasive placement.[8,22,25,26] It is important for clients to know that conversion to an open procedure and the need for traditional surgical techniques may be required in a small percentage of dogs whereby the obstruction cannot be bypassed endoscopically.[22,25] Frequent long-term follow-up is also paramount for the management of stent associated complications. Clients should additionally be aware of the potential need for stent exchange due to stent occlusion, migration, recurrent UTI, or the potential for the stent to be replaced with a SUB device.[22] If needed, stents can be removed or exchanged endoscopically in most patients.[8,25,27] Additional studies in larger populations may be helpful in further understanding the long-term management of stent placement in dogs.

SUBCUTANEOUS URETERAL BYPASS DEVICE

The SUB was designed to alleviate the previous challenges of ureteral obstruction management in cats. A SUB device is a system that bypasses the ureteral obstruction by creating a synthetic ureter in the form of a locking loop pigtail nephrostomy tube connected to a cystostomy tube by a subcutaneous access port (**Fig. 4**).[2] SUB placement usually requires specialty equipment; however, studies have shown that placement can be performed without fluoroscopic guidance and therefore treatment can be considered at facilities with access to ultrasound alone.[11,20,21] One of these studies also demonstrated that ureterotomy performed in conjunction with SUB placement for stone removal increased the procedure duration and did not have the benefit of decreasing complications or improving outcome.[20] While it is tempting to remove solitary stones for a definitive diagnosis, this study illustrated that is it not necessary or recommended.

The evolution of the commercially available SUB device[b] has lessened several initial SUB placement complications, such as leakage of urine associated with nephropexy or cystopexy, kinking of a catheter, and postoperative occlusion when the cystotomy

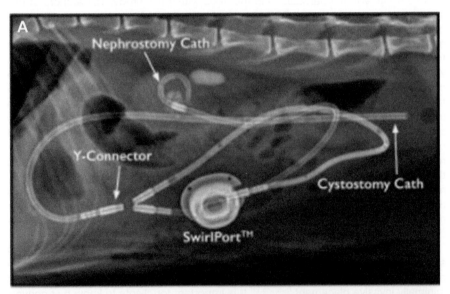

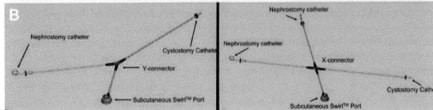

Fig. 4. Subcutaneous ureteral bypass (SUB) device. (A) Lateral radiographic image of a cat after the placement of the SUB 3.0 device showing the updated connecter, swivel port, and straight urinary catheter. (B) The SUB 3.0 device was put together outside of the patient. The Y-connector is for unilateral placement and the X-connector is for bilateral placement. (*Courtesy of* Norfolk Vet Products, Skokie, IL; with permission.)

catheters were made from silicone.[19] The SUB device catheters are currently made of polyurethane. The newest or third version of the commercially available device, SUB 3.0, consists of a locking loop pigtail catheter for placement in the affected kidney, one straight catheter placed within the bladder, and an updated connector securing the catheters to the subcutaneous port. Leaving too much catheter coiled within the urinary bladder causes irritation; therefore, this catheter was returned to a straight conformation to limit the amount within the bladder. A Dacron cuff adheres to the short urinary catheter at the level of the bladder to prevent too much or too little catheter being placed within the urinary bladder. Urine flows from the catheter within the affected kidney to the portion of the Y connector which then goes directly to the urinary bladder. With this version, urine no longer flows through the port. The Y connector helps prevent the kinking of the catheter as only 1 port (the SwivelPort[b]) attachment is outside of the body wall. The port outside the body wall is whereby urine can be sampled or used to flush the system as needed. A nephropexy or cystopexy are not performed using the commercially available SUB device as a Dacron cuff is used to prevent urine leakage by adhering the catheter to the renal capsule or serosal surface of the bladder.[19] Unlike a ureteral stent, urine must flow within these catheters (not around them), therefore, complications leading to the obstruction of the SUB device, such as mineralization or blood clots, may require SUB exchange (**Fig. 5**; **Table 3**).[19] The most common long-term complication, in one study, was blockage as a result of mineralization of the SUB device in 24% of patients.[19] Since this study, the infusion of tetrasodium ethylenediaminetetraacetic acid (tEDTA) has been recommended to restore patency in obstructed mineralized SUB devices. There is also a recommended tEDTA device irrigation protocol to both prevent and treat biofilm-related infections (see **Table 3**).[12,19,28] Alteplase, a synthetic tissue plasminogen activator, has also

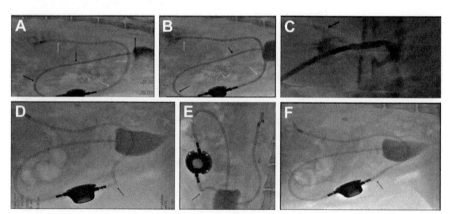

Fig. 5. Fluoroscopic images showing complications that can be seen with the SUB 2.0 device. (*A*) During fluoroscopic flushing, at the end of the procedure, the cystostomy catheter (*black arrows*) is seen to fill with contrast but the nephrostomy tube (*white arrows*) is not filling. This was due to a severe pyonephrosis; with serial flushing the catheter eventually cleared and started flowing. (*B*) If this occurs, recommendations are to drain the entire system completely and then flush again, as it can be that the renal pelvis is too full to allow more flush. (*C*) Leakage (*black arrow*) of contrast seen at the cranial pole of the kidney. This was due to inadvertent guide wire puncture of the renal calix which was of no clinical consequence. (*D* and *E*) A kinked (*red arrow*) SUB device in a cat. (*F*) After fixing the insertion hole of the catheter, the kink resolved. (*Courtesy of* Norfolk Vet Products, Skokie, IL; with permission.)

Table 3
Treatment options for SUB device obstruction

Complication	Treatment Option(s)	Recommended Protocol
Blood clot in kidney or bladder	Infuse TPA into port Device exchange	Protocol not fully established. Infuse 0.5 - 2 mg through the SUB port or intravesicular infusion, for clot within the kidney or bladder, respectively. Infusion can be repeated if needed.
Mineralization of the device	Infuse tEDTA into port Device exchange	Flush with 2% tETDA (T-FloLoc™) before discharge, 1 wk post-op, 1 mo, then every 3 mo thereafter to prevent mineralization. If mineralization is present, flush 1.5 mLs of 2% tETDA twice daily to twice weekly the first week, then weekly to every other week, then monthly, then every 3 mo
Catheter kinks	Device exchange	
Chronic UTI	Antimicrobials	Based on clinical signs, bacterial type, sensitivity. Antibiotics are stopped on week 5 of tEDTA infusions for recurrent UTI.
	Infuse tEDTA into port	Flush with 2% tETDA before discharge, 1 wk post-op, 1 mo, then every 3 mo thereafter to prevent UTI. If recurrent UTI is present, do not add more than 6–10 mLs after emptying the bladder - infused twice daily for 5 d, then once weekly for 5 weeks, then every other week, then monthly, then every 3 mo.
	Device exchange	

been infused into obstructed SUB devices secondary to blood clot formation, reestablishing patency.[19,29] Catheter kinks, either during or after placement, most commonly occur whereby the catheter crosses to the abdominal wall. Movement of the tissues near the port and excessive tubing are causes alone or in conjunction which lead to kinking. Kinking of previously appropriate tubing has been visualized during awake fluoroscopic/radiographic imaging of cats, especially when crouching/sitting in a sternal position. By changing the technique to have minimal tubing in the subcutaneous space with a gentle bending of the tubing, catheter kinks have been reduced from 13% to 2% in one study.[12]

The SUB has become the first choice for the treatment of feline ureteral obstruction that does not respond to medical management regardless of cause.[11] The mortality rate associated with SUB placement (4%–20.8%)[19–21] is typically less than with traditional surgical techniques and stent placement; however, the mortality rate and complications are variable with some remaining high (see **Table 1**).[18,21] Development of positive urine cultures in the postoperative period is common as biofilms may form on urinary implants, which can make clearance of bacteria difficult, as well as increase antibiotic resistance.[21,30] There is currently no standardization for perioperative or postoperative antibiotic use. The use of antibiotics for a median of 5 days significantly decreased the risk of positive urine culture in the postoperative follow-up period in one study.[30] The risks of recurrent UTIs versus unnecessary antibiotic use leading to further antibiotic resistance must be considered and frequent monitoring is recommended.

As newer standardized protocols become available (flushing with tEDTA and a tissue plasminogen activator) in addition to the standardization of technique for SUB placement, one would expect major complications requiring additional surgical intervention to lessen. With the placement of an implant in a population with underlying comorbidities, such as chronic kidney disease, UTI, and predisposition to stone formation, management of long-term complications may be unavoidable. Long-term maintenance of SUBs requires frequent examination and flushing after placement, then every 3 to 6 months for life, in addition to other diagnostic testing and imaging needed. Owners should be made aware of the financial and time commitment involved in the ongoing care associated with SUB placement. Further studies are needed to delineate best practices in case selection, postoperative management, and treatment of complications.

SUB devices are not placed commonly in dogs; therefore, outcomes and complications are not well described. Although ureteral stent placement in dogs is highly successful with good outcomes, one study noted a 16% need for stent exchange or placement of a SUB device due to stent occlusion, stent migration, or recurrent UTIs.[22] One study evaluating SUB device placement in dogs for benign ureteral obstruction, found most of the SUB devices were placed due to stricture or ureteritis associated with a previously placed stent.[13] All SUB devices were successfully placed; however, 50% of the devices became obstructed from mineralization at a median of 205 days, of which 33.3% required device exchange.[13] Because a large number of dogs that previously mineralized their stents went on to mineralize the SUB device, it is possible that their physiology may cause any device to obstruct.[13] Therefore, emphasis should be placed on frequent routine flushes to prevent stent or SUB device occlusion, especially in patients with underlying stone formation.[13] Caution is suggested regarding the placement of a SUB device in dogs with obstructive TCC. A cutaneous mass consistent with TCC was noted at the site of the subcutaneous access port of the SUB device in a dog whereby the percutaneous antegrade placement of ureteral stents was unsuccessful.[31] While SUBs are an option for dogs, this should only be considered after stent placement or if stent exchange is not possible.

INCONTINENCE ASSOCIATED WITH ECTOPIC URETERS

Ectopic ureters (EU) are a congenital condition whereby the ureteral orifice terminates caudal to the normal position in the trigone. EUs are most commonly intramural, whereby the ureter enters the bladder wall in the correct anatomic location but then tunnels below the submucosa and opens at a more distal location in the urethra, prostate, or vestibule.[4,5,8,32] The diagnostic approach for definitive diagnoses of EUs can be challenging as there is not one imaging modality alone which can assess both the upper and lower urinary tract for all anatomic and functional abnormalities. A noninvasive imaging modality, such as ultrasound, is often performed initially to evaluate the urinary tract. Identification of ureteral jets is difficult in most dogs during standard ultrasound.[33] Administration of either intravenous or subcutaneous furosemide significantly improves the ability to detect ureteral jets with ultrasound in normal dogs.[33] However, the effectiveness of furosemide to identify ureteral jets in dogs with ureteral pathology or renal insufficiency is not known.[33] Historically, excretory urography and ultrasonography combined, correctly identified 91% of EUs, although, disagreement between traditional imaging and surgical findings has led to the increased use of CT.[34] Computed tomography excretory urography (CTEU) is the imaging modality of choice for the detection of EUs, as it has a sensitivity reported between 91% and 100%.[34,35] CTEU avoids superimposition, allows the generation of 3D reconstructions, and provides additional information on renal anatomy compared with other imaging modalities; however, vestibular/vaginal abnormalities are usually not identified.[34,35] Cystoscopy is superior to CT in identifying vestibular/vaginal abnormalities, which are present in up 93% of female dogs with EUs.[34] A highly experienced operator can identify EUs via cystoscopy with 100% sensitivity and treat them in addition to other lower urinary tract anatomic abnormalities during the same anesthetic event in most cases.[34] One disadvantage of cystoscopy is the inability to assess the upper urinary tract for concurrent diseases such as unilateral renal agenesis, hydronephrosis, hydroureter, and pyelonephritis.[36] The difference between intra versus extramural EUs is important as it changes the surgical treatment dramatically. Intraoperative fluoroscopy can be used during cystoscopy to visualize guidewires within the ureter to add information regarding the conformation of the EU (intramural vs extramural). In doing so, the operator hopefully avoids the transection of an extramural ureter causing inadvertent entrance into the abdomen (uroabdomen) during cystoscopic treatment. Therefore, another imaging modality, ideally CTEU, is recommended before or in conjunction with cystoscopy.[34]

Persistent or recurrent incontinence after traditional surgical techniques without adjunctive treatment has been reported in up to 78% of dogs.[34,37,38] Although this may be attributed to several factors, such as UTI or recanalization of the ligated ureter, it has largely been attributed to USMI due to the improvement of continence with additional medication.[34,37] Disappointing rates of full continence with many traditional surgical techniques, in addition to the intramural nature of most EUs makes cystoscopic-guided laser ablation (CLA) an excellent option.[5,39,40]

CLA involves the resection/ablation of the medial aspect of the intraurethral ureteral wall, under cystoscopic guidance (**Fig. 6**). This is most commonly performed using endoscopic lasers (diode or holmium yttrium aluminum garnet) until the neoureteral orifice is within the bladder lumen at a similar location to a normal contralateral UVJ or when the ureter transitions from intramural to extramural.[38] The most important advantages of CLA are the minimally invasive nature and the excellent visualization (and magnification) that occurs during cystoscopy. This technique can be used for the diagnosis and treatment of EU and other lower urinary tract anomalies (hymenal remnant, paramesonephric septal remnant, vestibulovaginal stenosis) simultaneously, avoiding the need for multiple anesthetic episodes.[5,41] One study showed that CLA is safe and at least as effective as traditional surgical techniques previously reported in female dogs, with a continence rate of 47% at 6 weeks, which increased to 77% with the addition of medical management, collagen injections, or placement of a hydraulic occluder (HO).[40] Another study showed similar results with complete resolution of incontinence in 25% with CLA alone and an additional 31% achieving continence with the addition of medication.[36] A more recent study in female dogs with a minimum follow-up of 12 months, showed a good long-term outcome (postprocedure continence score of >9/10) in 72% of dogs with CLA alone, and 81% with the inclusion of additional medical or surgical management.[38] In contrast to female dogs, a study using CLA in 4 male dogs showed 100% postoperative continence rate.[42]

While most reported complications of CLA are considered minor (dysuria, hematuria, UTI), major complications have been reported in up to 6% of patients in one study.[38] Major complications included urethral tearing, uroabdomen, and encrusting cystitis with suspected ureteral obstruction, some of which required repeat procedures and/or led to death/euthanasia.[38,43] CLA offers a beneficial alternative to

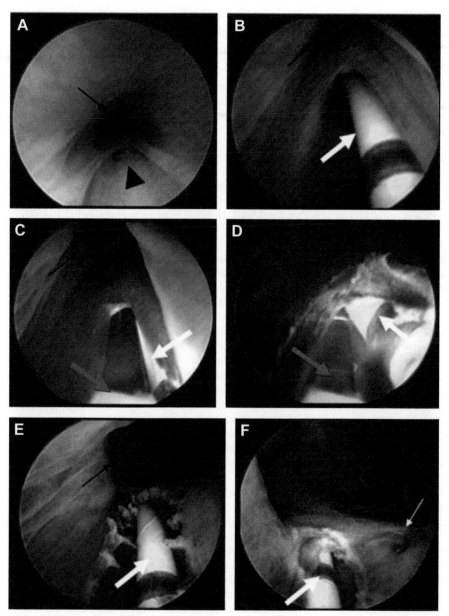

Fig. 6. Endoscopic images of the lower urinary tract in a female dog with a right-sided intra-mural ectopic ureter. The patient is in dorsal recumbency while undergoing CLA-EU. (*A*) The ectopic ureteral opening (*black arrowhead*) and urethral opening (*black arrow*) are evident. (*B*) An open-ended ureteral catheter (*white arrow*) is placed within the ureteral lumen; notice this placement in relation to the urethral opening (*black arrow*). (*C*) The diode laser fiber (*red arrow*) is positioned at the ectopic ureteral orifice. Notice the ureteral catheter (*white arrow*) and urethral opening (*black arrow*). (*D*) The ectopic tunnel is cut with the laser (*red arrow*), and the ureteral catheter (*white arrow*) is protecting the lateral ureteral wall. (*E*) Notice the ureteral catheter (*white arrow*) after the ureteral segment of the ectopic ureter is cut. The urethrovesicular junction (*black arrow*) is evident. (*F*) The neoureteral

traditional invasive surgical techniques, due to its minimally invasive nature, short hospitalization times, and acceptable complication rate.[36–38,40]

REFRACTORY URINARY INCONTINENCE

For animals that have refractory urinary incontinence after appropriate treatment of all anatomic abnormalities (EU, paramesonephric septal remnant, and so forth) and failure of medical and/or surgical management, additional treatments, such as cystoscopic transurethral bulking agents and HO can be considered.

TRANSURETHRAL BULKING AGENTS

Endoscopic injection of a biocompatible material into the submucosa of the proximal urethra is a minimally invasive alternative to surgery or an additional option if incontinence is refractory to previous treatment. Urethral closure is improved at the site of the injections as the deposits bulge into the urethral lumen (Videos 1 and 2).[44] Although not completely understood, the main effects of injecting certain bulking agents (polytef, bovine glutaraldehyde cross-linked collagen (GAX), dextranomer/hyaluronic acid copolymer (DEX), porcine gelatin), within the urethral submucosa are an increase in the central urethral volume, which both narrows the urethral lumen for more effective urethral closure and stretches the urethral muscle fibers increasing their force of contraction.[4,45] Polytef is no longer recommended due to the rejection of the material and recurrence of incontinence and GAX agents are not readily available due to hypersensitivity reactions described in people.[44,46,47] DEX and gelatin as bulking agents are biocompatible and create scaffolds for the stimulation of connective tissue cells at the injection site, which may lead to less loss of the deposits over time.[46,47] In a large study evaluating the injection of bovine collagen in female dogs with USMI, incontinence initially resolved in 68% with injection alone and an additional 15% were continent with the addition of medication (phenylpropanolamine, ephedrine hydrochloride, or both).[44] During the first 12 months there was a progressive deterioration in one-third of the dogs that were initially considered continent.[44] Another study showed variable duration of efficacy, with a median of 8 months of full continence in dogs treated for USMI compared with a median of 3.5 months of improved continence in dogs treated for EUs with collagen injection alone.[45] A more recent study evaluating the use of gelatin as a bulking agent achieved continence in 87% of dogs after the first injection for an average of 11.1 months.[47] One study comparing 2 different bulking agents found a mean duration of continence of 45.8 months in the GAX group versus 20.5 months for dogs in the DEX group.[46] Deterioration of results may occur due to the loss of volume of the bulking agents over time.[44,46] Although there is no reported standardization, the procedure can be repeated. In one study 5/15 (33.3%) dogs received a second injection between 3 and 13 months due to the recurrence of incontinence or failure to achieve continence after the first injection.[47] Because the duration of continence with urethral bulking agents is highly variable, the use of HO has been investigated.

───────────◄───────────────────────────────────

orifice with a ureteral catheter (*white arrow*) inside the lumen as it enters the urinary bladder. Notice the location of the right neoureteral orifice is even with the normal contralateral left ureteral orifice (*yellow arrow*). (From Berent A, et al. Evaluation of cystoscopic-guided laser ablation of intramural ectopic ureters in female dogs. J Am Vet Med Assoc 2012;240:716–725 with permission.)

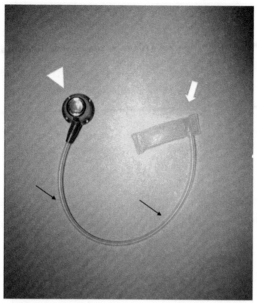

Fig. 7. Image of a hydraulic occluder device. The inflatable HO incomplete silicone cuff (white arrow) is placed around the proximal urethra and forms a ring once closed using suture through the eyelets at the ends of the cuff. The actuating tubing (black arrows) attaches the cuff to the subcutaneous metallic infusion port (white arrowhead) that can be injected with the use of a noncoring Huber needle.

HYDRAULIC OCCLUDERS

A static hydraulic urethral sphincter, also called an artificial urethral sphincter or HO, is an incomplete silicone ring that is surgically placed around the proximal urethra and attached to a subcutaneous port (**Fig. 7**). Once a section of the proximal urethra is dissected (2–3 cm caudal to the bladder neck in females and 2 cm caudal to the prostate in males) the outer urethral circumference is estimated by measuring a piece of suture material or Penrose drain passed loosely around the intended cuff placement site.[48,49] Per Currao and colleagues the HO size is calculated by dividing the outer urethral diameter (in millimeters) by 50% because the luminal diameter of the device, when it is a circle, is half of the outer urethral circumference.[50] Different devices may have alternative measuring protocols as Rose and colleagues, describes the measurement of the HO device to be equal to the outside urethral circumference at the pelvic urethra.[51] HO devices (AUS[TM])[c] are sized by the luminal diameter of 4, 6, 8, 10, 12, 14, and 16 mm and cuff widths of 11 and 14 mm for cats and dogs, respectively. The goal is not to have detectable compression of the urethra at the time of placement. The device can allow ongoing adjustment of the urethral diameter in a minimally invasive fashion by either inflation or deflation of the cuff via the subcutaneous port.[50,52]

The first pilot study evaluating a custom-designed percutaneously adjustable HO for the treatment of refractory USMI improved urinary incontinence for greater than 2 years in all 4 female dogs.[51] Three of these dogs were continent without any occluder injection for 18 months.[51] Although dogs did develop temporary incontinence with UTI, this resolved with appropriate antibiotic therapy.[51] In a larger study, placement of an HO in both male (3) and female (24) dogs was effective in the

Table 4
Hydraulic occluder outcomes and complications

Author	Species Sex	Procedure(s)	Incontinence Scores Pre-op (Median) out of 10	Incontinence Scores Post-Op (Median and Mean)	Median Follow-up Time - Months	% Not Requiring Inflation of the HO	% UTI Prior to sx	%UTI Post-Op	Post-op Obstruction	Other Complications
Currao et al,[50] 2013	Canine 18 Female	HO placement; Cystour-ethroscopy 56%; Cystopexy 44%;	2.8	At 6 wk 9.8 and 8.0; At last follow-up 10 and 8.9	32	33	78%	61% at some point	17% required removal and/or stent placement	
Reeves et al,[48] 2013	Canine 24 Female 3 Male	HO placement; 2 Cystoscopy 14.8%; Episioplasty 11.1%; Neoureterostomy 3.7%; Cystotomy 3.7%; OHE 7.4%	2	Median 9	12.5	45	15% (3/20) Diagnosed at time of surgery	None diagnosed	7.4% - required removal in 1 and euthanasia in 1	Minor - temporary worsening of incontinence 18.5%; mild stranguria 7.4%; seroma over port 11.1% - all resolved within 1 mo of surgery
Rose et al,[51] 2009	Canine 4 Female	HO placement 3		Median 9.5	26-30	75% for 18 mo; 2 required inflation at 24 mo	75%	50% at some point		Initial post op dysuria resolved in 2 weeks without treatment and required

Gomes et al,[52] 2018	Canine	20	Female	HO placement	3	At 6 and 12 mo, 8.5 and 9.0, respectively	39.6	35%	0% at the time of surgery	40% at some point	5% - 1 dog had an obstruction but resolved with deflation of the cuff	5% - 1 dog required removal of the device 28 mo post op due to persistent stranguria; Minor complications in 65% - stranguria, hematuria, prolonged duration of micturition, pain during urination or at the port site	removal of primer fluid in 1 dog. 1 dog had the port removed due to suspected infection.
Wilson et al,[53] 2016	Feline	3	Female	HO and cystoscopy	Cat 1–4; Cat 2–7; Cat 3–4	Cat 1–10; Cat 2–10; Cat 3 - initially 10/7.5 after HO removal	Cat 1 34 mo; Cat 2 73 mo	33.3%	0%	Cat 1 positive; Cat 3 positive 16 mo following	Urethral mucosal tear in cat 2 during cystoscopy requiring urinary		

(continued on next page)

Table 4
(continued)

Author	Species	Sex	Procedure(s)	Incontinence Scores Pre-op (Median) out of 10	Incontinence Scores Post-Op (Median and Mean)	Median Follow-up Time - Months	% Not Requiring Inflation of the HO	% UTI Prior to sx	% UTI Post-Op	Post-op Obstruction	Other Complications
									removal of the HO		catheter indwelling for 3 d; post-op hematuria in cat 2 resolved after 3 d; Cat 3 recurrent constipation and the HO was removed 14 wk after placement but constipation persisted and incontinence returned
Fournet et al,[54] 2021	Feline	1 Female	HO placement	3	9	18 mo	0	Recurrent but no infection at the time of surgery	Recurrent		Hematuria related to UTIs post op which resolved with antibiotic therapy

treatment of most congenital or acquired forms of urinary incontinence. Incontinence scores improved in all dogs with only 55% requiring HO inflation after surgery.[48] Progressive urethral obstruction developed in 2 dogs at 5 and 9 months after HO placement for which 1 dog was euthanized and one dog had the device surgically removed and remained continent.[48] In another study evaluating the placement of a percutaneously controlled urethral HO device for the treatment of refractory urinary incontinence in 18 female dogs with various urogenital anomalies, all dogs had improved continence scores and 33% did not require inflation of the occluder to achieve functional continence.[50] Three dogs (17%) developed urethral obstruction at 1.5, 2, and 23 months after device placement, which was treated with either occluder removal and/or stent placement. Cystourethroscopy was performed in 56% of dogs at the time of occluder placement and due to concern for urethral trauma which could lead to stricture, this was not continued in subsequent cases.[50] These studies show a high rate of continence is achieved, with most complications being minor in nature.[48,50–52] Clients must be aware of the possibility of urethral obstruction, even long term, as this could warrant the deflation of the cuff or removal of the device (**Table 4**).

Causes and outcome of urinary incontinence in cats are largely different than in dogs, with spinal cord disorders being the most common cause in cats.[55] Additional disparities between cats and dogs exist, including equal frequency of urinary incontinence in male and female cats, as well as, similar frequency of storage phase and voiding phase disorders.[55] Cats with spinal cord disorders also had a more favorable outcome compared with the bladder and urethral disorders.[55] In contrast to dogs, the feline urethra has more longitudinal smooth muscle and a narrower lumen, which may be why urethral disorders, are less common in cats. This may also explain why cats are less responsive to the effects of phenylpropanolamine. One cat developed urinary incontinence after the placement of a ureteral stent and SUB device to treat bilateral ureteral obstruction.[55]

Although incontinence in cats is uncommon, the use of a HO has been documented in 4 female cats, with the improvement of incontinence scores in all cats.[53,54] One cat did not require inflation of the HO to obtain complete continence.[53] Complications did not include urethral obstruction; however, one cat developed constipation after the placement of the HO which did not resolve with removal of the device 14 weeks after initial placement.[53] One cat experienced a urethral mucosal tear during cystoscopy, warranting an indwelling catheter for 3 days (see **Table 4**).[53] Continued studies to determine the success rates, complications, and outcome in a larger population of cats are needed.

Because an improvement of urinary incontinence after occluder placement without inflation is seen in a percentage of animals, placement of the occluder alone may help by creating a static increase in urethral resistance due to the semirigid implant.[51] Advantages of HOs are that they can be placed in both male and female dogs and in cats without advanced training or specialty equipment, they can be adjusted percutaneously by adding or removing saline to each patient's need, and they can be used to treat the causes of incontinence other than USMI, such as persistent or recurrence of incontinence after the treatment of EUs or transurethral bulking agents.[48,51–54] The ability to manage a case minimally invasively long term is an attractive advantage of the HO.

SUMMARY

Treatment of ureteral obstruction and urinary incontinence poses significant challenges in both dogs and cats. Minimally invasive techniques have increased the options available and have become more popular than traditional surgical techniques due to decreased major complications. Although these options have become more commonplace and specialty equipment is not always required, appropriate training and owner education about long-term costs and management are paramount. Additional studies are warranted to support a further increase in the success and reduction of complications with continued experience and standardization of minimally invasive techniques.

CLINICS CARE POINTS

- Although most ureteral stents in dogs can be placed minimally invasively, some patients will require an open procedure for placement. After placement, monitoring for stent occlusion, migration, or recurrent UTI is warranted as stent exchange may be warranted in these cases.
- After the placement of SUB devices in cats for ureteral obstruction, they require lifelong monitoring and care as most patients have underlying chronic kidney disease, UTI, and predisposition to stone formation which can lead to complications of recurrent/resistant UTI or obstruction of the SUB device.
- The diagnosis and treatment of EU can be difficult. CLA has advantages over traditional surgery; however, it is limited to treating intramural EUs and must be used in conjunction with another imaging modality to confirm intramural EUs and assess the upper urinary tract.
- Transurethral bulking agents may be used with refractory incontinence; however, they tend to lose their effectiveness over a variable amount of time. Repeat treatments can be considered depending on response to the initial treatment.
- HO placement can also be considered for refractory incontinence in both cats and dogs. Many patients do not require the inflation of the cuff. Urethral obstruction is a potential complication at any time point after placement.

SUPPLEMENTARY DATA

Supplementary data related to this article can be found online at https://doi.org/10.1016/j.cvsm.2021.12.003.

REFERENCES

1. Berent AC. Ureteral obstructions in dogs and cats: a review of traditional and new interventional diagnostic and therapeutic options. J Vet Emerg Crit Care (San Antonio) 2011;21(2):86–103.
2. Horowitz C, Berent AC, Weisse CW, et al. Predictors of outcome for cats with ureteral obstructions after interventional management using ureteral stents or a subcutaneous ureteral bypass device. J Feline Med Surg 2013;15(12):1052–62.
3. Berent A. New techniques on the horizon: interventional radiology and interventional endoscopy of the urinary tract ('endourology'). J Feline Med Surg 2014;16(1):51–65.
4. Acierno MJ, Labato MA. Canine incontinence. Vet Clin North Am Small Anim Pract 2019;49(2):125–40.
5. Berent AC. Interventional urology: endourology in small animal veterinary medicine. Vet Clin North Am Small Anim Pract 2015;45(4):825–55.
6. Roberts SF, Aronson LR, Brown DC. Postoperative mortality in cats after ureterolithotomy. Vet Surg 2011;40(4):438–43.

7. Kyles AE, Hardie EM, Wooden BG, et al. Management and outcome of cats with ureteral calculi: 153 cases (1984-2002). J Am Vet Med Assoc 2005;226(6): 937–44.

8. Gallagher A. Interventional radiology and interventional endoscopy in treatment of nephroureteral disease in the dog and cat. Vet Clin North Am Small Anim Pract 2018;48(5):843–62.

9. Berent AC, Weisse CW, Todd K, et al. Technical and clinical outcomes of ureteral stenting in cats with benign ureteral obstruction: 69 cases (2006-2010). J Am Vet Med Assoc 2014;244(5):559–76.

10. Snyder DM, Steffey MA, Mehler SJ, et al. Diagnosis and surgical management of ureteral calculi in dogs: 16 cases (1990-2003). N Z Vet J 2005;53(1):19–25.

11. Livet V, Pillard P, Goy-Thollot I, et al. Placement of subcutaneous ureteral bypasses without fluoroscopic guidance in cats with ureteral obstruction: 19 cases (2014-2016). J Feline Med Surg 2017;19(10):1030–9.

12. Kulendra NJ, Borgeat K, Syme H, et al. Survival and complications in cats treated with subcutaneous ureteral bypass. J Small Anim Pract 2021;62(1):4–11.

13. Milligan ML, Berent AC, Weisse CW, et al. Outcome of SUB placement for the treatment of benign ureteral obstruction in dogs: nine dogs and 12 renal units (2013 to 2017). J Small Anim Pract 2020;61(7):428–35.

14. Aronson LR, Kyles AE, Preston A, et al. Renal transplantation in cats with calcium oxalate urolithiasis: 19 cases (1997-2004). J Am Vet Med Assoc 2006;228(5): 743–9.

15. Manassero M, Decambron A, Viateau V, et al. Indwelling double pigtail ureteral stent combined or not with surgery for feline ureterolithiasis: complications and outcome in 15 cases. J Feline Med Surg 2014;16(8):623–30.

16. Wormser C, Clarke DL, Aronson LR. Outcomes of ureteral surgery and ureteral stenting in cats: 117 cases (2006-2014). J Am Vet Med Assoc 2016;248(5): 518–25.

17. Kulendra NJ, Syme H, Benigni L, et al. Feline double pigtail ureteric stents for management of ureteric obstruction: short- and long-term follow-up of 26 cats. J Feline Med Surg 2014;16(12):985–91.

18. Deroy C, Rossetti D, Ragetly G, et al. Comparison between double-pigtail ureteral stents and ureteral bypass devices for treatment of ureterolithiasis in cats. J Am Vet Med Assoc 2017;251(4):429–37.

19. Berent AC, Weisse CW, Bagley DH, et al. Use of a subcutaneous ureteral bypass device for treatment of benign ureteral obstruction in cats: 174 ureters in 134 cats (2009-2015). J Am Vet Med Assoc 2018;253(10):1309–27.

20. Butty EM, Labato MA. Subcutaneous ureteral bypass device placement with intraoperative ultrasound guidance, with or without microsurgical ureterotomy, in 24 cats. J Feline Med Surg 2021;23(12):1183–91.

21. Vrijsen E, Devriendt N, Mortier F, et al. Complications and survival after subcutaneous ureteral bypass device placement in 24 cats: a retrospective study (2016-2019). J Feline Med Surg 2021;23(8):759–69.

22. Pavia PR, Berent AC, Weisse CW, et al. Outcome of ureteral stent placement for treatment of benign ureteral obstruction in dogs: 44 cases (2010-2013). J Am Vet Med Assoc 2018;252(6):721–31.

23. Wormser C, Clarke DL, Aronson LR. End-to-end ureteral anastomosis and double-pigtail ureteral stent placement for treatment of iatrogenic ureteral trauma in two dogs. J Am Vet Med Assoc 2015;247(1):92–7.

24. Lam NK, Berent AC, Weisse CW, et al. Endoscopic placement of ureteral stents for treatment of congenital bilateral ureteral stenosis in a dog. J Am Vet Med Assoc 2012;240(8):983–90.

25. Kuntz JA, Berent AC, Weisse CW, et al. Double pigtail ureteral stenting and renal pelvic lavage for renal-sparing treatment of obstructive pyonephrosis in dogs: 13 cases (2008-2012). J Am Vet Med Assoc 2015;246(2):216–25.

26. Berent AC, Weisse CW, Beal MW, et al. Use of indwelling, double-pigtail stents for treatment of malignant ureteral obstruction in dogs: 12 cases (2006-2009). J Am Vet Med Assoc 2011;238(8):1017–25.

27. Gibson EA, Culp WTN, Palm CA, et al. Removal and repositioning of urinary tract implants by use of an endovascular snare system in dogs and cats (2013-2019). J Am Vet Med Assoc 2021;258(9):983–90.

28. Chik C, Berent AC, Weisse CW, et al. Therapeutic use of tetrasodium ethylenediaminetetraacetic acid solution for treatment of subcutaneous ureteral bypass device mineralization in cats. J Vet Intern Med 2019;33(5):2124–32.

29. Dropkin CA, Burdick SK, Berent AC, et al. Use of tissue plasminogen activator to alleviate postoperative subcutaneous ureteral bypass obstruction secondary to blood clot in seven cats. J Feline Med Surg 2021;23(10):996–1004.

30. Kopecny L, Palm CA, Drobatz KJ, et al. Risk factors for positive urine cultures in cats with subcutaneous ureteral bypass and ureteral stents (2010-2016). J Vet Intern Med 2019;33(1):178–83.

31. Merickel JL, Lawrence J, Young SJ, et al. Cutaneous seeding of transitional cell carcinoma of the urinary bladder after placement of a subcutaneous ureteral bypass device in a dog with bilateral ureteral obstruction. J Am Vet Med Assoc 2021;258(8):877–82.

32. Reichler IM, Specker CE, Hubler M, et al. Ectopic ureters in dogs: clinical features, surgical techniques and outcome. Vet Surg 2012;41(4):515–22.

33. Gremillion C, Cohen EB, Vaden S, et al. Optimization of ultrasonographic ureteral jet detection and normal ureteral jet morphology in dogs. Vet Radiol Ultrasound 2021;62(5):583–90.

34. Owen LJ. Ureteral ectopia and urethral sphincter mechanism incompetence: an update on diagnosis and management options. J Small Anim Pract 2019;60(1):3–17.

35. Fox AJ, Sharma A, Secrest SA. Computed tomographic excretory urography features of intramural ectopic ureters in 10 dogs. J Small Anim Pract 2016;57(4):210–3.

36. Smith AL, Radlinsky MG, Rawlings CA. Cystoscopic diagnosis and treatment of ectopic ureters in female dogs: 16 cases (2005-2008). J Am Vet Med Assoc 2010;237(2):191–5.

37. Noël SM, Claeys S, Hamaide AJ. Surgical management of ectopic ureters in dogs: Clinical outcome and prognostic factors for long-term continence. Vet Surg 2017;46(5):631–41.

38. Hoey C, Friend E, Meakin LB, et al. Long-term outcome of female dogs treated for intramural ectopic ureters with cystoscopic-guided laser ablation. Vet Surg 2021;50(7):1449–62.

39. Ho LK, Troy GC, Waldron DR. Clinical outcomes of surgically managed ectopic ureters in 33 dogs. J Am Anim Hosp Assoc 2011;47(3):196–202.

40. Berent AC, Weisse CW, Mayhew PD, et al. Evaluation of cystoscopic-guided laser ablation of intramural ectopic ureters in female dogs. J Am Vet Med Assoc 2012;240(6):716–25.

41. Cannizzo KL, McLoughlin MA, Mattoon JS, et al. Evaluation of transurethral cystoscopy and excretory urography for diagnosis of ectopic ureters in female dogs: 25 cases (1992-2000). J Am Vet Med Assoc 2003;223(4):475–81.

42. Berent AC, Mayhew PD, Porat-Mosenco Y. Use of cystoscopic-guided laser ablation for treatment of intramural ureteral ectopia in male dogs: four cases (2006-2007). J Am Vet Med Assoc 2008;232(7):1026–34.

43. Duffy M, Gallagher A. Encrusted cystitis with suspected ureteral obstruction following cystoscopic-guided laser ablation of ectopic ureters in a dog. J Am Anim Hosp Assoc 2018;54(2):117–23.

44. Barth A, Reichler IM, Hubler M, et al. Evaluation of long-term effects of endoscopic injection of collagen into the urethral submucosa for treatment of urethral sphincter incompetence in female dogs: 40 cases (1993-2000). J Am Vet Med Assoc 2005;226(1):73–6.

45. Byron JK, Chew DJ, McLoughlin ML. Retrospective evaluation of urethral bovine cross-linked collagen implantation for treatment of urinary incontinence in female dogs. J Vet Intern Med 2011;25(5):980–4.

46. Lüttmann K, Merle R, Nickel R. Retrospective analysis after endoscopic urethral injections of glutaraldehyde-cross-linked-collagen or dextranomer/hyaluronic acid copolymer in bitches with urinary incontinence. J Small Anim Pract 2019;60(2):96–101.

47. Chen H, Shipov A, Segev G. Evaluation of cross-linked gelatin as a bulking agent for the management of urinary sphincter mechanism incompetence in female dogs. J Vet Intern Med 2020;34(5):1914–9.

48. Reeves L, Adin C, McLoughlin M, et al. Outcome after placement of an artificial urethral sphincter in 27 dogs. Vet Surg 2013;42(1):12–8.

49. Adin CA, Farese JP, Cross AR, et al. Urodynamic effects of a percutaneously controlled static hydraulic urethral sphincter in canine cadavers. Am J Vet Res 2004;65(3):283–8.

50. Currao RL, Berent AC, Weisse CW, et al. Use of a percutaneously controlled urethral hydraulic occluder for treatment of refractory urinary incontinence in 18 female dogs. Vet Surg 2013;42(4):440–7.

51. Rose SA, Adin CA, Ellison GW, et al. Long-term efficacy of a percutaneously adjustable hydraulic urethral sphincter for treatment of urinary incontinence in four dogs. Vet Surg 2009;38(6):747–53.

52. Gomes C, Doran I, Friend E, et al. Long-term outcome of female dogs treated with static hydraulic urethral sphincter for urethral sphincter mechanism incompetence. J Am Anim Hosp Assoc 2018;54(5):276–84.

53. Wilson KE, Berent AC, Weisse CW. Use of a percutaneously controlled hydraulic occluder for treatment of refractory urinary incontinence in three female cats. J Am Vet Med Assoc 2016;248(5):544–51.

54. Fournet A, Maurey C, Decambron A, et al. Treatment of urinary incontinence in a cat with genitourinary dysplasia using an urethral sphincter occluder. J Small Anim Pract 2021;62(5):391–6.

55. Lonc KM, Kaneene JB, Carneiro PAM, et al. Retrospective analysis of diagnoses and outcomes of 45 cats with micturition disorders presenting as urinary incontinence. J Vet Intern Med 2020;34(1):216–26.

Concepts in Sterilization

Sarah J. Marvel, DVM, MS

KEYWORDS

- Castration • Ovariectomy • Ovariohysterectomy • Hysterectomy • Vasectomy
- Gonadectomy

KEY POINTS

- Ovariectomy has the potential for fewer complications when compared with ovariohysterectomy and is an acceptable method of sterilization given the low incidence of uterine pathology once sex hormones have been removed.
- Early gonadectomy may affect the risk of certain cancers and joint diseases in some breeds of dogs.
- Gonad sparing sterilization surgeries maintain sex hormones while rendering animals infertile and include hysterectomy and salpingectomy in females and vasectomy in males.
- Determining recommendations for the timing of sterilization in dogs is complex and a balanced approach is necessary. Consideration should be given to the breed or size of mixed-breed dogs, known risk of neoplasia and joint disease, behavioral concerns, longevity, and risk of unwanted mating/pregnancy.

INTRODUCTION

There are many controversies surrounding surgical sterilization in small animals, including the type of procedure that is performed and the timing of that procedure. To prevent overpopulation, early spay and neuter has been advocated in cats and dogs, particularly in the United States where approximately 86% of owned dogs are spayed or neutered.[1] Traditional sterilization techniques involve the removal of gonads, which in turn eliminates sex hormones. In the United States, sterilization of female companion animals was routinely performed by ovariohysterectomy (OHE) through an open mini-laparotomy. Recommendations on the timing of OHE in female dogs from nonshelter/rescue settings were historically based on a study by Schneider and colleagues. This study found that OHE before the first estrus cycle yielded a relative risk of 0.5% for developing mammary tumors, whereas those dogs undergoing OHE after their first heat cycle had a relative risk of 8% for developing mammary tumors and those with OHE after their second heat cycle had a relative risk of 26% of developing mammary tumors.[2] There was no protective effect of OHE for developing mammary tumors after the second heat cycle. Therefore, many dogs had an OHE before their first heat cycle to minimize the risk of mammary tumors. In male dogs,

Department of Clinical Sciences, Colorado State University, 300 West Drake Road, Fort Collins, CO 80523, USA
E-mail address: Sarah.Marvel@colostate.edu

Vet Clin Small Anim 52 (2022) 419–436
https://doi.org/10.1016/j.cvsm.2021.11.003
0195-5616/22/© 2021 Elsevier Inc. All rights reserved.

castration or orchidectomy has been the traditional method of sterilization, and timing was often based on achieving avoidance of unwanted behaviors linked to breeding, urination, and aggression.

Over time, 2 major developments occurred, which have altered recommendations on the procedure type and timing of sterilization, particularly in female dogs. The first was the increasing popularity of minimally invasive surgery. As laparoscopic sterilization became increasingly popular, so did a shift toward ovariectomy (OVE) as this is considered less technically challenging than a laparoscopic OHE.[3] Ovariectomy has been the preferred procedure for sterilization in many European countries for decades.[4] The second major development that occurred was additional research on the effects of timing of gonadectomy in relation to various orthopedic, oncologic, and other miscellaneous conditions. These studies have generated discussion regarding our historical recommendations on both timing and technique of sterilization.[4–32] In addition to delaying neutering in the nonshelter population, sterilization techniques that spare the gonads have recently been reported, including vasectomy and hysterectomy. Limited information is available on the long-term consequences of these procedures.

OVE VERSUS OHE

Both OVE and OHE are considered acceptable methods of sterilization in female cats and dogs. Although the American Veterinary Medical Association and the American College of Theriogenologists promote elective neuter for animals that are not intended for breeding, neither association recommends a specific procedure.[33,34] Recent literature review studies suggest OVE (**Fig. 1**) may be superior[4,35]; however, direct comparison of these 2 techniques has not yielded a significant benefit of one technique over another.[36] Proposed benefits of OVE include shorter surgical times; less potential for hemorrhage, urinary complications, and ovarian remnants; smaller incisions and therefore possibly reduced postoperative pain.[4,35] Many of these proposed benefits result from a more cranial abdominal incision centered over the ovaries rather than equidistant between the ovaries and the uterine body as is the case for OVH. This theoretically allows for improved visualization of the ovaries and surrounding anatomy. Improved visualization may decrease the risk of ovarian remnant syndrome (**Fig. 2**). With OVE, there are fewer structures encountered that can lead to potential hemorrhage (ovarian vasculature vs ovarian vasculature, broad ligament, and uterine vasculature). OVE also theoretically decreases the risk of urinary complications as inadvertent ureteral ligation should only occur near the kidney. Without removal of the uterus, caudal ureteral ligation should not occur. Another theoretic benefit is reduced pain, as fewer parts of the reproductive tract are manipulated and dissected with an OVE. During OHE, significant traction is applied to the ovaries and uterus to mobilize them toward the incision. During OVE, it is not necessary to tear or ligate the broad ligament. Not only is this a potential reduced source of hemorrhage, but also a potential reduced source of pain.

One of the main arguments for removal of the uterus is to avoid long-term complications from uterine disease. However, dogs that undergo OVE are not at an increased risk of cystic endometrial hyperplasia or pyometra as long as the hormone source has been removed and there is no exposure to exogenous hormones. In addition, the incidence of uterine neoplasia is low 0.03% and many of these tumors are benign leading to a 0.003% chance of developing a malignant uterine tumor.[37] When considering uterine pathology, it is important to take into consideration that in most cases of OVH, the entire uterus is not removed and endometrial tissue is often left behind unless the entire cervix is removed.[28]

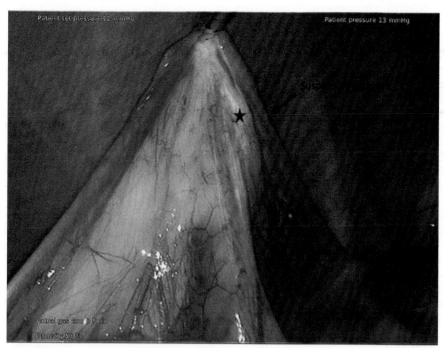

Fig. 1. A laparoscopic approach for an ovariectomy. The proper ligament has been grasped with 5-mm Babcock forceps to expose the ovary and ovarian pedicle. The black star denotes the ovary.

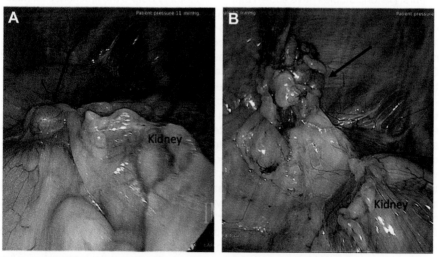

Fig. 2. A laparoscopic approach for ovarian remnant removal located caudal to the right kidney. The black arrow points to the ovarian remnant before (*A*) and during dissection (*B*). A 5-mm grasping forcep is used to elevate the remnant ventrally (*B*).

CONTROVERSIES SURROUNDING TIMING OF GONADECTOMY

In recent years, timing of sterilization has become a topic of discussion. This controversy stems from recent studies evaluating the risk of certain disease processes in relation to hormone status and timing of gonadectomy. Interpretation of this data is difficult as many of these studies are breed or species-specific, making it challenging to extrapolate across small animal companion medicine where significant diversity exists between breeds and species. Another potential source of bias is the study population. Although some studies include large numbers in the study population, they often use the Veterinary Medical Database (VMDB) and surveys from breed clubs. Studies using the VMDB reflect only those patients at referral hospitals and those from breed clubs represent a different population than those of typical pet owners. Another potential source of bias is the disproportionate number of animals that are spayed and neutered in the United States. As a result, there are often fewer intact animals represented in studies, which has the potential to result in an overinterpretation of neutered animals being higher risk for certain conditions.

There are 3 main categories of disease processes that have been looked at in relation to the timing of gonadectomy. These include the risk of neoplasia, orthopedic disease, and miscellaneous conditions such as inflammation/infection, urinary incontinence, obesity, and so forth. When considering the timing of gonadectomy, the risk of these conditions must be balanced along with the effects of gonadectomy on population management and lifespan in companion animals.

Neoplasia

There are many factors that contribute to the development of neoplasia, including genetics, age, environment, body condition, and sex hormone status. Although early gonadectomy supports minimizing the risk of reproductive tumors in females, it may potentially increase the risk of other cancers in certain breeds (**Table 1**). The degree of malignancy and incidence of the tumor type must be taken into consideration when making decisions about the timing of gonadectomy for the prevention of certain tumors. Historic studies have shown that gonadectomy before the first heat essentially eliminates the risk of mammary neoplasia (0.05%).[2] Gonadectomy also eliminates the risk of ovarian cancer and cysts in females and decreases the risk of uterine, vaginal, and vulvar tumors.[38,39] In male dogs, testicular tumors account for 16% to 27% of tumors in sexually intact male dogs; however, castration eliminates this risk.[40] Conversely, castration appears to increase the risk for prostatic carcinoma, but this tumor is rare (0.29%-0.6%) and the risk seems to vary among breeds.[40]

Multiple studies have evaluated gonadectomy status and/or the timing of gonadectomy on the risk of nonreproductive tumors in dogs, including lymphoma, mast cell tumors, hemangiosarcoma (HSA), and osteosarcoma (OSA).[6–9,11–13,29,41,42] A large study using the VMDB found that intact male dogs and neutered male and female dogs were twice as likely to develop lymphoma than intact females.[29] Timing of neuter was not evaluated in this study. However, when looking specifically at Vizslas, neutered males and females were 4.3 times as likely to have lymphoma compared with intact Vizslas.[11] Conversely, gonadectomy performed at any time did not affect the risk of lymphoma in either sex in Labrador Retrievers or German Shepherds.[8,9] Male Golden Retrievers neutered before a year of age were 3 times more likely to develop lymphoma than those that were intact.[12] Both male and female Golden Retrievers neutered between 6 and 11 months were found to be at increased risk of lymphoma.[9]

Mast cell tumors (MCTs) are more common in gonadectomized female dogs compared with intact female dogs; however, many studies do not take into account

Table 1
Risk of cancer in relation to timing of neuter in male and female dogs[2,8,9-13,29, 38-42]

Cancer Type	Breed	Effect of Neutering on Risk in Females	Effect of Neutering on Risk in Males	Timing of Neuter Evaluated[a]	Effect of Timing of Neuter
Mammary	Many	Decreased	N/A	Yes	Before first heat results in the greatest benefit
	Golden Retriever	None	N/A	Yes	Not significant
	German Shepherd	None	N/A	Yes	Not significant
	Labrador Retriever	None	N/A	Yes	Not significant
Ovarian, Uterine, and Vaginal	Many	Decreased	N/A	No	Not assessed
Testicular	Many	N/A	Decreased	No	Not assessed
Prostatic	Many	N/A	Increased	No	Not assessed
Lymphoma	Golden Retriever	Increased	Increased	Yes	Females and males neutered 6–11 mo
	German Shepherd	None	None	Yes	Not significant
	Labrador Retriever	None	None	Yes	Not significant
	Vizsla	Increased	Increased	Yes	Increased risk when neutered at all time frames
Mast Cell Tumors	Golden Retriever	Increased	None	Yes	Females neutered <6 mo, 1 y, 2–8 y
	German Shepherd	None	None	Yes	Not significant
	Labrador Retriever	None	None	Yes	Not significant
	Vizsla	Increased	Increased	Yes	Increased risk when neutered at all time frames
Hemangiosarcoma	Golden Retriever	None	None	Yes	Not significant
	German Shepherd	None	None	Yes	Not significant
	Labrador Retriever	None	None	Yes	Not significant
	Vizsla	Increased	Increased	Yes	Females neutered ≤12 mo and >12 mo; males neutered >12 mo

(continued on next page)

Table 1
(continued)

Cancer Type	Breed	Effect of Neutering on Risk in Females	Effect of Neutering on Risk in Males	Timing of Neuter Evaluated[a]	Effect of Timing of Neuter
Splenic Hemangiosarcoma	Many [b]	Increased	Increased	No	Not assessed
Cardiac Hemangiosarcoma	Many [c]	None	None	No	Not assessed
Osteosarcoma	Many	Increased	Increased	No	Not assessed
	German Shepherd	None	None	Yes	Not significant
	Rottweiler	Increased	Increased	Yes[d]	Females and males neutered <1 y

[a] Timing of neuter evaluated for Golden Retrievers, Labrador Retrievers, and German Shepherds: less than 6 months. 6 to 11 months, 1 year, and 2 to 8 years. Timing of neuter evaluated for Vizslas: ≦12 months, greater than 12 months.
[b] Overrepresented breeds: German Shepherd, Golden Retriever, American Cocker Spaniel, and Miniature Poodle.
[c] Overrepresented breeds: Golden Retriever.
[d] Timing of neuter evaluated: less than 1 year, ≥1 year.

the timing of spay and neuter.[41,43] When looking at breed-specific studies, there is a trend toward female gonadectomized dogs having an increased risk of MCT. Gonadectomized Vizslas were 3.5 times more likely to develop an MCT than those that were sexually intact.[11] Timing of neuter in both males and females was evaluated and neutering of both sexes and any time frame appeared to increase the risk of mast cell tumors in Vizslas. Gonad status and timing of gonadectomy did not appear to affect the risk of MCT in either sex for German Shepherds and Labrador Retrievers or male Golden Retrievers.[8,9,12] Female Golden Retrievers were more likely to develop MCT when they were spayed less than 6 months, at 1 year, or between 2 and 8 years.[9]

HSA is a highly malignant tumor associated with a poor prognosis. A large VMDB study looked at 5736 dogs diagnosed with HSA found that spayed females had an odds ratio (OR) of 1.72 for HSA and castrated males had an OR of 1.14 compared with their intact counterparts. All cases were matched to control for age and the period since the study period spanned almost 40 years.[10] When cardiac HSA was separated from splenic HSA cases, the risk of cardiac HSA did not appear to be associated with gonadectomy status. Several breed-specific studies have evaluated gonadectomy status as a risk factor for HSA. When looking at the overall gonadectomy status for male Vizslas, there did not appear to be a risk for the development of HSA.[11] However, when the timing of gonadectomy was considered, male and female Vizslas neutered after 12 months of age were more likely to develop HSA (OR, 5.3 and 11.5, respectively) and female Vizslas neutered before 12 months of age were also more likely to develop HSA (OR 6.0) compared with intact dogs.[11] An increased risk for HSA in female dogs neutered after a year of age was also seen in Golden Retrievers in one study,[12] but a follow-up study did not find an increased risk in neutered dogs of either sex for HSA in Golden Retrievers or Labrador Retrievers.[9] Similarly, neutered male and female German Shepherds were not found to have an increased risk for HSA.[8]

Gonadectomy status has also been evaluated as a risk factor for OSA. In an older case-controlled retrospective study using the VMDB, gonadectomized dogs were 2 times more likely compared with intact dogs to develop OSA.[42] Timing of gonadectomy was not considered in this study. In a breed-specific study on Rottweilers, male and female dogs neutered before 1 year of age were at increased risk of developing OSA.[13] Conversely, gonadectomy status did not appear to be a risk factor for OSA in German Shepherds.[8]

Age is likely a major confounding factor in many of these studies. When looking specifically at Golden Retrievers, which have a high incidence of cancer-related mortality, age appeared to be the most important variable associated with cancer-related death.[44] Kent and colleagues evaluated 655 Golden Retrievers that underwent a necropsy examination and found that 65% of dogs died of cancer; however, reproductive status had no effect on the risk of death from neoplasia, and increasing age was an independent risk factor for cancer-related death.[44]

Orthopedic Disease

It is well documented that sex hormones play an important role in musculoskeletal development. Gonadectomizing dogs before skeletal maturity delays physeal closure, leading to increased long bone growth, which may predispose some dogs to future joint disease.[6–9,12,14–19] Although many of these studies contain confounding factors that are difficult to tease out, including genetics, breed predispositions, body weight, body condition, lifestyle, and so forth, multiple studies have shown a link between gonadectomy and orthopedic disease. The most common diseases noted are hip dysplasia, elbow dysplasia, and cranial cruciate ligament rupture. Gonadectomized dogs have been shown to have an increased risk of cranial cruciate ligament injury.[14–17,19] Although some studies show a higher risk in spayed female dogs,[14,17] others have shown both neutered males and females have a higher risk of cranial cruciate ligament rupture.[15]

Breed-specific studies in Boxers, German Shepherds, Golden and Labrador Retrievers found an increased incidence of orthopedic disease in gonadectomized dogs; however, the risk differs substantially between breeds (**Table 2**).[8,9,12,18,19] The incidence of one or more joint disorders (hip dysplasia, elbow dysplasia, cranial cruciate ligament rupture) in Labrador Retrievers doubled in both males and females when they were neutered before 6 months of age.[9] When Golden Retrievers were neutered before 6 months of age, the incidence of a joint disease was 4 to 5 times higher compared with intact dogs.[9] A study looking at German Shepherds found that the incidence of joint disease (mostly cranial cruciate ligament rupture) was higher in both males and females neutered before a year of age.[8]

The risk of hip dysplasia was evaluated in Boxers and it was found that those neutered at least 6 months before the diagnosis of hip dysplasia were 1.5 times more likely to develop hip dysplasia (median age at gonadectomy was 3 years) compared with those that were intact.[18] In other studies, there was no association between timing of gonadectomy and hip or elbow dysplasia in German Shepherds,[8] but both male and female Golden Retrievers neutered before 1 year of age were at higher risk of hip dysplasia,[9] and only female Labrador Retrievers neutered before a year of age had a higher incidence of hip dysplasia.[9]

Table 2
Risk of orthopedic disease in relation to timing of neuter in male and female dogs[8,9,18]

Orthopedic Condition	Breed	Effect of Neutering on Risk in Females	Effect of Neutering on Risk in Males	Timing of Neuter Evaluated[a]	Effect of Timing of Neuter
Hip Dysplasia	Boxer	Increased	Increased	Yes	Males and females neutered 6 mo before diagnosis
	German Shepherd	None	None	Yes	Not significant
	Golden Retriever	None	Increased	Yes	Males neutered <6 mo, 6–11 mo, 2–8 y
	Labrador Retriever	Increased	None	Yes	Females neutered <6 mo, 6–11 mo, 1 y
Elbow Dysplasia	German Shepherd	None	None	Yes	Not significant
	Golden Retriever	None	None	Yes	Not significant
	Labrador Retriever	None	Increased	Yes	Males neutered <6 mo and 2–8 y
Cranial Cruciate Ligament Rupture	German Shepherd	Increased	Increased	Yes	Females and males neutered <12 mo
	Golden Retriever	Increased	Increased	Yes	Females and males neutered <6 mo, 6–11 mo, 2–8 y
	Labrador Retriever	None	Increased	Yes	Males neutered <6 mo

[a] Timing of neuter evaluated for Golden Retrievers, Labrador Retrievers, and German Shepherds: less than 6 months, 6 to 11 months, 1 year, and 2 to 8 years.

Miscellaneous Conditions

Another factor to consider regarding timing and technique of sterilization in female dogs is urinary incontinence. Urinary incontinence following spay appears to be at highest risk in larger breed dogs gonadectomized before 3 months of age.[20] Studies looking at the risk of incontinence when spayed between 4 and 6 months versus waiting until after the first heat cycle did not reveal an increased risk of incontinence.[20,21] A more recent study suggests that heavier dogs have a higher risk of urethral sphincter mechanism incompetence following neuter and recommend delaying neuter to closer to a year of age in dogs whose adult weight is anticipated to be >25 kg.[22] A breed-specific study looking at German Shepherds found that urinary incontinence was much less likely to occur in intact females versus females spayed between 6 and 11 months.[8]

Vulvar conformation may also be affected by the timing of spay. Although there are no data that the author is aware of regarding the timing of spay and its effect on vulvar conformation, there is anecdotal evidence to suggest that prepubertal spay may contribute to a recessed vulvar conformation, which could contribute to perivulvar dermatitis. As a result of this, some recommend delaying gonadectomy in female dogs until after their first heat cycle. The risks of mammary neoplasia should be discussed with owners considering this delay.

In male dogs, sterilization impacts the occurrence of prostatic disease, perineal hernias, and perianal tumors. Castration eliminates the occurrence of benign prostatic hyperplasia and reduces the risk of prostatic abscessation/prostatitis, and prostatic cysts.[45,46] Other sex-hormone-driven conditions like perineal hernia and perianal adenomas are much less likely to occur in castrated dogs. Conversely, prostatic neoplasia is more common in castrated male dogs, but this tumor is rare (0.29%-0.6%)[40] and may have less of an impact on decision making for timing of neuter in male dogs than other more prevalent conditions.

Obesity is common in companion animals and is estimated to affect 24% to 30% of the pet population in the United States.[47] Although it is unclear if age at the time of sterilization contributes to obesity, studies consistently document obesity in neutered animals versus those that are sexually intact.[23–25] Obesity is confounded by environmental factors and other medical problems; therefore, a recommendation on timing of sterilization based solely on this condition is difficult to make.

Studies document that removal of sex hormones with gonadectomy leads to decreased roaming, hormonal aggression, and urine marking.[25,48,49] Other behaviors including noise phobias, fear, and anxiety have been evaluated, but the effects of early gonadectomy on these behaviors appear to be inconsistent across studies.[11,20] Spain and colleagues[20] found that dogs neutered before 5.5 months were more likely to have noise phobias and to display sexual behaviors and less likely to have separation anxiety and inappropriate urination due to fear. Meanwhile, a breed-specific study in Vizslas found that those neutered before 6 months of age appeared more fearful and more anxious.[11]

Despite numerous recent studies documenting associations between gonadectomy and timing of gonadectomy in relation to the development of cancer,[6–13,29,42] studies also show that gonadectomized animals live longer.[25–27] A study using the VMDB found that spayed females live 26.3% longer and castrated males live 13.8% longer than their intact counterparts.[26] Sterilized animals also had different causes of death than intact animals. Those that were intact were more likely to die from infectious disease and trauma compared with those that were neutered were more likely to die from cancer and immune-mediated disease.[26] A retrospective study of 927 military working dogs found that castrated males lived longer than intact males and spayed females (intact females were not evaluated). The leading cause of death was due to degenerative joint disease, neoplasia, and spinal cord disease.[27]

GONAD SPARING STERILIZATION

Given the recent body of literature suggesting possible connections to certain disease processes and timing of gonadectomy, there has been interest in sterilization procedures that spare the gonads and therefore maintains the sex hormone source. In males, vasectomy, which prevents sperm from reaching the semen and therefore rendering them infertile, has gained popularity. In female dogs, hysterectomy and salpingectomy are options for ovarian sparing sterilization. Hysterectomy requires the complete removal of the uterus and endometrium, whereas salpingectomy involves surgical removal of the fallopian tubes and has been described in the veterinary literature.[50] Hysterectomy is more widespread and therefore will be discussed here. Both hysterectomy and vasectomy can be performed through an open or laparoscopic approach.[30,31,41–55]

Hysterectomy

Limited information is available on hysterectomy in dogs.[28,30,51] Criticism of this procedure surrounds the fact that the entire endometrial lining must be removed to prevent a stump pyometra from occurring given that dogs still maintain their hormone source (**Figs. 3** and **4**). A cadaveric study evaluated the feasibility of this procedure in dogs and found that ligation and transection of the uterus caudal to the cervix allowed for complete removal of glandular tissue from the caudal aspect of the uterus; however, half of the uterine horns, which were transected at the proper ligament had glandular tissue noted at the cut margin, which could be a risk for pyometra in the future.[28] As the risk of pyometra increases with age, many of the younger dogs undergoing hysterectomy may not develop clinical signs associated with this potential risk until later in life. Another consequence of complete removal of the uterus and cervix

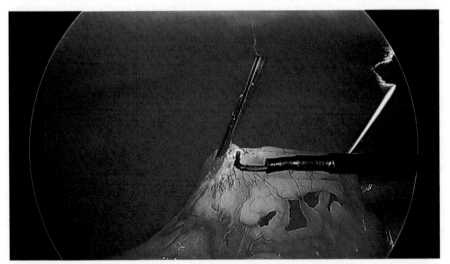

Fig. 3. Laparoscopic-assisted ovarian sparing hysterectomy performed in a dog. The ovary (*left*) and the uterine horn (*right*) have been suspended to allow for dissection at the proper ligament with the J-hook electrocautery. Separation of the uterine horn is performed as close as possible to the ovary. (*Image courtesy of* Dr Boel Fransson.)

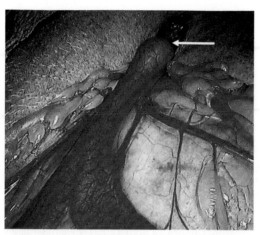

Fig. 4. Laparoscopic-assisted ovarian sparing hysterectomy performed in a dog. The ovaries have been spared and the uterus has been dissected and exteriorized out through the body wall incision. The white arrow denotes the cervix. Ligation is performed on the vaginal side of the cervix to ensure all endometrium has been removed. (*Image courtesy of* Dr Boel Fransson.)

while maintaining sex hormones is that female dogs continue to cycle, attract males, and are at risk of being mated. There are anecdotal reports of these dogs having weakened and altered vaginal vaults leading to perforation of the remaining vagina resulting in life-threatening injury.[51] A small case series evaluated laparoscopic sterilization techniques in dogs including 17 dogs that underwent hysterectomy. They found that 24% of dogs continued to have mild nonhemorrhagic vaginal discharge during their heat cycles and 29% of dogs had behavioral changes during heat. Although one dog went on to get ovariectomized, none of the dogs developed medical conditions related to maintaining their gonads 34 months (±13) after hysterectomy.[30]

Vasectomy

Vasectomy can be performed through an inguinal approach[51,52] (**Fig. 5**) or a laparoscopic approach[30–32,53](**Fig. 6**). During vasectomy, the blood supply to the testicles

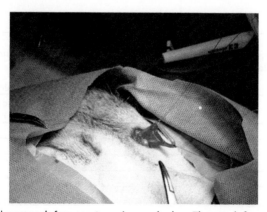

Fig. 5. An inguinal approach for vasectomy in a male dog. The vas deferens has been double ligated before removing a small segment between the 2 sutures. (*Image courtesy of* Dr Dan Smeak.)

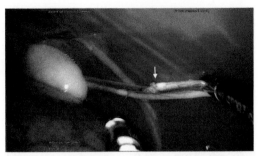

Fig. 6. A laparoscopic approach for vasectomy in a male dog. The vas deferens has been sealed and transected with a 5-mm vessel sealant device. The white arrow points to the sealed end of the vas deferens. (*Image courtesy of* Dr Eric Monnet.)

can be perserved,[30,53] which allows for sterilization while maintaining sex hormones or the blood supply to the testicles can be ligated removing the hormone source.[31,32] Recently, laparoscopic vasectomy was performed on 8 dogs. Sixty-three percent of those dogs went on to have a castration performed due to behavioral challenges associated with their intact status.[30] Although very few dogs were reported in this abstract, results suggest that counseling owners on the behavioral implications of gonad sparing sterilization surgery in male dogs is important. Other important considerations are the long-term disease implications of sex hormones in male dogs discussed previously.

Libermann and colleagues recently described laparoscopic castration in 17 dogs where in addition to sealing and transecting the vas deferens (as is performed during vasectomy), the blood supply to the testicles was also sealed and transected. Testosterone levels were measured up to 12 months postoperatively and were not significantly different from those dogs that had traditional orchidectomy, showing that laparoscopic castration without removal of the testicles achieves testosterone suppression in addition to sterilization.[31] This technique deserves further investigation, but it is important to note that it would not be considered a hormone sparing procedure because testosterone levels were similar to those dogs with traditional orchidectomy.

Table 3
Suggested guidelines considering joint disease and cancers for age of neutering 5 mixed-breed groups of dogs

	Males				Females			
	Leave Intact	Choice	Beyond 11 mo	Beyond 23 mo	Leave Intact	Choice	Beyond 11 mo	Beyond 23 mo
<10 kg	✓				✓			
10–19 kg	✓				✓			
20–29 kg		✓					✓	
30–39 kg		✓					✓	
>40 kg			✓				✓[a]	

[a] Consider neutering beyond 11 months due to weight "Choice" means there was no increased risk for any age of neutering.
Adapted from Hart et al.[7]

Table 4
Authors' suggested timing of sterilization based on adult weight

Adult Weight (kg)	Suggested Timing of Sterilization (mo)
<10	6
10–20	6–8
21–30	9–12
31–40	10–14
>40	12–24

SUMMARY
Recommendations on Timing and Sterilization Technique in Dogs

Given that there are numerous factors that affect decision making for timing of sterilization, including whether the animal is going to be bred, population control, behavioral concerns, lifespan, breed, size, risk for orthopedic disease, risk for development of malignant cancers, urinary incontinence, and so forth, many organizations are reluctant to make recommendations for timing of sterilization in dogs. The American Veterinary Medical Association does not take a stance on when to perform surgical sterilization in dogs or which procedure to perform. Instead, it provides veterinarians with resources to determine which procedure (OVE, OHE, hysterectomy, orchidectomy, vasectomy) is appropriate for the patient/client.[33] This is similar to the American College of Theriogenologists and the Society for Theriogenology, which states that the method and age of sterilization should be made on a case-by-case basis.[34]

Recently, 2 studies were published regarding recommendations on timing of gonadectomy in relation to risk factors for particular breeds and mixed-breeds.[6,7] The first study evaluated pure-breed dogs and their risk for joint disorders (hip and elbow dysplasia, and cranial cruciate ligament rupture), neoplasia (lymphoma, mast cell tumor, HSA, and OSA), and urinary incontinence. Most breeds evaluated did not have an increased risk of joint disorders or cancers in relation to timing of neutering. However, this is not true for all breeds.[6] They also found that in some breeds, the risk of joint disorders and cancers was different between for males and females. These results emphasize the difficulty with applying data from breed-specific studies across all breeds or making blanket recommendations for timing of gonadectomy for all breeds and sexes. Instead, veterinarians can reference this information when they are helping clients decide on timing of gonadectomy for the specific breeds and disease processes evaluated in that study. The second study evaluated the timing of gonadectomy on similar joint and neoplastic disease processes in a population of mixed-breed dogs divided into 5 weight categories. Interestingly, there was no significant risk of occurrence of cancer in mixed breed neutered dogs in any weight category compared with intact dogs. However, they found that dogs that weighed ≥20 kg and were neutered before a year of age were at higher risk for one or more joint diseases.[7] Suggested guidelines from this study for age of neutering mixed-breed dogs based on body weight are recommended in **Table 3**.[7] These recommendations for mixed-breed dogs only take into consideration certain cancers and joint disease and do not consider behavior, longevity, obesity, environmental factors, and the risk of accidental breeding/pregnancy. The studies from Hart and colleagues can aid in decision making[6,7]; however, when breed-specific data are not available, the author uses **Table 4** as a guideline to aid in decision making on timing of gonadectomy.

Given the lack of information supporting the need to remove the uterus, the author prefers OVE (laparoscopic or open) for sterilization of females, but also supports OHE (laparoscopic or open) as an acceptable means of sterilization. There is a lack of large prospective data on hysterectomy in dogs for both short-term and long-term complications; therefore, the author does not recommend hysterectomy in dogs at this time. Vasectomy is a routine surgical procedure, which allows for sterilization while maintaining sex hormones and appears to be an acceptable method of sterilization in male dogs. In some pure-breed dogs with increased risk of malignant cancers or joint disease with gonadectomy, vasectomy may be an appropriate option for certain clients and their dogs. Pet owners should be counseled that vasectomy will not alleviate sex-hormone-related behaviors and can leave dogs predisposed to BPH, prostatic cysts and abscesses as well as perineal hernias and perianal gland and testicular tumors.

Recommendations on Timing and Sterilization Technique in Cats

Cats are induced ovulators and therefore very efficient breeders. In an effort to reduce overpopulation and unwanted litters the Veterinary Task Force on Feline Sterilization Recommendations for Age of Spay and Neuter Surgery recommend sterilization of cats by 5 months of age if they are not intended for breeding.[56] This recommendation is endorsed by the American Veterinary Medical Association and stems from both behavioral and medical issues. Unintended pregnancies can occur in cats as early as 4 months of age. Gonadectomizing cats before their first estrous cycle decreases their risk of mammary carcinoma,[57] eliminates the risk of pyometra and dystocia, and has the potential to decrease behavioral problems which have been linked to relinquishment in cats.[58] Many of the controversies (oncologic and orthopedic) surrounding timing of gonadectomy in dogs have not been studied in cats. A retrospective study in 26 cats found that overweight male neutered cats appeared to be at higher risk of capital femoral physeal fractures.[59] Twenty-five of the cats were neutered males, but timing of neuter was only known in 16 of the cats. Fourteen cats were neutered before 6 months of age. Bodyweight may be a confounding factor in this study and additional prospective research is needed in cats to determine if similar links to orthopedic and neoplastic conditions are affected by timing of gonadectomy. Both OVE and OHE are considered acceptable methods of sterilization in females. There are currently no data regarding gonad sparing surgeries in male or female cats.

CLINICS CARE POINTS

- Timing of gonadectomy in mixed-breed dogs may increase the risk of joint-related conditions in dogs greater than 20 kg.

- Timing of gonadectomy in certain pure-breed dogs may increase the risk of certain neoplastic and joint conditions, but there are significant differences among breeds and sexes.

- When performing hysterectomy alone it is essential that all the glandular epithelium is removed.

- There are no long-term studies determining the consequences of hysterectomy alone in the dog and further research is needed to determine the risk of pyometra and vaginal rupture as a result of accidental breeding.

DISCLOSURE

The author has nothing to disclose.

REFERENCES

1. American Pet Products Association. Dog ownership. In: *APPA national pet owners survey 2015–2016*. Greenwich, Conn: American Pet Products Association Inc; 2016. p. 63–175.
2. Schneider R, Dorn CR, Taylor DO. Factors influencing canine mammary cancer development and postsurgical survival. J Natl Cancer Inst 1969;43(6):1249–61.
3. Gower S, Mayhew P. Canine laparoscopic and laparoscopic-assisted ovariohysterectomy and ovariectomy. Compend Contin Educ Vet 2008;30(8):430–40.
4. van Goethem B, Schaefers-Okkens A, Kirpensteijn J. Making a rational choice between ovariectomy and ovariohysterectomy in the dog: a discussion of the benefits of either technique. Vet Surg 2006;35(2):136–43.
5. Houlihan KE. A literature review on the welfare implications of gonadectomy of dogs. J Am Vet Med Assoc 2017;250(10):1155–66.
6. Hart BL, Hart LA, Thigpen AP, et al. Assisting decision-making on age of neutering for 35 breeds of dogs: associated joint disorders, cancers, and urinary incontinence. Front Vet Sci 2020;7:388.
7. Hart BL, Hart LA, Thigpen AP, et al. Assisting decision-making on age of neutering for mixed breed dogs of five weight categories: associated joint disorders and cancers. Front Vet Sci 2020;7:472.
8. Hart BL, Hart LA, Thigpen AP, et al. Neutering of German Shepherd Dogs: associated joint disorders, cancers and urinary incontinence. Vet Med Sci 2016;2(3):191–9.
9. Hart BL, Hart LA, Thigpen AP, et al. Long-term health effects of neutering dogs: comparison of labrador retrievers with golden retrievers. PLoS One 2014;9(7):e102241.
10. Robinson KL, Bryan ME, Atkinison ES, et al. Neutering is assoociated with developing hemangiosarcoma in dogs in the Veteriniary Medical Database: an age and time-period matched case-conotrol study (1964-2003). Can Vet J 2020;61:499–504.
11. Zink MC, Farhoody P, Elser SE, et al. Evaluation of the risk and age of onset of cancer and behavioral disorders in gonadectomized Vizslas. J Am Vet Med Assoc 2014;244(3):309–19.
12. Torres de la Riva G, Hart BL, Farver TB, et al. Neutering dogs: effects on joint disorders and cancers in golden retrievers. PLoS One 2013;8(2):e55937.
13. Cooley DM, Beranek BC, Schlittler DL, et al. Endogenous gonadal hormone exposure and bone sarcoma risk. Cancer Epidemiol Biomarkers Prev 2002;11(11):1434–40.
14. Slauterbeck JR, Pankratz K, Xu KT, et al. Canine ovariohysterectomy and orchiectomy increases the prevalence of ACL injury. Clin Orthop Relat Res 2004;429:301–5.
15. Witsberger TH, Villamil JA, Schultz LG, et al. Prevalence of and risk factors for hip dysplasia and cranial cruciate ligament deficiency in dogs. J Am Vet Med Assoc 2008;232(12):1818–24.
16. Duval JM, Budsberg SC, Flo GL, et al. Breed, sex, and body weight as risk factors for rupture of the cranial cruciate ligament in young dogs. J Am Vet Med Assoc 1999;215(6):811–4.

17. Whitehair JG, Vasseur PB, Willits NH. Epidemiology of cranial cruciate ligament rupture in dogs. J Am Vet Med Assoc 1993;203(7):1016–9.

18. van Hagen MA, Ducro BJ, van den Broek J, et al. Incidence, risk factors, and heritability estimates of hind limb lameness caused by hip dysplasia in a birth cohort of boxers. Am J Vet Res 2005;66(2):307–12.

19. Simpson M, Albright S, Wolfe B, et al. Age at gonadectomy and risk of overweight/obesity and orthopedic injury in a cohort of Golden Retrievers. PLoS One 2019;14(7):e0209131.

20. Spain CV, Scarlett JM, Houpt KA. Long-term risks and benefits of early-age gonadectomy in dogs. J Am Vet Med Assoc 2004;224(3):380–7.

21. de Bleser B, Brodbelt DC, Gregory NG, et al. The association between acquired urinary sphincter mechanism incompetence in bitches and early spaying: a case-control study. Vet J 2011;187(1):42–7.

22. Byron JK, Taylor KH, Phillips GS, et al. Urethral sphincter mechanism incompetence in 163 neutered female dogs: diagnosis, treatment, and relationship of weight and age at neuter to development of disease. J Vet Intern Med 2017; 31(2):442–8.

23. Lefebvre SL, Yang M, Wang M, et al. Effect of age at gonadectomy on the probability of dogs becoming overweight. J Am Vet Med Assoc 2013;243(2):236–43.

24. Kustritz MV. Determining the optimal age for gonadectomy of dogs and cats. J Am Vet Med Assoc 2007;231(11):1665–75.

25. Root Kustritz MV. Effects of surgical sterilization on canine and feline health and on society. Reprod Domest Anim 2012;47(Suppl 4):214–22.

26. Hoffman JM, Creevy KE, Promislow DEL. Reproductive capability is associated with lifespan and cause of death in companion dogs. PLoS One 2013;8(4): e61082–7.

27. Moore GE, Burkman KD, Carter MN, et al. Causes of death or reasons for euthanasia in military working dogs: 927 cases (1993-1996). J Am Vet Med Assoc 2001;219(2):209–14.

28. Mejia S, Duncan C, Iodence A, et al. Evaluation of completeness of resection of the glandular portion of the uterus with hysterectomy in dogs - A pilot study. Anim Reprod Sci 2020;219:106527.

29. Villamil JA, Henry CJ, Hahn AW, et al. Hormonal and sex impact on the epidemiology of canine lymphoma. J Cancer Epidemiol 2009;2009:591753.

30. Fransson, B. Laparoscopic Alternative Sterilization Surgeries in 17 Female and 8 Male Dogs. Scientific Presentation Abstracts: ACVS Surgery Summit; October 17-19, 2019;Las Vegas, NV.

31. Libermann S, Etchepareborde S, Gautherot A, et al. Laparoscopic castration in dogs: complications, outcomes, and long-term follow-up. Rev Vét Clin 2020; 55:1–10.

32. Mathon DH, Palierne S, Meynaud-Collard P, et al. Laparoscopic-assisted colopexy and sterilization in male dogs: short-term results and physiologic consequences. Vet Surg 2011;40:500–8.

33. American Veterinary Medical Association. Spaying and neutering. Available at: https://www.avma.org/resources/pet-owners/petcare/spaying-and-neutering. Accessed August 29, 2021.

34. American College of Theriogenologists. Mandatory spay/neuter. Available at: https://www.theriogenology.org/page/PositionStatements#SpayNeuter. Accessed August 29, 2021.

35. DeTora M, McCarthy RJ. Ovariohysterectomy versus ovariectomy for elective sterilization of female dogs and cats: is removal of the uterus necessary? J Am Vet Med Assoc 2011;239(11):1409–12.

3C. Peeters ME, Klrpensteijn J. Comparison of surgical variables and short-term postoperative complications in healthy dogs undergoing ovariohysterectomy or ovariectomy. J Am Vet Med Assoc 2011;238(2):189–94.

37. Brodey RS, Roszel JF. Neoplasms of the canine uterus, vagina, and vulva: a clinicopathologic survey of 90 cases. J Am Vet Med Assoc 1967;151(10):1294–307.

38. Saba CF, Lawrence J. Tumors of the female reproductive system. In: Vail D, Withrow S, editors. Withrow and MacEwen's small animal clinical oncology. 5th edition. St. Louis: Elsevier; 2013. p. 532–6.

39. Arlt SP, Haimerl P. Cystic ovaries and ovarian neoplasia in the female dog - a systematic review. Reprod Domest Anim 2016;51:3–11.

40. Lawrence J, CF S. Tumors of the male reproductive system. In: Vail D, Withrow S, editors. Withrow and MacEwen's small animal clinical oncology. 5th edition. St. Louis: Elsevier; 2013. p. 557–65.

41. White CR, Hohenhaus AE, Kelsey J, et al. Cutaneous MCTs: associations with spay/neuter status, breed, body size, and phylogenetic cluster. J Am Anim Hosp Assoc 2011;47(3):210–6.

42. Ru G, Terracini B, Glickman LT. Host related risk factors for canine osteosarcoma. Vet J 1998;156(1):31–9.

43. London C, Thamm D. Mast cell tumors. In: Vail D, Withrow S, editors. Withrow and MacEwen's small animal clinical oncology. 5th edition. St. Louis: Elsevier; 2013. p. 335–55.

44. Kent MS, Burton JH, Dank G, et al. Association of cancer-related mortality, age and gonadectomy in golden retriever dogs at a veterinary academic center (1989-2016). PLoS One 2018;13(2):e0192578.

45. Smith J. Canine prostatic disease: a review of anatomy, pathology, diagnosis, and treatment. Theriogenology 2008;70(3):375–83.

46. Johnston SD, Kamolpatana K, Root-Kustritz MV, et al. Prostatic disorders in the dog. Anim Reprod Sci 2000;60-61:405–15.

47. Remillard R. Obesity, a disease to be recognized and managed. In: Ettinger S, Feldman E, eds. Textbook of veterinary Internal medicine. vol. 1. 6th edition.2005.

48. Hart BL, Eckstein RA. The role of gonadal hormones in the occurrence of objectionable behaviours in dogs and cats. Appl Anim Behav Sci 1997;52(3):331–44.

49. Hopkins SG, Schubert TA, Hart BL. Castration of adult male dogs: effects on roaming, aggression, urine marking, and mounting. J Am Vet Med Assoc 1976; 168(12):1108–10.

50. Saxena OP. Ligature of fallopian tubes (salpingectomy) in bitches. Indian Vet J 1966;43(1):83–4.

51. Kutzler MA. Gonad-sparing surgical sterilization in dogs. Front Vet Sci 2020; 7:342.

52. Rubin LD, Maplesden DC. A technique for vasectomy in dogs. Vet Med Small Anim Clin 1977;72(4):579–81.

53. Clinton RL, Stump FJ, Wiggers KL. Canine vasectomy: a modern solution to an age-old problem. (A photographic essay). Vet Med Small Anim Clin 1972; 67(10):1097–9.

54. Silva LD, Onclin K, Donnay I, et al. Laparoscopic vasectomy in the male dog. J Reprod Fertil Suppl 1993;47:399–401.

55. Urfer SR, Kaeberlein M. Desexing dogs: a review of the current literature. Animals (Basel) 2019;9(12):1086.

56. Veterinary task force on feline sterilization. Recommendations for age of spay and neuter surgery. 2016. Available at: https://www.avma.org/resources-tools/animal-health-and-welfare/elective-spaying-and-neutering-pets. Accessed August 31, 2021.

57. Overley B, Shofer FS, Goldschmidt MH, et al. Association between ovarihysterectomy and feline mammary carcinoma. J Vet Intern Med 2005;19(4):560–3.

58. Patronek GJ, Glickman LT, Beck AM, et al. Risk factors for relinquishment of cats to an animal shelter. J Am Vet Med Assoc 1996;209(3):582–8.

59. McNicholas WT, Wilkens BE, Blevins WE, et al. Spontaneous femoral capital physeal fractures in adult cats: 26 cases (1996-2001). J Am Vet Med Assoc 2002;221(12):1731–6.

Current Concepts in Small Animal Gastrointestinal Surgery

Penny J. Regier, DVM, MS

KEYWORDS

- Gastrointestinal surgery • Surgical stapling • Handsewn anastomosis • Enterotomy
- Intestinal anastomosis • Intestinal dehiscence • Leak testing

KEY POINTS

- Intestinal dehiscence is a devastating consequence of intestinal surgery that requires surgical intervention, and a mortality rate as high as 85% has been reported.
- Handsewn and stapled anastomoses may be considered when performing an intestinal resection and anastomosis, with stapled anastomoses resulting in a shorter surgical time.
- Intestinal thickness should be considered when selecting staple size for intestinal anastomosis and may warrant use of larger staple size in order to achieve proper tissue engagement.
- Reinforcing techniques, such as oversewing at the transverse staple line of functional end-to-end stapled anastomosis, placement of a crotch suture, omental wraps, and serosal patches, may aid in reducing postoperative dehiscence.
- Intraoperative anastomotic leak testing, although unable to predict intestinal healing postoperatively, provides a means of acutely evaluating the surgical repair and is a valuable tool for surgeons in training.

 Video content accompanies this article at http://www.vetsmall.theclinics.com.

INTRODUCTION/BACKGROUND

Whether performing an intestinal biopsy, enterotomy, or enterectomy, intestinal wound closure requires precision, because intestinal leakage can have devastating consequences, such as peritonitis, sepsis, and death. Resection and anastomosis (R&A) is a common surgical procedure performed to remove diseased or nonviable tissue, and leakage at the anastomosis site is the most common cause of septic peritonitis, with dehiscence rates reported as high as 28%. Predisposing factors for anastomotic leakage include foreign body obstruction, hypoalbuminemia, intraoperative hypotension, preoperative peritonitis, inflammatory bowel disease, and anastomosis location

Department of Small Animal Clinical Sciences, College of Veterinary Medicine, University of Florida, PO Box 100126, 2015 Southwest 16th Avenue, Gainesville, FL 32610-0126, USA
E-mail address: pregier@ufl.edu

Vet Clin Small Anim 52 (2022) 437–454
https://doi.org/10.1016/j.cvsm.2021.11.002
0195-5616/22/© 2021 Elsevier Inc. All rights reserved.

vetsmall.theclinics.com

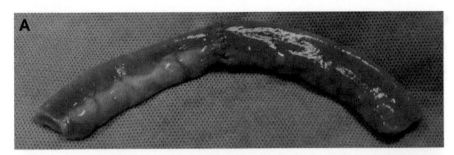

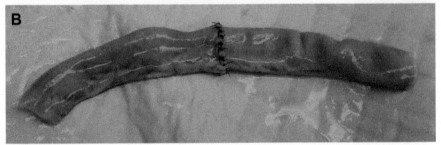

Fig. 1. Images of handsewn anastomosis constructs: (*A*) simple continuous anastomosis and (*B*) simple interrupted anastomosis.

as well as poor surgical technique.[1–6] Decreasing the risk of this potentially fatal complication is of great importance with respect to overall outcome after gastrointestinal (GI) surgery in small animal patients. The focus of this article is on current surgical techniques, primarily regarding small intestinal R&A, and surgeon decision making intraoperatively.

SURGICAL TECHNIQUES

Currently, intestinal anastomosis in small animals is dictated largely by surgeon preference and commonly is performed with either a traditional handsewn technique or a surgical stapling device. Variations of these techniques have been described with different suture patterns, suture materials, and types of stapling equipment along with benefits of surgical reinforcement techniques and leak testing.

Handsewn Techniques

Handsewn anastomosis techniques continue to be popular in veterinary medicine, likely due to ready availability of materials, decreased cost, and applicability in patients of varying sizes compared with stapling devices.[7–9] In an effort to minimize mucosal eversion, handsewn anastomoses (**Fig. 1**) are performed most commonly using an appositional pattern (ie, simple interrupted, simple continuous, or modified Gambee technique), with suture placement no more than 3 mm apart and 3 mm to 4 mm from the wound margin (Video 1).[10] Prior studies have shown that appositional suture patterns maintain intraluminal diameter and have comparable resistance to leakage,[11,12] with noncrushing approximating patterns resulting in less vascular disturbance to the anastomotic edges and less mucosal eversion than crushing patterns.[13]

Simple Interrupted Versus Simple Continuous

Both simple continuous (see **Fig. 1**A) and simple interrupted (see **Fig. 1**B) handsewn techniques commonly are used for intestinal surgery in veterinary medicine, but there is relatively little information directly comparing the 2 techniques. In the author's experience, simple interrupted techniques often are advocated for novice surgeons despite an absence of data demonstrating an increased risk of dehiscence with a simple continuous technique. Prior studies have reported no difference in dehiscence rates[1,14] and leak pressures that exceeded the maximum physiologic intraluminal peristaltic pressures (15–25 mm Hg),[15] when comparing simple interrupted and simple continuous techniques.[16] Simple continuous anastomoses are faster to complete, however, than simple interrupted anastomoses.[16] Based on findings from prior studies,[1,12–14,16] both simple interrupted and simple continuous approximating anastomoses are appropriate for use in a clinical setting, although the author believes that simple continuous anastomoses may be preferable due to more consistent tissue apposition and to decreased likelihood of mucosal eversion, which occurs more commonly when utilizing simple interrupted techniques and is associated with increased inflammation, delayed healing, and increased potential for adhesion formation.[13,14] The author recommends performing a simple continuous technique by placing 2 simple continuous suture lines, one starting at the mesenteric border and the second at the antimesenteric border, and completing the suture line for each strand with a square knot 180° from the start of the suture line. It also is of utmost importance that consistent tension must be maintained to ensure the suture does not loosen as the continuous line progresses and before the final knot is tied.

Suture Material

There is a paucity of literature comparing different suture materials and their efficacy for intestinal closure in small animals. Many different suture materials have been used in GI surgery, but prior studies have shown these materials to be inferior for the following reasons: chromic gut dissolves rapidly in the gut lumen, silk harbors bacteria and causes excessive inflammation, braided sutures (polyglactin 910 [Vicryl], Ethicon, Somerville, New Jersey) create tissue drag, and nonabsorbable sutures (polypropylene) remain in the tissue longer than needed and can cause foreign material adherence.[13,17–19] Synthetic monofilament absorbable sutures are used most commonly in veterinary medicine due to their many purported advantages, including ability to not harbor bacteria and ability to be absorbed by hydrolysis, which are ideal in a contaminated environment. Absorbable suture materials commonly used include polydioxanone (PDS II, Ethicon), glycomer 631 (Biosyn, Medtronic, Minneapolis, Minnesota), and poliglecaprone 25 (Monocryl, Ethicon) and are dictated largely by surgeon preference and estimated tensile strengths at 2 weeks (20% for poliglecaprone 25, 50% for gylcomer 631, and 80% for polydioxanone).[20] Studies evaluating suture size alone in handsewn techniques are lacking in the veterinary literature. The author recommends using a taper point needle with 4-0 suture material in cat and dog intestine and reserving 3-0 suture for larger dogs or dogs with edematous bowel and for use in the stomach.

Knotless Barbed Suture

Knotless sutures, also termed barbed sutures (**Fig. 2**), include V-Loc wound closure device (Medtronic), Quill knotless tissue-closure device (Surgical Specialties, Wyomissing, Pennsylvania), and Stratafix spiral knotless tissue control device (Ethicon). These sutures have protruding spurs along the surface of monofilament suture and are gaining widespread interest and use in veterinary medicine due to many purported advantages, including reduced surgical time, absence of terminal knot, consistent tissue apposition, and even distribution of tension along the wound margins, which reduce tissue ischemia.[21–25] There are few studies comparing knotless barbed sutures

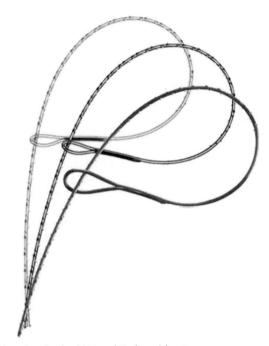

Fig. 2. Images of knotless barbed V-Loc (Medtronic) suture.

to monofilament sutures for intestinal surgery, although current studies have found that continuous barbed suture closure was performed faster with similar or higher leak pressures compared with monofilament sutures in canine jejunum.[26–29] In the author's experience and similar to a recent case report,[30] use of barbed suture for intestinal wound closure may lead to intestinal abscessation, but further in vivo studies are needed. Their current use in small animal GI surgery primarily is for intracorporeal laparoscopic gastropexies.[31–34]

Auto Stapling Devices

Intestinal anastomosis via stapling has been widely accepted in veterinary surgery. Functional end-to-end stapled anastomosis (FEESA) (**Fig. 3**) is the stapled anastomosis performed most commonly in dogs to remove diseased intestine and traditionally is constructed with a combination of a thoracoabdominal (TA) stapler (**Fig. 4**A) and GI anastomosis (GIA) stapler (**Fig. 4**B) (Medtronic),[35–40] although variations of the technique have been reported, including using the GIA stapler for both vertical and transverse staple lines (see **Fig. 3**C) as well as oversewing the TA staple line.[11,28,37,41,42] The staple sizes currently used in small animal patients for FEESA have been adopted from human medicine, but recent literature has recommended re-evaluation of staple size selection because the mural thickness of human intestine (1.5 mm) reportedly is less than that of dogs (2.06 mm).[43] A recent cadaveric study reported the mean mural thicknesses for the canine GI tract: stomach (3.99 mm), duodenum (2.34 mm), jejunum (2.49 mm), and ileum (2.30 mm), with the mean mural thicknesses of the duodenum, jejunum, and ileum 1.6-times greater than those of humans.[11] Currently, blue staple cartridges (open staple height, 3.5 mm), with a closed staple height of 1.5 mm and double overlapping row of titanium staples, are used most commonly for intestinal

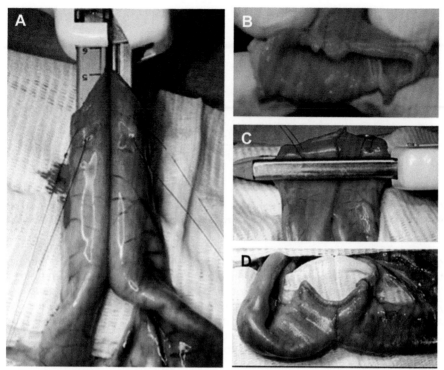

Fig. 3. FEESA. (*A*) GIA stapler placed in either end of the intestinal loop with stay sutures place on the mesenteric border to aid in placement of the bowel on the limbs of the stapler with the antimesenteric border apposed. (*B*) Partially offset GIA staple lines prior to placing the TA staple line. (*C*) GIA stapler used to close the transverse staple line. (*D*) Completed FEESA.

anastomosis in dogs with the larger green staples (closed staple height, 2 mm) reserved for gastric surgery.[35–40] The largest TA staple size, green, may be most appropriate for routine intestinal use in dogs, given the increased mural wall thickness compared with humans and that the thickness is doubled when the staple device is encompassing both lumen walls, which may compromise microvasculature. A recent

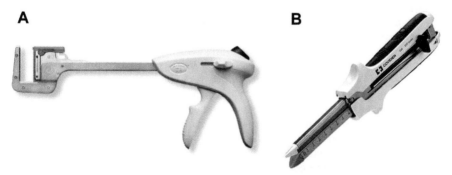

Fig. 4. Images of (*A*) TA stapler and (*B*) GIA stapler with DST series technology from Medtronic. ©2021 Medtronic. All rights reserved. Used with the permission of Medtronic.

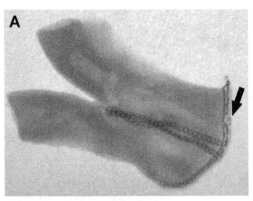
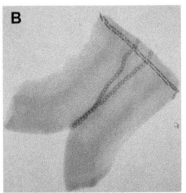

Fig. 5. Fluoroscopic images of the transverse staple line in a FEESA construct. (*A*) TA staple line with blue staple cartridge with malformation (*arrow*) of a single staple and (*B*) TA staple line with green staple cartridge.

study demonstrated similar leak pressures comparing the blue and green staple cartridges; however, serosal tearing and noncompressed staples in the transverse staple line were appreciated when using the blue cartridge (**Fig. 5**A) in canine cadaveric jejunum, which was not noted when using the green cartridge (**Fig. 5**B).[11] This is in support of previous studies demonstrating that edematous canine intestines have been noted to be thickened beyond the capacity of the 3.5-mm staples, which led to staple line failure,[38] and is similar to humans undergoing traumatic intestinal injuries.[7]

The transverse staple line of FEESA has been reported as the most common site of leakage or abscess formation in prior studies.[38,39,44,45] Although the GIA staple line is an inverting closure (**Fig. 6**A), the TA staple line is an everting closure (**Fig. 6**B), which is less ideal for mucosal healing and leads to a prolonged inflammatory response and promotes adhesion formation.[46] For this reason, many surgeons reinforce the transverse staple line with a suture oversew (**Figs. 7**). Although ex vivo studies evaluating oversewing of the transverse staple line have shown similar leak pressures[11,28] when using a suture oversew at the TA staple line versus not using a suture oversew, a recent retrospective study by Sumner and colleagues[41] concluded that oversewing the transverse staple line in FEESA was associated with a reduced occurrence of postoperative dehiscence (0%) compared with non-oversewn FEESA (14.6%). Based on these findings, oversewing of the transverse staple line may aid in preventing leakage at the transverse staple line. The crotch area also has been reported as a high-risk area for dehiscence, and a recommendation has been made to place a suture in this area to reduce tension.[35] Conversely, a different study did not see dehiscence in the crotch area.[38] It also is recommended to partially offset the GIA staple lines when placing the TA staple line (see **Fig. 3**B), because the GIA and TA staple line intersection also is a high risk area for dehiscence because of increased tissue thickness and decreased blood supply.[45] When performing FEESA, the author recommends evaluation of the intestinal thickness and use of a green staple cartridge for the transverse closure, especially with larger dogs, thickened bowel, or edematous bowel. The author routinely performs a suture oversew of the transverse staple line and recommends considering a suture oversew, especially when using a blue staple cartridge or if the surgeon is concerned about staple engagement of the tissue.

Current veterinary studies are under way to evaluate recent advances in stapling technology, which may provide further advantages to stapled anastomoses and

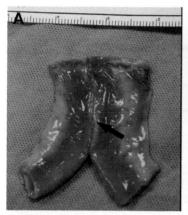
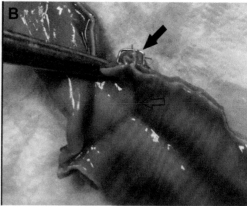

Fig. 6. Demonstration of inverting and everting anastomoses using canine cadaveric small intestine. (*A*) The vertical staple line (*arrow*) of the FEESA is inverted, precluding visualization of the staples extraluminally. (*B*) Cross-sectional intraluminal view of a skin-stapled anastomosis showing eversion of the anastomosed intestinal ends (*solid arrow*) and demonstration of mucosal-to-mucosal contact (*open arrow*).

may help alleviate some of the complications associated with staple malformation. Directional stapling technology (DST) (Medtronic) was developed to incorporate alterations in staple shape that allow staples to bend more consistently in the desired plane and has become more mainstream in veterinary medicine. Also, Tri-Staple (Medtronic) technology was developed with 3 rows of height progressive staples, rather than the conventional 2 rows, to decrease the incidence of staple line failure by creating less stress on the tissue on the outer staple line and also may preserve vasculature to the tissue.[47,48] Lastly, Ethicon-Endo Surgery (Cincinnati, Ohio) has developed the Linear Cutter (**Fig. 8**), which allows surgeons to select their preferred staple height by employing a novel 3-dimensional staple within a single cartridge containing 3 different staple heights. Further studies evaluating these stapling devices in veterinary medicine are under way.

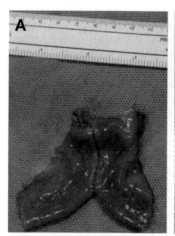
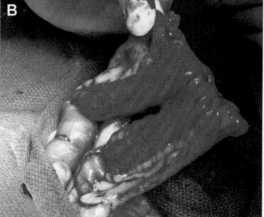

Fig. 7. Images (*A* and *B*) of oversewn FEESA. After completion of the stapled anastomosis, the transverse staple line was oversewn to invert the transverse staple line.

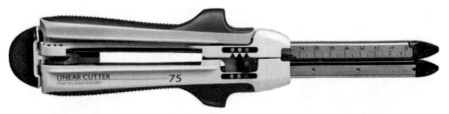

Fig. 8. Image of a Linear Cutter from Ethicon-Endo Surgery.

Skin Staples

Recent literature has described use of disposable skin staplers (Appose ULC disposable skin staplers [Medtronic]) to perform closures in both enterotomies and enterectomies (**Fig. 9**) with staples applied every 2 mm to 3 mm.[49–53] Prior studies evaluating stapled anastomoses have shown similar bursting strengths and faster surgical times compared with handsewn anastomoses,[50] with recent data revealing a dehiscence rate of 4.5% when evaluating disposable staplers used for intestinal anastomosis in 63 dogs.[51] Use of skin staplers also has been described with enterotomy closures, with a reported dehiscence rate of 1.2% in dogs and no dehiscence in a small group of cats.[52,53] The benefit of speed may be useful in certain clinical situations, such as unstable emergency cases, but further studies need to be performed to compare this technique to other anastomotic techniques.

Handsewn Versus Stapled Anastomosis

Surgical stapling devices increasingly are used in veterinary medicine due to many purported benefits, including reduced surgical time, ability to address lumen disparity, decreased tissue handling, improved blood supply, consistency and repeatability, and ease of use for inexperienced surgeons,[1,4,35,38] although they are limited in application due to fixed staple heights[4] and limited applicability in small dogs and cats.[1] Despite several benefits of stapled anastomotic techniques,[7–9] handsewn techniques remain popular, likely due to ready availability of materials, substantial cost differences, and applicability in patients of varying sizes compared with stapling devices.

Prior studies evaluating postoperative dehiscence of hand-sutured and stapled intestinal anastomosis in dogs have shown no differences in the frequency of dehiscence between the 2 techniques in the absence of septic peritonitis[1,5–8,50,54]; however, the duration of surgery was reduced when staples were used.[1,11,54] In conjunction with these findings, recent ex vivo studies have shown no differences in leak pressures between handsewn and stapled techniques.[11,28] A recent retrospective study, however, found that stapled anastomoses were less likely to have dehiscence (9.7%) compared with handsewn anastomoses (28.9%) in dogs with preoperative septic peritonitis.[6] A prior study by Jardel and colleagues[38] concluded that stapled anastomoses (FEESA) performed by nonexpert surgeons had outcomes comparable to those performed by experts, highlighting the ease of use of surgical stapling devices. In the human literature, stapled anastomoses were more than twice as likely to fail compared with handsewn during emergency trauma surgery, which is suspected to be due to the edematous nature of injured bowel.[8] This is similar to findings in dogs, where severely edematous bowel caused failure of the TA staple line in 2 cases.[38] This finding supports the current veterinary literature[11] recommending larger staple cartridges with larger dogs or dogs with thickened or edematous bowel.

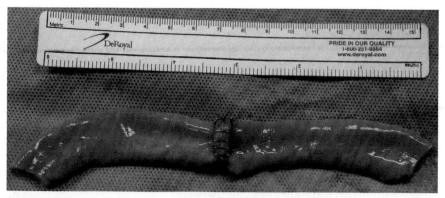

Fig. 9. Representative image of a canine cadaveric skin-stapled anastomosis construct.

When considering prior research and deciding whether to perform a handsewn or stapled anastomosis, many factors should be taken into consideration, including surgeon skill level, presence of septic peritonitis, surgery time, and thickness of the intestinal tissue.

Omentum Wrap/Serosal Patch

Reinforcement techniques at the surgery site, including serosal patch and omental wrap, have been recommended to prevent leakage after intestinal R&A.[4,39,55] The omentum has been evaluated experimentally in the past and has been coined the "abdominal policeman."[56] A vascularized omental pedicle should be used to protect an intestinal wound closure, because it helps seal the wound edge, restore blood supply, and facilitate lymphatic drainage.[57] The author recommends use of an omental wrap, with or without tacking sutures, for all intestinal wound closures (Videos 2 and 3). Serosal patching is another technique used to bolster the anastomosis, either in addition to omentum or often when the omentum is unavailable or contaminated. A prior cadaveric study showed that placement of a serosal patch around an intestinal anastomosis almost tripled the leak pressure.[55] In the author's experience, serosal patches should be performed with care in order to not create hairpin turns, which can cause subsequent obstructions and difficulty on repeat abdominal explores.

Leak Testing

Due to the potential for fatal complications with dehiscence of enterotomies or enterectomies, intraoperative leak testing (**Fig. 10**) commonly is performed in veterinary medicine to evaluate the integrity of the surgical repair.[36] Current recommended methods for leak testing involve occlusion of a 10-cm segment of intestine containing the surgical site followed by injection of 16 mL to 19 mL of sterile saline into the lumen with a 22-gauge hypodermic needle with visual observation for saline leakage from the suture line.[58,59] Intraoperative leak testing, although unable to predict the effect of perioperative and patient-dependent risk factors on intestinal healing, is able to evaluate the acute integrity of the surgical repair as well as serve as a valuable tool to surgeons in training. Although leak testing has been validated as a means of reducing postoperative leakage rates in human surgery,[60–66] a recent retrospective study evaluating postoperative dehiscence in dogs failed to establish an association between intraoperative anastomotic leak testing and reduction in the incidence of postoperative dehiscence in dogs undergoing R&A of the small intestine.[67] The author recommends use of intraoperative leak testing as a means of critically evaluating the

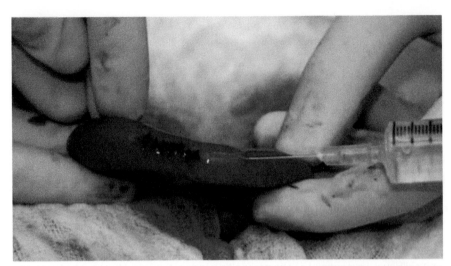

Fig. 10. Intraoperative leak testing performed by occluding a 10-cm segment of intestine containing the surgical site followed by injection of sterile saline into the lumen with a 22-gauge hypodermic needle.

surgical technique alone, especially for novice surgeons, to help eliminate poor surgical technique as a factor for dehiscence.

LAPAROSCOPIC AND LAPAROSCOPIC-ASSISTED GASTROINTESTINAL SURGERY

Traditionally, laparotomies have been used in veterinary medicine to perform abdominal exploratory surgery. This technique is associated, however, with greater morbidity, due to longer incisions and the potential for increased postoperative pain compared with laparoscopy, a minimally invasive technique.[68–71] With advances in both technology and experience, laparoendoscopic GI surgery has become the preferred method in many human GI procedures.[72,73] This minimally invasive approach also may be considered in dogs and cats with intestinal disease requiring an abdominal exploratory surgery; however, not all small animal patients are considered good candidates, and the surgeon must be thorough and willing to convert to a laparotomy if indicated.[74–80]

Patient selection is an important consideration when determining if laparoscopy would benefit a patient. In humans, contraindications for laparoscopic surgery include septic peritonitis, linear foreign bodies, presence of intraabdominal adhesions, and a patient unable to tolerate pneumoperitoneum.[68] There are similar recommendations in veterinary medicine, with additional considerations of intestinal lesion size and location, with lesions greater than 5 cm as well as lesions affecting the stomach, orad duodenum, or bowel aborad to the ileocecocolic junction less amicable to a minimally invasive approach.[74–77] There have been several recent reports of small animals, describing the use of diagnostic and therapeutic laparoscopic-assisted techniques in GI exploratory surgery using both multiport and single-port laparoscopic techniques, with reported excellent outcomes, and also reports of utilizing both intracorporeal and extracorporeal means of exploration.[74–80] Surgical procedures described using a laparoscopic or laparoscopic-assisted approach in small animal patients include intestinal biopsies, gastrotomies, enterotomies, resection, and anastomosis.[72–81] Reported complications using a laparoscopic approach to GI surgery

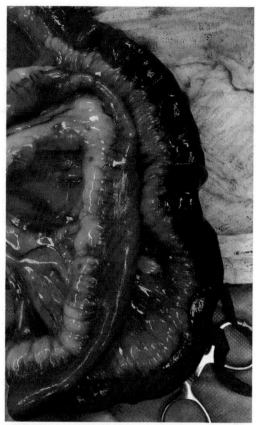

Fig. 11. Image of healthy canine small intestine alongside compromised canine bowel. Using intraoperative appearance of the bowel for determining the need for resection of devitalized tissue and evaluating intestinal color, thickness, presence of peristalsis, pulsations, and arterial bleeding.

include need for conversion to an open approach and inability to evaluate specific regions of the intestinal tract.[72,73] In conclusion, a minimally invasive approach may be used in small animal patients for both diagnostic and therapeutic indications in GI surgery, but factors, including surgeon experience, size and location of lesion, presence of peritonitis, presence of adhesions, willingness to convert, and other patient-dependent factors, should be considered.

TISSUE VIABILITY

Failure to resect devitalized small intestine can result in devastating consequences, including surgical site dehiscence, intestinal leakage, septic peritonitis, and death. Intestinal resection should be considered carefully, however, given the potential for adverse consequences, including short-bowel syndrome, need to reroute pancreatic and biliary ducts, and intestinal stricture formation postoperatively, as well as increased morbidity compared with an enterotomy alone.[36,82]

Traditionally, surgeons use experience and intraoperative appearance of the bowel for determining the need for resection of devitalized tissue and evaluate intestinal color, thickness, presence of peristalsis, pulsations, and arterial bleeding (**Fig. 11**).[83–85]

This method is highly subjective, and alternative methods have been described and include angiographic studies, infusion of arterial fluorescein dye, trans-serosal pulse oximetry, pulsed-wave Doppler ultrasonography, and laser Doppler flowmetry; but these methods have been found to have low sensitivity, specificity, and predictive values.[13,83,85–90] There is ongoing research in this field, including use of sidestream dark field videomicroscopy and real-time near-infrared fluorescence (NIRF), which may provide more sensitive and quantitative means of assessment. In humans, NIRF has become an increasingly popular intraoperative imaging modality, with extensive literature demonstrating its utility in gastroesophageal[91,92] and colorectal resections[93–97] and during emergency abdominal surgery.[98] Specifically, use of NIRF in emergency surgery modified a surgeon's operative strategy in 32% of patients.[98] Ultimately, there is a paucity of veterinary literature addressing accurate means of assessing GI viability intraoperatively. Utilization of these modalities has the potential to reduce the morbidity and mortality associated with emergent GI surgery in dogs significantly, and future studies to further evaluate these methods are needed in veterinary medicine.

SUMMARY

Intestinal dehiscence is a devastating consequence of intestinal surgery that requires surgical intervention, and mortality rates as high as 85% have been reported. Both handsewn and stapled anastomosis techniques commonly are used in veterinary medicine, with similar reported rates of dehiscence in the absence of septic peritonitis and stapled anastomoses resulting in shorter surgical time and reported ease of use in the hands of inexperienced surgeons. When performing FEESA, intestinal thickness should be considered when selecting staple size for anastomosis and may warrant use of larger staple size for proper tissue engagement as well as consideration for reinforcement techniques, such as oversewing the TA staple line and use of an omental wrap, which may aid in reducing postoperative dehiscence. Intraoperative anastomotic leak testing, although unable to predict intestinal healing postoperatively, provides a means to acutely evaluate the surgical repair and is a valuable tool for surgeons in training. A minimally invasive surgical approach may be used in small animal patients for both diagnostic and therapeutic indications in GI surgery. Patient selection is an important consideration, however, and surgeon experience and patient-dependent factors should be considered as well as willingness to convert. Determining when and where to resect compromised, and potentially devitalized, intestine is of utmost importance for patient outcome. Traditionally, surgeons use the subjective appearance of bowel for determining the needs for resection. Ongoing research is under way to determine more sensitive and quantitative methods to assess intestinal tissue viability, which may reduce the morbidity and mortality associated with emergent GI surgery in dogs significantly.

CLINICS CARE POINTS

- Surgical factors, such as surgical time, surgeon experience, presence of septic peritonitis, lumen disparity, location of anastomosis, and cost/availability of materials, all should be considered when deciding whether to perform a handsewn or stapled anastomosis for an intestinal R&A.
- Handsewn anastomoses are performed most commonly using an appositional pattern with suture placement no more than 3 mm apart and 3 mm to 4 mm from the wound margin

using monofilament, absorbable suture. FEESA traditionally is constructed with a combination of a TA stapler and GIA.

- When selecting staple size, intestinal thickness should be considered because mural thickness in canine intestine is 1.6-times greater than that of humans and may warrant use of a larger staple size in order to achieve proper tissue engagement. When performing FEESA, the author recommends evaluation of the intestinal thickness and use of a green staple cartridge for the transverse closure, especially with larger dogs, thickened bowel, or edematous bowel.

- The transverse staple line of FEESA and the crotch area have been reported as high-risk areas for dehiscence. Subsequently, reinforcing techniques, such as oversewing at the transverse staple line, omental wraps, and placing a suture in the crotch area, are recommended to aid in reducing postoperative dehiscence.

- Intraoperative leak testing is recommended as a means of critically evaluating the surgical technique alone, especially for novice surgeons, in order to help eliminate poor surgical technique as a factor for dehiscence; however, it is not able to predict intestinal healing postoperatively.

DISCLOSURE

The author has nothing to disclose.

SUPPLEMENTARY DATA

Supplementary data related to this article can be found online at https://doi.org/10.1016/j.cvsm.2021.11.002.

REFERENCES

1. Duell JR, Thieman Mankin KM, Rochat MC, et al. Frequency of Dehiscence in Hand-Sutured and Stapled Intestinal Anastomoses in Dogs. Vet Surg 2016; 45(1):100–3.
2. Ralphs SC, Jessen CR, Lipowitz AJ. Risk factors for leakage following intestinal anastomosis in dogs and cats. J Am Vet Med Assoc 2003;223:73–7.
3. Allen DA, Smeak DD, Schertel ER. Prevalence of small intestinal dehiscence and associated clinical factors: a retrospective study of 121 dogs. J Am Anim Hosp Assoc 1992;28:70–6.
4. Snowdon KA, Smeak DD, Chiang S. Risk factors for dehiscence of stapled functional end-to-end intestinal anastomoses in dogs: 53 cases (2001-2012). Vet Surg 2016;45(1):91–9.
5. DePompeo CM, Bond L, George YE, et al. Intra-abdominal complications following intestinal anastomoses by suture and staple techniques in dogs. J Am Vet Med Assoc 2018;253(4):437–43.
6. Davis DJ, Demianiuk RM, Musser J, et al. Influence of preoperative septic peritonitis and anastomotic technique on the dehiscence of enterectomy sites in dogs: A retrospective review of 210 anastomoses. Vet Surg 2018;47:125–9.
7. Brundage SI, Jurkovich GJ, Hoyt DB, et al. Stapled versus sutured gastrointestinal anastomosis in the trauma patient: a multicenter trial. J Trauma 2001;51: 1054–61.
8. Farrah JP, Lauer CW, Bray MS, et al. Stapled versus hand-sewn anastomoses in emergency general surgery: a retrospective review of outcomes in a unique patient population. J Trauma Acute Care Surg 2013;74:1187–92.

9. Ellison GW, Case JB, Regier PJ. Intestinal surgery in small animals: historical foundations, current thinking, and future horizons. Vet Surg 2019;48(7):1171–80.

10. Hardy KS. Suture anastomosis: an experimental study using limited suturing of the small bowel in the dog. Arch Surg 1968;97(4):586–9.

11. Mullen KM, Regier PJ, Waln M, et al. Gastrointestinal thickness, duration, and leak pressure of six intestinal anastomoses in dogs. Vet Surg 2020;49(7): 1315–25.

12. Kieves N, Krebs A, Zellner E. A Comparison of ex vivo leak pressures for four entertomy closures in a canine model. J Am Anim Hosp Assoc 2018;54:71–6.

13. Ellison GW, Jokinen MP, Park RD. End to end approximating anastomosis in the dog: a comparative fluorescein dye, angiographic and histopathologic evaluation. J Am Anim Hosp Assoc 1982;18(4):729–36.

14. Weisman DL, Smeak DD, Birchard SJ, et al. Comparison of a continuous suture pattern with a simple interrupted pattern for enteric closure in dogs and cats: 83 cases (1991–1997). J Am Vet Med Assoc 1999;214:1507–10.

15. Tasaka K, Farrar JT. Intraluminal pressure of the small intestine of the unanesthetized dog. Pflügers Arch 1976;364:35–44.

16. Fruehwald C, Regier PJ, Mullen K, et al. Comparison of gastrointestinal resection and anastomosis using simple interrupted and simple continuous patterns. Abst In: Society of Veterinary Soft Tissue Surgery; June 3-5, 2021; Online.

17. Van Winkle W, Hastings JC Jr. Considerations in the choice of suture material for various tissues. Surg Gynecol Obstet 1972;135:113–26.

18. M1 Milovancev, Weisman DL, Palmisano MP. Foreign body attachment to polypropylene suture material extruded into the small intestinal lumen after enteric closure in three dogs. J Am Vet Med Assoc 2004;225(11):1713–5.

19. Kirpensteijn J, Maarschalkerweerd RJ, van der Gaag I, et al. Comparison of three closure methods and two absorbable suture materials for closure of jejunal enterotomy incisions in healthy dogs. Vet Q 2001;23(2):67–70.

20. Schmiedt CW. Suture material, tissue staplers, ligation devices, and closure methods. In: Tobias KM, Johnston SA, editors. Veterinary surgery: small animal. 2nd edition. St Louis: Saunders; 2018. p. 210–24.

21. Paul MD. Bidirectional barbed sutures for wound closure: Evolution and applications. J Am Coll Certified Wound Specialists 2009;1:51–7.

22. Ruff G. Techniques and uses for absorbable barbed sutures. Aesth Surg J 2006; 26:620–8.

23. Matarasso A. Introduction to the barbed sutures supplement: The expanding applications of barbed sutures. Aesth Surg J 2012;33(3S):7S–11S.

24. Murtha A, Kaplan AL, Paglia MJ, et al. Evaluation of a novel technique for wound closure using a barbed suture. Plast Reconstr Surg 2006;117:1769–80.

25. Villa MT, White LE, Alam M, et al. Barbed sutures: a review of the literature. Plast Reconstr Surg 2008;121:102e–8e.

26. Ehrhart NP, Kaminskaya K, Miller JA, et al. In vivo assessment of absorbable knotless barbed suture for single layer gastrotomy and enterotomy closure. Vet Surg 2013;42:210–6.

27. Hansen L, Monnet EL. Evaluation of a novel suture material for closure of intestinal anastomoses in canine cadavers. Am J Vet Res 2012;73:1819–23.

28. Fealey MJ, Regier PJ, Steadman Bs C, et al. Initial leak pressures of four anastomosis techniques in cooled cadaveric canine jejunum. Vet Surg 2020;49(3): 480–6.

29. Miller J, Zaruby J, Kaminskaya K. Evaluation of a barbed suture device versus conventional suture in a canine enterotomy model. J Invest Surg 2012;25:107–11.

30. Smeak DD, Turner H, Hoon-Hanks L. Intramural abscess causing obstruction at a previous jejunal enterotomy site in a dog. J Am Anim Hosp Assoc 2018;54(5): 545–606.
31. Spah CE, Elkins AD, Wehrenberg A, et al. Evaluation of two novel self-anchoring barbed sutures in a prophylactic laparoscopic gastropexy compared with intracorporeal tied knots. Vet Surg 2013;42:932–42.
32. Arbaugh M, Case JB, Monnet E. Biomechanical comparison of glycomer 631 and glycomer 631 knotless for use in canine incisional gastropexy. Vet Surg 2013;42: 205–9.
33. Imhoff DJ, Cohen A, Monnet E. Biomechanical analysis of laparoscopic incisional gastropexy with intracorporeal suturing using knotless polyglyconate. Vet Surg 2015;44:39–43.
34. Takacs JD, Singh A, Case JB, et al. Total laparoscopic gastropexy using 1 simple continuous barbed suture line in 63 dogs. Vet Surg 2017;46(2):233–41.
35. Tobias KM. Surgical Stapling Devices in Veterinary Medicine: A Review. Vet Surg 2007;36:41–349.
36. Giuffrida MA, Brown DC. Small intestine. In: Tobias KM, Johnston SA, editors. Veterinary surgery: small animal. 2nd edition. St Louis: Saunders; 2018. p. 1730–60.
37. White RN. Modified functional end-to-end stapled intestinal anastomosis: technique and clinical results in 15 dogs. J Small Anim Pract 2008;49:274–81.
38. Jardel N, Hidalgo A, Leperlier D, et al. One stage functional end-to-end stapled intestinal anastomosis and resection performed by nonexpert surgeons for the treatment of small intestinal obstruction in 30 dogs. Vet Surg 2011;40(2):216–22.
39. Ullman SL, Pavletic MM, Clark GN. Open intestinal anastomosis with surgical stapling equipment in 24 dogs and cats. Vet Surg 1991;20:385–91.
40. Ullman SL. Surgical stapling of the small intestine. Vet Clin North Am: Small Anim Pract 1994;24:305–22.
41. Sumner SM, Regier PJ, Case JB, et al. Evaluation of suture reinforcement for stapled intestinal anastomoses: 77 dogs (2008-2018). Vet Surg 2019;48(7):1188–93.
42. Duffy DJ, Moore GE. Influence of oversewing the transverse staple line during functional end-to- end stapled intestinal anastomoses in dogs. Vet Surg 2020; 49(6):1221–9.
43. Sarria R, Latorre R, Henroteaux M, et al. Morphometric study of the layers of the canine small intestine at five sampling sites. Vet J 2012;192:498–502.
44. Ellison GW. Wound healing in the gastrointestinal tract. Semin Vet Med Surg Small Anim 1989;4:287–93.
45. Hansen LA, Smeak DD. In vitro comparison of leakage pressure and leakage location for various staple line offset configurations in functional end-to-end stapled small intestinal anastomoses of canine tissues. Am J Vet Res 2015;76(7): 644–8.
46. Ellison GW. Complications of gastrointestinal surgery in companion animals. Vet Clin North Am Small Anim Pract 2011;41(5):915–34, vi.
47. Novacek V, Trn TN, Klinge U, et al. Finite element modelling of stapled colorectal end-to-end anastomosis: advantages of variable height stapler design. J Biomech 2012;45:2693–7.
48. Sheppard CE. Laparoscopic sleeve gastrectomy with Tri-Staple™ reinforcement for severe obesity. Surg Curr Res 2013;03:144.
49. Coolman BR, Ehrhart N, Marretta SM. Use of skin staples for rapid closure of gastrointestinal incisions in the treatment of canine linear foreign bodies. J Am Anim Hosp Assoc 2000;36(6):542–7.

50. Coolman BR, Ehrhart N, Pijanowski G, et al. Comparison of skin staples with sutures for anastomosis of the small intestine in dogs. Vet Surg 2000;29(4):293–302.

51. Rosenbaum JM, Coolman BR, Davidson BL, et al. The use of disposable skin staples for intestinal resection and anastomosis in 63 dogs: 2000 to 2014. J Small Anim Pract 2016 Nov;57(11):631–6.

52. Schwartz Z, Coolman BR. Disposable skin staplers for closure of linear gastrointestinal incisions in dogs. Vet Surg 2018;47(2):285–92.

53. Schwartz Z, Coolman BR. Closure of gastrointestinal incisions using skin staples alone and in combination with suture in 29 cats. J Small Anim Pract 2018;59(5): 281–5.

54. Catena F, La Donna M, Gagliardi S, et al. Stapled versus hand-sewn anastomoses in emergency intestinal surgery: results of a prospective randomized study. Surg Today 2004;34:123–6.

55. Hansen LA, Monnet EL. Evaluation of serosal patch supplementation of surgical anastomoses in intestinal segments from canine cadavers. Am J Vet Res 2013; 74:1138–41.

56. Morison R. Remarks on some functions of the omentum. Br Med J 1906;1:76.

57. McLackin AD, Denton DW. Omental protection of intestinal anastomosis. Am J Surg 1973;125:134–40.

58. Saile K, Boothe HW, Boothe DM. Saline volume necessary to achieve predetermined intraluminal pressures during leak testing of small intestinal biopsy sites in the dog. Vet Surg 2010;39:900–3.

59. Brand KJ, Hess E, Risselada M. Effects of needle gauge and syringe size on small intestinal leakage at injection sites. Vet Surg 2019;48:1237–44.

60. Gilbert JM, Trapnell JE. Intraoperative testing of the integrity of left-sided colorectal anastomoses—a technique of value to the surgeon in training. Ann R Coll Surg Engl 1988;70:158–60.

61. Wu Z, van de Haar RC, Sparreboom CL, et al. Is the intraoperative air leak test effective in the prevention of colorectal anastomotic leakage? A systematic review and meta-analysis. Int J Colorectal Dis 2016;31:1409–17.

62. Allaix ME, Lena A, Degiuli M, et al. Intraoperative air leak test reduces the rate of postoperative anastomotic leak: analysis of 777 laparoscopic left-sided colon resections. Surg Endosc 2019;33:1592–9.

63. Wheeler JM, Gilbert JM. Controlled intraoperative water testing of left-sided colorectal anastomoses: are ileostomies avoidable? Ann R Coll Surg Engl 1999;81: 105–8.

64. Kwon S, Morris A, Billingham R, et al. Routine leak testing in colorectal surgery in the surgical care and outcomes assessment program. Arch Surg 2012;147: 345–51.

65. Beard JD, Nicholson ML, Sayers RD, et al. Intraoperative air testing of colorectal anastomoses: a prospective, randomized trial. Br J Surg 1990;77:1095–7.

66. Ricciardi R, Roberts PL, Marcello PW, et al. Anastomotic leak testing after colorectal resection: what are the data? Arch Surg 2009;144:407–12.

67. Mullen KM, Regier PJ, Fox-Alvarez WA, et al. Evaluation of intraoperative leak testing of small intestinal anastomoses performed by hand-sewn and stapled techniques in dogs: 131 cases (2008-2019). J Am Vet Med Assoc 2021;258(9): 991–8.

68. Litwin DE, Cahan M, Sneider EB. Laparoscopic treatment of disorders of the small bowel. In: Swanstrom LL, Soper NJ, editors. Mastery of Endoscopic and laparoscopic surgery. 4th edition. Williams, & Wilkins: Lippincott; 2014.

69. Case JB, Boscan PL, Monnet EL, et al. Comparison of surgical variables and pain in cats undergoing ovariohysterectomy, laparoscopic-assisted ovariohysterectomy, and laparoscopic ovariectomy. J Am Anim Hosp Assoc 2015;51:1–7.

70. Gauthier O, Holopherne-Doran D, Gendarme T, et al. Assessment of postoperative pain in cats after ovariectomy by laparoscopy, median celiotomy, or flank laparotomy. Vet Surg 2015;44:23–30.

71. Coisman JG, Case JB, Shih A, et al. Comparison of surgical variables in cats undergoing single incision laparoscopic ovariectomy using a LigaSure or extracorporeal suture versus open ovariectomy. Vet Surg 2014;43:38–44.

72. Khaikin M, Schneidereit N, Cera S, et al. Laparoscopic vs open surgery for acute adhesive small-bowel obstruction: patients' out- come and cost-effectiveness. Surg Endosc 2007;21(5):742–6.

73. Delaney CP, Chang E, Senagore AJ, et al. Clinical outcomes and resource utilization associated with laparoscopic and open colectomy using a large national database. Ann Surg 2008;247(5):819–24.

74. Gower SB, Mayhew PD. A wound retraction device for laparoscopic- assisted intestinal surgery in dogs and cats. Vet Surg 2011;40(4):485–8.

75. Case JB, Ellison G. Single incision laparoscopic-assisted intestinal surgery (SI-LAIS) in 7 dogs and 1 cat. Vet Surg 2013;42(5):629–34.

76. Mitterman L, Bonczynski J, Hearon K, et al. Comparison of perioperative and short-term postoperative complications of gastrointestinal biopsies via laparoscopic-assisted technique versus laparotomy. Can Vet J 2016;57(4):395–400.

77. Barry KS, Case JB, Winter MD, et al. Diagnostic usefulness of laparoscopy versus exploratory laparotomy dogs with suspected gastrointestinal obstruction. J Am Vet Med Assoc 2017;251:307–14.

78. Baron J, Giuffrida M, Mayhew PD, et al. Minimally invasive small intestinal exploration and targeted abdominal organ biopsy with a wound retraction device in 42 cats (2005-2015). Vet Surg 2017;46:925–32.

79. McClaran JK, Skerrett SC, Currao RL, et al. Com- parison of laparoscopic-assisted technique and open laparotomy for gastrointestinal biopsy in cats. Vet Surg 2017;46:821–8.

80. Otomo A, Singh A, Valverde A, et al. Comparison of outcome in dogs undergoing single-incision laparoscopic-assisted intestinal surgery and open laparotomy for simple small intestinal foreign body removal. Vet Surg 2018;48(S1):O83–90.

81. Lew M, Jalynski M, Brzeski W. Laparoscopic removal of gastric foreign bodies in dogs—comparison of manual suturing and stapling viscerosynthesis. Pol J Vet Sci 2005;8(2):147–53.

82. Willard M. Short bowel syndrome. In: Bojrab MJ, Monnet E, editors. Mechanisms of disease in small animal surgery. 3rd edition. Jackson, Wyo: Teton NewMedia; 2010. p. 196–9.

83. Erikoglu M, Kaynak A, Beyatli EA, et al. Intraoperative determination of intestinal viability: a comparison with transserosal pulse oximetry and histopathological examination. J Surg Res 2005;128:66–9.

84. Karliczek A, Harlaar NJ, Zeebregts CJ, et al. Surgeons lack predictive accuracy for anastomotic leakage in gastrointestinal surgery. Int J Colorectal Dis 2009;24:569–76.

85. Bulkley GB, Zuidema GD, Hamilton SR, et al. Intraoperative determination of small intestinal viability following ischemic injury: a prospective, controlled trial of two adjuvant methods (Doppler and fluorescein) compared with standard clinical judgment. Ann Surg 1981;193:628–37.

86. Urbanavicius L, Pattyn P, de Putte DV, et al. How to assess intestinal viability during surgery: a review of techniques. World J Gastrointest Surg 2011;3:59–69.
87. Monnet E, Pelsue D, MacPhail C. Evaluation of laser Doppler flowmetry for measurement of capillary blood flow in the stomach wall of dogs during gastric dilatation-volvulus. Vet Surg 2006;35:198–205.
88. Smith CR, Cokelet GR, Adams JT, et al. Vascularity of gastrointestinal staple lines demonstrated with silicone rubber injection. Am J Surg 1981;142:563–6.
89. Horgan PG, Gorey TF. Operative assessment of intestinal viability. Surg Clin North Am 1992;72:143–55.
90. Tuŕkyilmaz Z, Söhmez K, Bacaklar AC, et al. Assessment of anastomotic reliability with pulse oximetry in graded intestinal ischemia: an experimental study in dogs. J Pediatr Surg 1997;32:1728–31.
91. Ishige F, Nabeya Y, Hoshino I, et al. Quantitative Assessment of the Blood Perfusion of the Gastric Conduit by Indocyanine Green Imaging. J Surg Res 2019;234: 303–10.
92. Ohi M, Toiyama Y, Mohri Y, et al. Prevalence of anastomotic leak and the impact of indocyanine green fluorescein imaging for evaluating blood flow in the gastric conduit following esophageal cancer surgery. Esophagus 2017;14:351–9.
93. Degett TH, Andersen HS, Gogenur I. Indocyanine green fluorescence angiography for intraoperative assessment of gastrointestinal anastomotic perfusion: a systematic review of clinical trials. Langenbecks Arch Surg 2016;401:767–75.
94. Protyniak B, Dinallo AM, Boyan WP Jr, et al. Intraoperative indocyanine green fluorescence angiography–an objective evaluation of anastomotic perfusion in colorectal surgery. Am Surg 2015;81:580–4.
95. Kudszus S, Roesel C, Schachtrupp A, et al. Intraoperative laser fluorescence angiography in colorectal surgery: a noninvasive analysis to reduce the rate of anastomotic leakage. Langenbecks Arch Surg 2010;395:1025–30.
96. Shen R, Zhang Y, Wang T. Indocyanine Green Fluorescence Angiography and the Incidence of Anastomotic Leak After Colorectal Resection for Colorectal Cancer: A Meta-analysis. Dis Colon Rectum 2018;61:1228–34.
97. De Nardi P, Elmore U, Maggi G, et al. Intraoperative angiography with indocyanine green to assess anastomosis perfusion in patients undergoing laparoscopic colorectal resection: results of a multicenter randomized controlled trial. Surg Endosc 2020;34:53–60.
98. Liot E, Assalino M, Buchs NC, et al. Does near-infrared (NIR) fluorescence angiography modify operative strategy during emergency procedures? Surg Endosc 2018;32:4351–6.

Current Concepts in Parathyroid/Thyroid Surgery

Katy L. Townsend, BVSc(hons), MS, DACVS[a],*,
Kathleen M. Ham, DVM, MS, DACVS-SA[b]

KEYWORDS

- Thyroid • Dog • Cat • Hypercalcemia • Primary hyperparathyroidism
- Functional testing • Staging • Surgery

KEY POINTS

- Approximately 40% of patients that have primary hyperparathyroidism is asymptomatic, and hypercalcemia is detected incidentally on laboratory work. Concurrent hypercalcemia with parathyroid hormone concentrations within reference ranges or elevated is consistent with autonomous hyperfunctional parathyroid tissue.
- Surgery is the most successful treatment modality for primary hyperparathyroidism with a good prognosis, and hypocalcemia is the most common complication requiring treatment.
- Dogs should undergo functional testing when diagnosed with a thyroid tumor because of higher rates of functional tumors than previously reported.
- Thyroidectomy should be considered for dogs even with advanced disease because of potential long-term control. Local lymph nodes should be removed during surgery.
- Hemorrhage is the most common complication with thyroidectomy, and hemostatic devices should be used.

PARATHYROID SURGERY
Introduction and History

Primary disease of the parathyroid glands in dogs and cats is relatively uncommon compared with the incidence in people, although, over the last few decades, the incidence of primary hyperparathyroidism (PHPT) has increased in both.[1,2] The most common parathyroid disease in dogs and cats is PHPT, a condition causing hypercalcemia that occurs when one or more parathyroid glands become hyperfunctional and secrete

[a] Veterinary Clinical Sciences, Carlson College of Veterinary Medicine, Oregon State University, 277 Magruder Hall, Corvallis, OR 97330, USA; [b] Department of Small Animal Clinical Sciences, University of Florida, 2089 Southwest 16th Avenue, Gainesville, FL 32608, USA
* Corresponding.
E-mail address: katy.townsend@oregonstate.edu

Vet Clin Small Anim 52 (2022) 455–471
https://doi.org/10.1016/j.cvsm.2021.12.004
0195-5616/22/© 2021 Elsevier Inc. All rights reserved.

parathyroid hormone (PTH) with no response to feedback loops. Treatment with surgery or glandular ablation is strongly recommended, as the prognosis is very good.

Increased emphasis on the human-animal bond has led to an increased emphasis on animal health and improvement in diagnostic and therapeutic options. Asymptomatic detection of hypercalcemia has increased, likely because of routine blood screening tests for age or peri–anesthesia events.[1,2]

Definitions

PHPT is a functional disease of the parathyroid glands that can be caused by solitary adenomas, multiple adenomas, hyperplasia, or carcinomas, and the distinction has been based on histopathology and surgical and clinical findings. Most animals have sporadic PHPT, whereas some Keeshonds have a genetically transmitted form of PHPT, and there are case reports of animals with multiple endocrine neoplasia.[3,4]

A single adenoma is the most common cause of PHTP in dogs with a reported incidence of 60% to 90% in retrospective studies and multiglandular disease 10% to 40% of the time.[5–7] Parathyroid carcinomas are less common. One case reported metastasis to a mediastinal lymph node, whereas a larger study in 19 dogs had no evidence of metastasis at the time of surgery with surgical excision of the tumor providing an excellent prognosis.[8,9] Primary hyperplasia of the parathyroid glands has been defined as proliferation of multiple parathyroid glands with no known stimulus.[10] This disease has been reported, although the reports find that patients have similar outcomes to those with an adenoma.[11] Histopathology to discriminate hyperplasia versus adenoma may present a challenge, as immunohistochemistry labeling found similar uptake with both hyperplasia and adenoma.[12] Patients with PHPT should be monitored after treatment; recurrence is approximately 7% to 10%.[13,14]

Secondary hyperparathyroidism (SHPT) is characterized by increased PTH concentrations and low or normal calcium. Conditions that lead to SHPT include renal failure, vitamin D deficiency, decreased calcium intake, and malabsorption. Tertiary hyperparathyroidism (THPT) is a condition reflecting the development of abnormal parathyroid function following a period of SHPT resulting in increased concentrations of PTH and ionized calcium. Patients with THPT typically have hypercalcemia, hyperphosphatemia, and increased PTH concentrations. Treatment of the primary or underlying condition should be attempted, and if unable to control the hypercalcemia, surgery to remove some or all of the parathyroid glands may be recommended.

There are many differentials for hypercalcemia in dogs and cats with the most common being hypercalcemia of malignancy, PHPT, renal disease, Addison, and idiopathic (specifically in cats).[15] Humoral hypercalcemia of malignancy can lead to parathyroid hormone related protein (PTHrP) secretion, which causes calcium resorption and phosphorus excretion, increased osteoclastic bone resorption, and overall reduced renal calcium excretion.[10] Neoplastic diseases that can cause hypercalcemia include apocrine gland anal sac adenocarcinoma, lymphoma, thymoma, multiple myeloma, carcinomas, and several other reported cancers.

Epidemiology and Genetics

The mean reported age of dogs diagnosed with PHPT is 11.2 years (range, 4 to 17 years).[1] There is no sex predilection detected in retrospective studies. Keeshonds have an odds ratio of 50.7 for developing PHPT, and they tend to be younger at diagnosis and more likely to have recurrence.[3,14] Segregation analysis was used to determine that PHPT in Keeshonds is an autosomal dominant genetically transmitted disease. Keeshonds can be screened for the PHPT gene, allowing monitoring if positive for the PHPT gene and responsible breeding.[16]

Clinical Presentation and Diagnostics

Patients presenting with PHPT tend to have mild insidious clinical signs, with duration varying from 0 days to 2.5 years.[1] Approximately 40% of patients diagnosed with PHPT are asymptomatic or presenting for reasons unrelated to hypercalcemia[1]; however, owners could decipher clinical signs with specific prompts. The clinical manifestations of PHPT are caused by hypercalcemia and tend to affect the gastrointestinal, urinary, and musculoskeletal systems (**Box 1**). Physical examination findings are often unremarkable, and it is almost impossible to palpate the abnormal parathyroid gland. Along with a careful and thorough physical examination, emphasis should be placed on peripheral lymph node and anal sac palpation (**Box 2**).

Complete blood counts are often normal but may show changes consistent with dehydration. A chemistry profile will reveal hypercalcemia and a low or low normal phosphorus most commonly. PTH acts on the kidney to increase renal excretion of phosphorus, increase tubular calcium reabsorption, and create calcitriol. Feldman and Miner[13] evaluated 185 dogs and found the mean (range) of total calcium, 14.5 mg/dL (12.1–23.4); ionized calcium, 1.71 mmol/L (1.22–2.41); and phosphorus, 2.8 mg/dL (1.3–6.1) in dogs with PHTP. Identifying low or normal phosphorus can help rule out renal disease and SHPT, as phosphorus is typically elevated with those disease processes. Renal failure in dogs with PHPT has been reported but is relatively uncommon most likely because of the low calcium phosphorus product. Dogs with hyperphosphatemia and an elevated calcium phosphorus product develop calcium phosphate precipitation in the renal interstitium, leading to interstitial fibrosis and tubular atrophy and progression of kidney failure.[17] Urinalysis should be evaluated, and urine culture should be submitted, as approximately 29% of dogs had urinary tract infections and 31% of dogs had urolithiasis[1] at time of diagnosis. It is common to find isosthenuria, hyposthenuria, crystalluria, bacteriuria, and pyuria.

Following detection of elevated ionized calcium, a malignancy panel will further help diagnose the cause of hypercalcemia. Evaluation of PTH and PTHrP must be performed with a concurrent ionized calcium to establish a relationship between the calcium and PTH. Extracellular calcium will bind to calcium-sensing receptors in the parathyroid glands and provide feedback for synthesis and secretion of PTH. When extracellular calcium is high, PTH secretion should be significantly reduced or

---

Box 1
Clinical manifestations of dogs with primary hyperparathyroidism

Gastrointestinal
- Vomiting
- Inappetence

Musculoskeletal
- Lethargy
- Decreased activity
- Weakness
- Difficulty rising
- Muscle wasting
- Shivering/shaking

Urinary
- Polyuria/polydipsia
- Stranguria
- Pollakiuria
- Incontinence

Box 2	
Recommended workup for suspect primary hyperparathyroidism	
Diagnostics	**Results consistent with PHPT**
Physical exam • Lymph node and anal sac palpation	Unremarkable
Complete blood count and biochemical profile	Hypercalcemia, low normal phosphorus
Urinalysis	Low urinary specific gravity, +/- calcium oxalate crystals, +/- bacteria
Urine culture	+/- infection
PTH malignancy panel	Hypercalcemia, normal or elevated PTH, 0 PTHrP
Thoracic and abdominal imaging	+/- urinary stones
Cervical ultrasound	Enlarged parathyroid gland(s)

stopped. Therefore, PTH concentrations that are normal or high with concurrent hypercalcemia are consistent with PHPT; parathyroid glands autonomously make PTH regardless of negative feedback. Patients with PHPT should have no PTHrP, but the absence of PTHrP does not exclude hypercalcemia of malignancy.

Thoracic radiographs are used to assess the cranial mediastinum, thoracic lymph nodes, bones, and lung. Patients with a cranial mediastinal mass, lymphadenopathy, or pulmonary metastasis are more likely to have hypercalcemia of malignancy. Abdominal radiographs can assess the bones, liver, and spleen, which may be enlarged with lymphoma, the abdominal lymph nodes, and the urinary tract for the presence of calculi. If a patient has urinary calculi and PHPT, cystotomy at the time of parathyroidectomy would be indicated.

Parathyroid Gland Imaging

Assessment of the parathyroid glands and localization of the abnormal gland are strongly recommended before surgery to reduce morbidity and improve success. In people, nuclear scintigraphy is commonly used before and during surgery, but was not found to be reliable in dogs.[10,18] The use of computed tomography (CT) in normal dogs having cervical imaging has made parathyroid detection a challenge with poor visibility, although there have been no studies specifically using CT for detection of abnormal parathyroid glands.[19] Ultrasound is recognized as the most reliable imaging modality for parathyroid assessment and localization, with varying reported sensitivity and specificity[5,6,20] (**Fig. 1**). One ultrasound study evaluated the size of the gland to correlate that to the histopathologic diagnosis.[20] In a large retrospective study of 142 masses from a single institution, ultrasound found the median greatest diameter of 6 mm (range, 3–23 mm), with 85 of the masses being 4 to 6 mm.[1] Another study found that parathyroid carcinomas were less homogenous and usually larger, but ultrasound size should not be used as the sole criterion for differentiating hyperplasia from neoplasia and normal versus abnormal parathyroid glands owing to the wide range in size.[21] Comparison of ultrasound and surgery found agreement in the number of glands at 65.9% and side of the affected gland at 72.3% of the time.[22]

Treatment and Outcome

Patients with PHPT do not typically require medical or acute therapies for their hypercalcemia; the severity of hypercalcemia is mild to moderate. The surgical technique for parathyroidectomy is well described and allows for visual and tactile evaluation. Most animals will have 2 parathyroid glands external to the thyroid capsule near the cranial

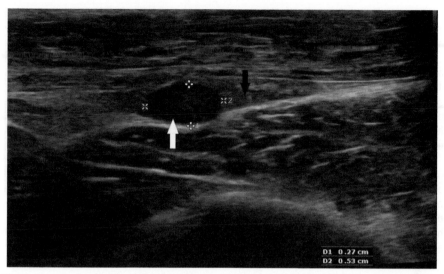

Fig. 1. Longitudinal view of the thyroid lobe (*black arrow*) with a 0.27 cm × 0.53 cm hypo-echoic parathyroid nodule (*white arrow*).

pole of the thyroid lobe and 2 parathyroid glands internal to the thyroid capsule. Abnormal parathyroid glands are often round, pink, red, or tan and firm (**Fig. 2**). After careful evaluation of each thyroid lobe, the abnormal parathyroid gland or glands should be removed, being careful to prevent iatrogenic injury to the remaining

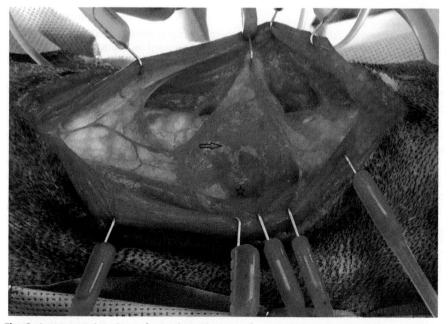

Fig. 2. Intraoperative view of parathyroidectomy for a parathyroid adenoma. Star shows enlarged parathyroid gland adjacent to thyroid lobe labeled with large open arrow.

parathyroid glands. Use of magnification, bipolar cautery, and fine instruments can aid in meticulous dissection to avoid damaging structures, such as the recurrent laryngeal nerve and carotid sheath. The reported success rate of surgery is 92% to 95%.[5]

Intraoperative PTH monitoring is a common tool used in people to confirm removal of all hyperfunctional tissue before ending surgery.[10] PTH has a short half-life, lending itself to rapid intraoperative measurement using a rapid point-of-care chemilumines-cent assay. The concentration of PTH will have a greater than 50% decrease between preoperative and postoperative concentration 10 minutes after excision of the hyper-functional gland, and this has been used in dogs to confirm removal of hyperfunctional tissue.[5]

Alternatives to surgery include glandular ablation with heat or ethanol. Both tech-niques use ultrasound guidance to identify the abnormal gland and observe the cath-eter or stylet insertion into the gland. Dogs with concurrent hypothyroidism or a large parathyroid nodular size have been found to be associated with failure of heat abla-tion.[23] Ethanol ablation has a reported success rate of 72% to 85%.[24] Heat ablation has a reported success rate of 72% to 90%.[23] These procedures typically still require anesthesia and may require multiple treatments, and reported complications include laryngeal paralysis, Horner syndrome, pneumonia, change in bark, cough, persistent hypercalcemia, and hypocalcemia.[25,26]

Long-term medical management for dogs with PHPT is not recommended, as the success rates with surgery are good and the options for medical management are so limited.

Although PHPT is even less common in cats, the workup and approach are similar, along with surgery being treatment of choice with a good prognosis. Parathyroid masses may be more likely cystic in cats[27] (**Fig. 3**).

Complications

Hypercalcemia

Dogs can have persistent or recurrent hypercalcemia following treatment. Persistent hypercalcemia occurs within 4 to 6 months of treatment and is typically thought to be unresolved disease.[5,10] Differentials for failed therapy include failure to detect the correct hyperfunctional gland such as removing thyroid tissue, lymphoid tissue, removing the wrong parathyroid gland, or dogs with multiglandular disease whereby one or more glands were missed at the initial operation. Parathyroid ectopia is another reason for surgical failure and persistent hypercalcemia. Parathyroid tissue may span from the base of the tongue to the cranial mediastinum. Ectopic parathyroid glands are known to occur in dogs and cats, but the incidence is not known, and the clinical sig-nificance has not been investigated.[28] If persistent disease occurs, repeating initial di-agnostics to include a malignancy panel to confirm the diagnosis, cervical ultrasound, or additional imaging, such as CT or MRI, should also be considered.[9,10] Additional imaging and modalities that have been reported in people include SPECT-CT (sin-gle-photon emission computed tomography-CT), PET-CT, 4-dimensional CT, and fluorescence-guided imaging.[10,29] Selective venous sampling to localize the hyper-functional tissue with serial PTH concentration assessments using fluoroscopic guid-ance is used in people and has been described in dogs.[10,30]

Hypercalcemia that is from a separate disease process, also considered recurrent hypercalcemia occurring after 6 months from the surgical intervention, may be due to a second autonomously hyperfunctional gland, primary hyperplasia, or carcinoma metastasis. It is also more likely in Keeshonds.[14] The workup should be similar to the initial workup, as it is presumed there is another parathyroid gland that is diseased.

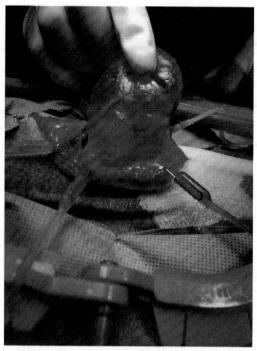

Fig. 3. Intraoperative photograph of a parathyroid cyst in a cat.

Surgery to remove additional hyperfunctional tissue can produce a good outcome and is recommended if an abnormal gland is localized.[5]

Hypocalcemia

Postoperative hypocalcemia is the most common complication and has been reported to occur frequently, ranging from 30% to 58% following treatment.[6] Hypocalcemia typically occurs within the first 1 to 3 days after surgery, but calcium may continue to drop for a week or longer.[13] Clinical signs of hypocalcemia include anxiety, rubbing of the face or extremities, muscle fasciculations, panting, ataxia, and seizures. Hypocalcemia can result in increased expenses associated with treatment, and increased morbidity, such as emergency hypocalcemia treatments, death, and prolonged hospitalization. Some texts and studies describe an increased risk of developing hypocalcemia if the total calcium concentration is greater than 14 mg/dL or with high preoperative ionized calcium greater than 1.75 mmol/L.[13,31] Many studies have not been able to elucidate definite risk factors for developing hypocalcemia.[32] One study of 62 dogs found that preoperative total calcium concentration was not predictive, but that a history of weakness, PTH concentrations above reference ranges, low serum calcium phosphorus product, and high blood urea nitrogen was associated with low postoperative calcium.[6] Newer studies have further defined subclinical hypocalcemia as those patients that have low ionized calcium concentrations and no clinical manifestations versus having clinical signs.[22] This study was not able to explain risk factors for either group but found that a preoperative iCa ≥1.75 mEq/L was associated with postoperative hypocalcemia.

If postoperative hypocalcemia occurs, PTH, phosphorus, vitamin D metabolites, and magnesium concentrations should be evaluated to help discern the mechanism.

If the PTH is low or absent, then the patient is experiencing some type of hypoparathyroidism. The primary mechanism for postoperative hypocalcemia is thought to be from suppression of the normal parathyroid tissue; these glands should recover function, but the time of recovery is different for each case. Surgical or iatrogenic damage can be classified as transient or permanent and occurs with radical cervical surgeries, complete thyroidectomy, or inadvertent damage to the normal parathyroid glands or blood supply. If the PTH is elevated, the patient may have hungry bone syndrome especially if they presented with bone disease before parathyroidectomy. This develops when calcium is rapidly deposited into the bone following surgery. Although this is rare, in people, risk factors for hungry bone syndrome include old age, radiographic evidence of bone disease, high alkaline phosphatase, and vitamin D deficiency.[10] Some patients may have concurrent hypomagnesemia for other reasons; if so, the magnesium should be corrected, as patients with hypomagnesemia have inhibition of PTH secretion and peripheral PTH resistance.[10]

Supplemental treatment is needed for patients that become hypocalcemic, patients that are clinical for hypocalcemia, or if the calcium is falling rapidly to prevent serious complications of hypocalcemia. The timing of treatment has not been validated, and one study found that prophylactic treatment with calcitriol did not provide any protection from developing hypocalcemia.[7] Supplementation can be provided parentally with calcium gluconate or ideally enterally with calcium carbonate and calcitriol. Intravenous infusion can be associated with risks of cardiac arrhythmias (bradycardia) and tissue necrosis if extravasated and should only be used in urgent or emergent situations (**Fig. 4**). Strict rest after surgery is recommended to limit calcium requirement for muscle metabolism. Patients can be hospitalized to monitor iCa every 8 to 12 hours until the calcium concentration plateaus with or without supplementation, or prophylactic supplementation can be provided, and the patient can be managed as an outpatient. Once supplementation is initiated, ideally it is tapered over weeks to months as needed for each patient.

In the authors' practice, ionized calcium is monitored every 12 hours after surgery. If the iCa drops $\geq$0.3 within a 12-hour interval, or if the iCa does not plateau within 48 hours after surgery, calcitriol supplementation is started. The initial dose is 20 to 30 ng/kg twice a day for 3 to 5 days with a recheck of iCa in 3 to 5 days. If calcium is high or normal, the dose is tapered to 10 to 15 ng/kg twice a day for 1 week with a recheck of iCa within 1 week. If the calcium is high or normal, the dose is tapered to 5 to 10 ng/kg twice a day for 1 week, with a recheck of iCa within 1 week. If the calcium is high or normal, the dose is tapered to 5 ng/kg per day for 1 week, then 5 ng/kg every other day for 1 week. Some cases may require higher dosing of calcitriol for longer intervals or supplemental calcium carbonate. The dose for calcium carbonate is 30 to 60 mg/kg once to twice daily, and the authors' preferred calcium product is Caltrate Bone. If the patient is still requiring supplementation within 3 months, PTH and vitamin D concentrations are assessed to further define the differentiate the problem.

Parathyroid Summary

PHPT is an uncommon disease but a common cause of hypercalcemia.[15] Most patients are older at the time of diagnosis; many are asymptomatic, and urinary stones and urinary tract infections are common. Treatment is recommended, as the prognosis is usually excellent regardless of the histopathologic diagnosis. Complications can occur with hypocalcemia being the most frequent, but this is easily managed with supplementation and monitoring. Current areas needing additional research include localization, histopathology, risk factors for hypocalcemia, and standardization of supplementation.

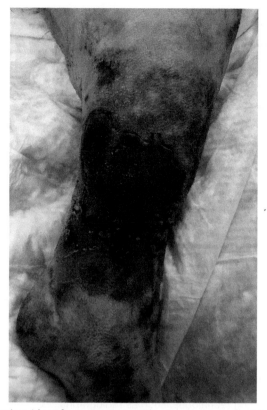

Fig. 4. Tissue necrosis evident from a patient with extravasation of calcium.

THYROID SURGERY
Introduction

Thyroid tumors in dogs are the most common endocrine neoplasms.[33] They have a prevalence of 1% to 4%, depending on age and breed, and represent 1.1% to 3.8% of canine cancers.[33] Thyroid carcinomas can arise from thyroid follicular cells (follicular cell thyroid carcinoma [FTC] most common) or parafollicular cells (C cell; medullary thyroid carcinomas). Follicular cell carcinomas are further subclassified into follicular, compact, or solid, follicular-compact (the most common subclassification), papillary, or undifferentiated. Parafollicular (medullary) tumors may be underdiagnosed because of the inability to differentiate from FTC. Immunohistochemistry (calcitonin and neuroendocrine tissue markers) is needed for differentiation.[34]

Preoperative Workup

Dogs with thyroid tumors are typically older[35]; therefore, patients should have a minimum data base, including complete blood count, biochemical profile, and urinalysis. Because of the highly vascular nature of thyroid tumors, a coagulation panel, blood type, and cross-match to available blood products should be considered to mitigate hemorrhage as a complication.

Functionality testing

Historically, thyroid tumors in dogs were thought to be mainly nonfunctional. Recent studies have shown that dogs with functional thyroid tumors may be more common, showing a rate of functionality to be up to 41%.[36] Dogs with functional thyroid tumors have clinical signs consistent with hyperthyroidism[37,38] (**Box 3**). Dogs with functional thyroid tumors had a median total thyroxine (TT4) level 56% above the upper reference range.[37] This study found that all dogs had elevated TT4; 9/10 had elevated free thyroxine (T4), and 11/12 had low thyrotropin. After surgical resection for functional thyroid tumors, approximately 64% of dogs developed hypothyroidism.[37] After resection of a functional thyroid tumor, testing for hypothyroidism postoperatively should be considered within 1 to 3 weeks after surgery, along with treatment, including levothyroxine after diagnosis or prophylactically. In one study, 30% of dogs with functional thyroid tumors treated prophylactically with hormone supplementations still became hypothyroid after surgery.[37]

Imaging and staging

Advanced imaging, such as CT, is useful to determine staging, malignant potential, and surgical resectability of the tumor (**Fig. 5**). The World Health Organization (WHO) staging for dogs with thyroid tumors is listed in **Table 1**. In the literature, there is a wide reported rate of metastasis at the time of diagnosis or necropsy ranging from 6% to 60%. This broad range may be dependent on the type of imaging and sampling technique used to appropriately stage these dogs. Staging criteria have both tumor size and status of metastatic disease as factors contributing to stage of disease. Therefore, differentiating between higher stages owing to these 2 factors is difficult to assess in the literature. A study assessing CT staging showed that 10% are stage I, 50% are stage II, 9% are stage III, and 31% are stage IV.[39] This likely represents the more sensitive nature of CT imaging to detect pulmonary metastases compared with more standard imaging techniques, such as radiographs.[40] CT assessment to determine metastatic lymph nodes in the head and neck has historically been poor,[41] although recently this has been shown to have a better correlation.[39] Because of this discrepancy, sampling of lymph nodes through cytology or histopathology should be performed for accurate staging.

CT imaging parameters of the thyroid mass to determine malignancy in dogs have also been assessed.[42] Mineralization, vascular invasion, and tissue invasion were only detected when tumors were malignant and when the presence of intratumoral vascularization was significantly associated with presence of malignancy.

To determine resectability on imaging studies, vascular invasion can be assessed. In a study of 73 dogs with gross vascular invasion, only approximately 50% of these dogs had evidence of tumor thrombus on CT images.[43] Gross vascular invasion may correspond to "fixed" tumors clinically, and because of the discrepancy of imaging

---

Box 3
Clinical signs of dogs with functional thyroid tumors[34,35]

- Polyuria (31%–56%)
- Polydipsia (31%–56%)
- Weight loss (24%–44%)
- Polyphagia (10%–22%)
- Excessive panting (10%–19%)

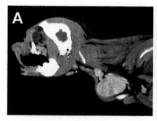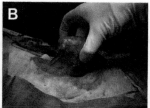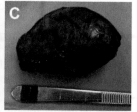

Fig. 5. (*A*) Preoperative CT of a dog with a left thyroid carcinoma. (*B*) Intraoperative images showing a well-encapsulated mobile thyroid mass. (*C*) Thyroid mass after excision.

studies versus intraoperative findings, the authors often find the only way to determine resectability is to surgically explore the cervical region, as CT may underestimate disease. Incidental thyroid tumors can be found with imaging obtained unrelated to the thyroid gland and has a prevalence of 0.76%.[42] Among these "incidentalomas," 70.6% of these tumors were malignant, so the authors recommend surgical removal of any thyroid mass found on advanced nonthyroid imaging.

Cytology and preoperative biopsy
Cytology of the tumor can often determine that it is of neuroendocrine or thyroid origin but it can be challenging to determine if it is benign or malignant. Because of vascularity of thyroid tumors, Tru-Cut biopsy is not recommended because of the risk of severe, sometimes fatal hemorrhage.

Surgery and complications
Surgery is the treatment of choice for thyroid tumors and allows for the best survival. Surgical candidates for dogs with thyroid masses typically are freely movable, which has been described as movement of greater than 1 cm in all planes during palpation.[44] Single or bilateral thyroid tumors are both considered surgical candidates; however, postoperatively, bilateral thyroidectomies have ongoing thyroid and calcium supplementation needs.[44] Fixed or nonmobile masses have typically been thought to not be candidates for surgical resection; however, advanced imaging, such as CT and MRI, can help determine the degree of invasion. Fixed tumors have a 5.4 times higher rate of complication than mobile tumors[45]; however, as surgery is the treatment of

Table 1
World Health Organization's clinical staging system for dogs with thyroid tumors

Stage	Primary Tumor	Regional LN	Distant Metastases
I	T_1 a, b	N_0	M_0
II	T_0	N_1	M_0
	T_1 a, b	N_1	M_0
	T_2 a, b	N_0 or N_1 a	M_0
III	T_3	Any N	M_0
	Any T	N_1 b or N2 b	
IV	Any T	Any N	M_1

Abbreviations: a, freely movable; b, fixed; LN, lymph node; M_0, no evidence of distant metastasis; M_1, evidence of distant metastases; N_0, no lymph node involvement; N_1, ipsilateral lymph node involvement; N_2, bilateral lymph node involvement; T_0, microscopic residual disease; T_1, <2 cm; T_2, 2 to 5 cm; T_3, >5 cm.

choice and provides a longer median survival time, thyroidectomy should be pursued if safe.[37,39]

At induction, it may be helpful to determine if there is any evidence of laryngeal paralysis. The recurrent laryngeal nerves are positioned dorsally and medial to the thyroid glands. Damage to the recurrent laryngeal nerve clinically causes paralysis of the larynx, which has potential sequelae of aspiration pneumonia, reported as a complication of thyroidectomy.[45] Laryngeal examination presurgery and postsurgery may identify dogs with laryngeal paralysis. In more recent studies,[45] laryngeal examinations have been performed preoperatively and postoperatively especially in large or fixed tumors to determine if paralysis is present and showed preoperative concurrent laryngeal paralysis in 6.4% of cases.

For surgery, the dog is placed in dorsal recumbency, and a towel under the neck can help facilitate exposure. A standard ventral midline cervical approach is performed (see **Fig. 5**). The vascular supply to the thyroid gland is through the cranial and caudal thyroid arteries. Venous return is primarily through the cranial and caudal thyroid veins. The caudal thyroid vein empties into the internal jugular vein. This is clinically significant because of the potential for tumor thrombi in these vessels.[43] Excessive hemorrhage can occur during surgery because of the presence of a fragile weblike vascular supply overlying and supplying these tumors. Hemorrhage is the most common complication of thyroidectomy, and in one study, packed cell volume (PCV) dropped 10% after surgery.[43] In people, the gold-standard instrumentation is vessel-sealing devices to minimize hemorrhage.[46] This has been advocated for canine patients, with one study showing shorter surgery times, no increase in complications, and no hemorrhage complications occurring with use of a vessel-sealing device.[47]

The thyroid gland's lymphatic drainage is to the cranial deep cervical lymph node from the cranial portion of the gland and into the caudal deep cervical lymph node from the caudal portion of the glands.[36] The cranial and caudal deep cervical lymph nodes typically only measure a few millimeters in diameter, with the cranial deep cervical lymph node lying between the medial retropharyngeal (MRP) and the thyroid gland, and the caudal deep cervical lymph nodes can vary in number and are located at the ventral aspect of the caudal third of the trachea. These may be difficult to locate intraoperatively, in which drainage is thought to be to the MRP lymph nodes. Lymph node metastasis has been reported in 7.1% to 45%[36,43] of dogs with thyroid tumors, although methods of identification and staging have not been routinely established in veterinary medicine. Contralateral lymph node metastasis has also been identified in canine thyroid tumors.[36,43]

If bilateral thyroidectomies are performed, hypothyroidism occurs in approximately 40% of dogs,[44] and T4 supplementation is needed in those patients with low T4 concentrations. It is presumed there is ectopic thyroid tissue in patients that maintain a normal T4. In addition, hypoparathyroidism with associated hypocalcemia should be expected and treated accordingly. Parathyroid tissue has been shown to be successfully reimplanted to avoid long-term supplementation for hypoparathyroidism.[44] Caution should be used to avoid seeding neoplastic cells if performing a parathyroid reimplantation.

Nonsurgical options

A variety of radiation options can be used for patients with thyroid tumors deemed inoperable.[48,49] There have been mixed results ranging from MST of 170 to 455 days,[48,49] with response to radiation, either complete or partial being the best indicator of having a significantly longer MST. Radioactive iodine can also be used for nonresectable functional or nonfunctional follicular thyroid tumors with good long-term outcomes reached.[50] Because of the need for high doses for this treatment modality and specialized isolation, only a few centers offer this as a treatment option. Parafollicular (or medullary) tumors are unable to be treated with radioactive iodine, as the cells have to uptake iodine.

Prognosis

Dogs with benign thyroid tumors represent 9% to 50%[35] of dogs with thyroid tumors and have an excellent prognosis that can be cured with surgery alone. The prognosis for malignant thyroid tumors depends on several factors, including mobility and size of the tumor, surgical treatment and complications, pathology, and stage of disease (**Box 4**).

The mobility and size have been shown to affect prognosis for thyroid tumors. As mobile versus fixed tumor classification is often subjective, vascular or local invasion is commonly associated with "fixed" tumors. Tumor diameter, tumor volume, ectopic location, and follicular cell origin are associated with local invasiveness.[34] Fixed tumors have a median survival time range of 6 to 12 months versus a median survival time of mobile tumors of 3 years. Increased maximal tumor dimensions have been shown to have a shorter disease-free interval,[45] although other studies show that size or tumor volume has no effect on survival.[43] Size can be a negative prognostic indicator for likelihood of metastasis, with larger tumors having a higher rate of metastases.[34,35] As many "fixed" and large tumors can be surgically resected,[43] these 2 factors should not deter a clinician from surgery, as surgical resection is a positive prognostic indicator.[37,39] Surgical complications are associated with shorter median survival times.[45]

Pathology prognostic indicators include vascular invasion having a negative prognosis for survival[34]; however tumor type does not affect survival.[34] Parafollicular tumors are less likely to be locally invasive, corresponding with less "fixed" tumors clinically. Immunohistochemical markers, such as Ki-67, have been used to assess aggressive markers of thyroid tumors, such as in dogs, and is associated with local invasiveness, tumor size and bilateral location, and time to metastases.[34] Higher mitotic index has been shown to be negatively associated with shorter disease-free interval and median survival times.[45]

Higher stages of disease generally correlate with poorer prognosis. In a recent study assessing the WHO staging criteria, staging did not correlate with overall survival

---

Box 4
Negative prognostic indicators for dogs with thyroid tumors[34,35,37,39,43,45]

- Fixed tumors or locally invasive
  - Factors associated with local invasiveness include increased size and follicular origin
- Size of tumor increases risk of metastases, which decreases disease-free interval
- Surgically unresectable
- Metastases or increased stage of disease
- Pathology
  - Malignant
  - Vascular invasion
  - Increased mitotic index
  - Positive Ki-67 immunohistochemical marker

time[39]; however, higher stages trended toward reduced survival times. There are many negative prognostic indicators for metastasis, including tumor diameter, tumor volume, and bilateral location.[34]

Functional tumors do not appear to be associated with a poor prognosis.[37,38] Dogs with functional thyroid tumors have reported median survival times of greater than 35 months with surgery.[37,38]

Ectopic thyroid tissue is common in the dog and cat and can be found from the base of the tongue to the thoracic inlet, mediastinum, and along the descending aorta in approximately 50% of dogs on necropsy examination. Ectopic thyroid tumors are thought to be approximately 13% of dogs with thyroid neoplasia and are not associated with a negative prognosis.[51]

Thyroid Summary

Thyroidectomy for canine thyroid tumors remains the treatment of choice even for dogs with advanced stages of disease. CT is useful for staging, assessing malignant potential, and assessing whether it is surgically resectable. Functional testing in the preoperative phase is useful to determine if the tumor is functional. Resecting lymph nodes at the time of surgery should be performed ipsilaterally, even if they appear to be unaffected on CT. Ectopic thyroid tissue can also be located anywhere from the base of the tongue to the thoracic cavity, and surgical excision still is the best option for survival.

CLINICS CARE POINTS

- Hypercalcemia is always a significant abnormality even if mildly elevated. If elevated iCa is detected, the patient should have a workup to diagnose the cause of hypercalcemia and include imaging to localize the parathyroid gland before surgery.

- Older dogs develop parathyroid disease, and surgery should always be strongly considered given the good prognosis and minimal morbidity associated with surgery.

- Thyroid functional testing preoperatively should be performed in dogs with thyroid tumors owing to higher than reported rates of functional tumors.

- Advanced imaging, such as computed tomography, is useful in dogs with thyroid cancer to determine staging, malignant potential, and surgical resectability of the tumor, although cervical exploration may be necessary to determine if the tumor is resectable.

- Surgery is considered treatment of choice for thyroid cancer even in dogs with high stages of disease and dogs with bilateral tumors, as it prolongs survival. Ipsilateral lymphadenectomy should be performed at time of surgery, and the use of a vessel sealant device is recommended to minimize hemorrhage.

DISCLOSURE

The authors have nothing to disclose.

REFERENCES

1. Feldman EC, Hoar B, Pollard R, et al. Pretreatment clinical and laboratory findings in dogs with primary hyperparathyroidism: 210 cases (1987-2004). J Am Vet Med Assoc 2005;227(5):756–61.
2. Griebeler ML, Kearns AE, Ryu E, et al. Secular trends in the incidence of primary hyperparathyroidism over five decades (1965-2010). Bone 2015;73:1–7.

3. Goldstein RE, Atwater DZ, Cazolli DM, et al. Inheritance, mode of inheritance, and candidate genes for primary hyperparathyroidism in Keeshonden. J Vet Intern Med 2007;21(1):199–203.

4. Arias EA, Castillo VA, Trigo RH, et al. Multiple endocrine neoplasia similar to human subtype 2A in a dog: medullary thyroid carcinoma, bilateral pheochromocytoma and parathyroid adenoma. Open Vet J 2016;6(3):165–71.

5. Ham K, Greenfield CL, Barger A, et al. Validation of a rapid parathyroid hormone assay and intraoperative measurement of parathyroid hormone in dogs with benign naturally occurring primary hyperparathyroidism. Vet Surg 2009;38(1):122–32.

6. Milovancev M, Schmiedt CW. Preoperative factors associated with postoperative hypocalcemia in dogs with primary hyperparathyroidism that underwent parathyroidectomy: 62 cases (2004-2009). J Am Vet Med Assoc 2013;242(4):507–15.

7. Armstrong AJ, Hauptman JG, Stanley BJ, et al. Effect of prophylactic calcitriol administration on serum ionized calcium concentrations after parathyroidectomy: 78 cases (2005-2015). J Vet Intern Med 2018;32(1):99–106.

8. Sawyer ES, Northrup NC, Schmiedt CW, et al. Outcome of 19 dogs with parathyroid carcinoma after surgical excision. Vet Comp Oncol 2012;10(1):57–64.

9. Kishi EN, Holmes SP, Abbott JR, et al. Functional metastatic parathyroid adenocarcinoma in a dog. Can Vet J 2014;55(4):383–8.

10. Bilezikian JP, Marcus R, Levine MA, et al. The parathyroids: basic and clinical concepts. 3rd edition. Elsevier: San Diego (CA); 2015. p. 919, xxv.

11. DeVries SE, Feldman EC, Nelson RW, et al. Primary parathyroid gland hyperplasia in dogs: six cases (1982-1991). J Am Vet Med Assoc 1993;202(7):1132–6.

12. van Vonderen IK, Kooistra HS, Peeters ME, et al. Parathyroid hormone immunohistochemistry in dogs with primary and secondary hyperparathyroidism: the question of adenoma and primary hyperplasia. J Comp Pathol 2003;129(1):61–9.

13. Feldman EC, Miner A. Canine and feline endocrinology. 4th edition. St. Louis (MO): Elsevier; 2015.

14. Thompson D, Skelly B. Prevalence of canine primary hyperparathyroidism recurrence in Keeshond and non-Keeshond dogs after curative parathyroidectomy. Vet Rec 2020;187(11):e93.

15. Coady M, Fletcher DJ, Goggs R. Severity of ionized hypercalcemia and hypocalcemia is associated with etiology in dogs and cats. Front Vet Sci 2019;6:276.

16. https://www.vet.cornell.edu/animal-health-diagnostic-center/testing/protocols/PHPT.

17. Lucero MC, Duque FJ, Gil M, et al. A plasma calcium-phosphorus product can be used to predict the lifespan of dogs with chronic kidney disease. Can Vet J 2019;60(12):1319–25.

18. Matwichuk CL, Taylor SM, Daniel GB, et al. Double-phase parathyroid scintigraphy in dogs using technetium-99M-sestamibi. Vet Radiol Ultrasound 2000;41(5):461–9.

19. Taeymans O, Schwarz T, Duchateau L, et al. Computed tomographic features of the normal canine thyroid gland. Vet Radiol Ultrasound 2008;49(1):13–9.

20. Wisner ER, Penninck D, Biller DS, et al. High-resolution parathyroid sonography. Vet Radiol Ultrasound 1997;38(6):462–6.

21. Secrest S, Grimes J. Ultrasonographic size of the canine parathyroid gland may not correlate with histopathology. Vet Radiol Ultrasound 2019;60(6):729–33.

22. Burkhardt SJ, Sumner JP, Mann S. Ambidirectional cohort study on the agreement of ultrasonography and surgery in the identification of parathyroid pathology, and predictors of postoperative hypocalcemia in 47 dogs undergoing

parathyroidectomy due to primary hyperparathyroidism. Vet Surg 2021. https://doi.org/10.1111/vsu.13707.

23. Bucy D, Pollard R, Nelson R. Analysis of factors affecting outcome of ultrasound-guided radiofrequency heat ablation for treatment of primary hyperparathyroidism in dogs. Vet Radiol Ultrasound 2017;58(1):83–9.

24. Guttin T, Knox VW, Diroff JS. Outcomes for dogs with primary hyperparathyroidism following treatment with percutaneous ultrasound-guided ethanol ablation of presumed functional parathyroid nodules: 27 cases (2008-2011). J Am Vet Med Assoc 2015;247(7):771–7.

25. Rasor L, Pollard R, Feldman EC. Retrospective evaluation of three treatment methods for primary hyperparathyroidism in dogs. J Am Anim Hosp Assoc 2007;43(2):70–7.

26. Leal RO, Frau Pascual L, Hernandez J. The use of percutaneous ultrasound-guided radiofrequency heat ablation for treatment of primary hyperparathyroidism in eight dogs: outcome and complications. Vet Sci 2018;5(4). https://doi.org/10.3390/vetsci5040091.

27. Singh A, Giuffrida MA, Thomson CB, et al. Perioperative characteristics, histological diagnosis, and outcome in cats undergoing surgical treatment of primary hyperparathyroidism. Vet Surg 2019;48(3):367–74.

28. Flanders JA, Neth S, Erb HN, et al. Functional analysis of ectopic parathyroid activity in cats. Am J Vet Res 1991;52(8):1336–40.

29. Chakedis JM, Maser C, Brumund KT, et al. Indocyanine green fluorescence-guided redo parathyroidectomy. BMJ Case Rep 2015;2015. https://doi.org/10.1136/bcr-2015-211778.

30. Howard J, Ham K. Parathyroid localization using parathyroid hormone concentration and fluoroscopy. 2017.

31. Dear JD, Kass PH, Della Maggiore AM, et al. Association of hypercalcemia before treatment with hypocalcemia after treatment in dogs with primary hyperparathyroidism. J Vet Intern Med 2017;31(2):349–54.

32. Arbaugh M, Smeak D, Monnet E. Evaluation of preoperative serum concentrations of ionized calcium and parathyroid hormone as predictors of hypocalcemia following parathyroidectomy in dogs with primary hyperparathyroidism: 17 cases (2001-2009). J Am Vet Med Assoc 2012;241(2):233–6.

33. Liptak JM. Canine thyroid carcinoma. Clin Tech Small Anim Pract 2007;22(2):75–81.

34. Campos M, Ducatelle R, Rutteman G, et al. Clinical, pathologic, and immunohistochemical prognostic factors in dogs with thyroid carcinoma. J Vet Intern Med 2014;28(6):1805–13.

35. Wucherer KL, Wilke V. Thyroid cancer in dogs: an update based on 638 cases (1995-2005). J Am Anim Hosp Assoc 2010;46(4):249–54.

36. Skinner OT, Souza CHM, Kim DY. Metastasis to ipsilateral medial retropharyngeal and deep cervical lymph nodes in 22 dogs with thyroid carcinoma. Vet Surg 2021;50(1):150–7.

37. Scharf VF, Oblak ML, Hoffman K, et al. Clinical features and outcome of functional thyroid tumours in 70 dogs. J Small Anim Pract 2020;61(8):504–11.

38. Frederick AN, Pardo AD, Schmiedt CW, et al. Outcomes for dogs with functional thyroid tumors treated by surgical excision alone. J Am Vet Med Assoc 2020;256(4):444–8.

39. Giannasi C, Rushton S, Rook A, et al. Canine thyroid carcinoma prognosis following the utilisation of computed tomography assisted staging. Vet Rec 2021;189(1):e55.

40. Eberle N, Fork M, von Babo V, et al. Comparison of examination of thoracic radiographs and thoracic computed tomography in dogs with appendicular osteosarcoma. Vet Comp Oncol 2011;9(2):131–40.
41. Skinner OT, Boston SE, Giglio RF, et al. Diagnostic accuracy of contrast-enhanced computed tomography for assessment of mandibular and medial retropharyngeal lymph node metastasis in dogs with oral and nasal cancer. Vet Comp Oncol 2018;16(4):562–70.
42. Bertolini G, Drigo M, Angeloni L, et al. Incidental and nonincidental canine thyroid tumors assessed by multidetector row computed tomography: a single-centre cross sectional study in 4520 dogs. Vet Radiol Ultrasound 2017;58(3):304–14.
43. Latifi M, Skinner OT, Spoldi E, et al. Outcome and postoperative complications in 73 dogs with thyroid carcinoma with gross vascular invasion managed with thyroidectomy. Vet Comp Oncol 2021. https://doi.org/10.1111/vco.12739.
44. Tuohy JL, Worley DR, Withrow SJ. Outcome following simultaneous bilateral thyroid lobectomy for treatment of thyroid gland carcinoma in dogs: 15 cases (1994-2010). J Am Vet Med Assoc 2012;241(1):95–103.
45. Reagan JK, Selmic LE, Fallon C, et al. Complications and outcomes associated with unilateral thyroidectomy in dogs with naturally occurring thyroid tumors: 156 cases (2003-2015). J Am Vet Med Assoc 2019;255(8):926–32.
46. Yao HS, Wang Q, Wang WJ, et al. Prospective clinical trials of thyroidectomy with LigaSure vs conventional vessel ligation: a systematic review and meta-analysis. Arch Surg 2009;144(12):1167–74.
47. Lorange M, De Arburn Parent R, Huneault L, et al. Use of a vessel-sealing device versus conventional hemostatic techniques in dogs undergoing thyroidectomy because of suspected thyroid carcinoma. J Am Vet Med Assoc 2019;254(10): 1186–91.
48. Lee BI, LaRue SM, Seguin B, et al. Safety and efficacy of stereotactic body radiation therapy (SBRT) for the treatment of canine thyroid carcinoma. Vet Comp Oncol 2020;18(4):843–53.
49. Tsimbas K, Turek M, Christensen N, et al. Short survival time following palliative-intent hypofractionated radiotherapy for non-resectable canine thyroid carcinoma: a retrospective analysis of 20 dogs. Vet Radiol Ultrasound 2019; 60(1):93–9.
50. Worth AJ, Zuber RM, Hocking M. Radioiodide (131I) therapy for the treatment of canine thyroid carcinoma. Aust Vet J 2005;83(4):208–14.
51. Broome MR, Peterson ME, Walker JR. Clinical features and treatment outcomes of 41 dogs with sublingual ectopic thyroid neoplasia. J Vet Intern Med 2014; 28(5):1560–8.

Update on Adrenalectomy

Galina Hayes, PhD, DVSc, BVSc, DACVECC, DACVS

KEYWORDS

- Adrenalectomy • Adrenal • Dogs • Surgery • Pheochromocytoma
- Cortical adenocarcinoma

KEY POINTS

- Adrenal masses larger than 2.0 cm are highly likely to be malignant
- Advanced imaging using CTA or contrast ultrasound, FNA cytology, or urine biochemical testing may provide additional information to identify malignancies when smaller than 2.0 cm and distinguish cortical tumors from pheocromocytoma; however, no test has 100% accuracy, and mixed endocrine tumors secreting both cortisol and catecholamines have been reported
- Pretreatment of pheochromocytoma with phenoxybenzamine before surgery is associated with a 35% mortality risk reduction
- Laparoscopic adrenalectomy is safe with appropriate case selection
- Successful removal of adrenal masses with substantial invasion is highly feasible; however, success relies on good coordination and communication with the surgical and anesthesia team, forward planning, and surgical experience

PREOPERATIVE WORKUP AND IMAGING

Adrenal tumors are most commonly identified in dogs either during diagnostic workup of adrenal-dependent hyperadrenocorticism, hypertension, or during abdominal ultrasonography performed for nonspecific clinical signs such as weakness, anorexia, and vomiting. Although ultrasound assessment provides a readily accessible method of adrenal gland interrogation, the clinical significance of minor adrenal gland enlargement can be elusive. An adrenal gland width greater than 10 mm in the longitudinal plane is considered to be enlarged[1] beyond a degree consistent solely with physiologic stress. More recently, bodyweight-specific measurements for adrenal gland width that differentiate between normal tissue or hyperplastic/neoplastic disease have been reported.[2]

Distinguishing Hyperplasia from Neoplastic Disease

Differential diagnoses for adrenal gland enlargement include adrenal hyperplasia, adrenal adenoma, adrenal adenocarcinoma, pheochromocytoma, and other neoplasms

Department of Small Animal Surgery, Cornell University, 930 Campus Road, Ithaca, NY, USA
E-mail address: Gmh59@cornell.edu

Vet Clin Small Anim 52 (2022) 473–487
https://doi.org/10.1016/j.cvsm.2021.12.005
0195-5616/22/Published by Elsevier Inc.

vetsmall.theclinics.com

including metastatic disease. In general, only adrenal neoplasia is considered a surgical disease. A diagnostic cut point of a lesion diameter of greater than 20 mm has been suggested for distinguishing between nonneoplastic and neoplastic disease. A study in 119 dogs that received abdominal ultrasonography and subsequently underwent necropsy or adrenalectomy found that all 12 ultrasonographic adrenal lesions greater than 2.0 cm diameter were ultimately diagnosed as cortical carcinoma or pheochromocytoma, providing a specificity of 100%.[3] However, at this cut point a total of 26 malignant neoplasms were missed, providing a meager 32% sensitivity.

As surgical resection of smaller (<2.0 cm) lesions is less challenging and lower risk than large tumors, it would be helpful if the diagnosis of adrenal neoplasia, particularly cortical adenocarcinoma and pheochromocytoma, could be made while the lesions are still small, rather than allowing an aggressive growth pattern to dictate surgical intervention.

Cytology has been investigated for accurate preoperative diagnosis of adrenal masses and has been found to allow cortical lesions (adrenocortical hyperplasia, adenoma, adenocarcinoma) to be readily distinguished from medullary lesions (pheochromocytoma) but does not allow for differentiation of level of malignancy within the cortical group.[4] Clinicians may be reluctant to perform fine-needle aspiration cytology of adrenal lesions, particularly when small, due to their challenging location, proximity to large vessels, and risk of inciting hemodynamic instability. Two studies investigating the safety of this intervention in clinical populations totaling 69 dogs found a risk percentage of 7%, including ventricular tachycardia, hemorrhage, and respiratory crisis resulting in euthanasia,[5,6] alongside a somewhat disappointing diagnostic yield of 70%.[5] These issues have prompted investigation of additional screening tools that might facilitate preoperative diagnosis of adrenal neoplasia with greater sensitivity, lower risk, and higher yield.

Distinguishing Different Neoplastic Types Preoperatively

Pheochromocytoma manipulation is likely to result in a greater degree of intraoperative hemodynamic instability than removal of an adrenal adenoma or adenocarcinoma and thus exerts a greater imperative for both preoperative and intraoperative adrenal blockade. Conversely, cortisol- or sex steroid-secreting tumors may predispose to a hypercoagulable presentation and benefit from the use of anticoagulants in the face of cytokine exacerbation following surgical trauma and/or venotomy. Thus, preoperative diagnosis of the neoplastic type may directly prompt changes in subsequent management and allow greater individualization of treatment.

Complicating matters, polymorphic endocrine activity from adrenal tumors is well reported, ranging from pheochromocytomas secreting ectopic cortisol,[7] neuroendocrine tumors secreting adrenocorticotropic hormone,[8] to adrenocortical carcinomas secreting catecholamines[9] or mineralocorticoids[10] with resulting mixing of the clinical endocrine picture. Neoplastic masses consisting histologically of different tumor types, for example, pheochromocytoma and cortical carcinoma have been identified.[4] Finally, bilateral metastatic adrenal neoplasia compromising normal cortisol secretion with resulting addisonian crisis has also been reported.[11-13] The presence of such diverse functionality within the canine tumor population may limit attempts at highly specific preoperative tissue diagnosis; however, both contrast computed tomography (CT) and contrast-enhanced ultrasonography have been investigated with this goal in mind.

Contrast-enhanced ultrasonography using perflubutane and assessing mean transit time found an area under the receiver operator curve (AUROC) of 0.91 with a sensitivity of 69% and a specificity of 94% for distinguishing pheochromocytoma from adrenocortical tumors when using a measurement of less than 6225 milliseconds as indicating pheochromocytoma.[14] A study investigating triple-phase CT for distinguishing different adrenal tumor types in dogs described different patterns of contrast uptake and washout between the different tumor types over the different phases. In cortical adenomas, contrast enhancement typically increased to its maximum level in the venous phase and was then reduced in the delayed phase. In cortical adenocarcinomas, contrast enhancement increased gradually from the arterial to the venous phase and was maintained into the delayed phase. In pheochromocytomas, contrast enhancement was very pronounced in the arterial phase and then decreased steadily over the venous and delayed phases.[15]

Several biochemical tests that attempt to distinguish pheochromocytoma from other adrenal tumors are available. Urine vanillylmandelic acid:creatinine ratio has been found to be highly accurate for this purpose, with an AUROC of 0.92 (implying very few false-positives or false-negatives), and may be more readily available than urine metanephrine analysis.[16] Urine normetanephrine:creatinine ratio was also identified to have high specificity for pheochromocytoma in a study of 7 dogs with this disease,[17] although false-negatives may be an issue due to both episodic secretion of catecholamines from the tumor and sample lability. Work is ongoing to overcome some of the technical challenges with laboratory measurement.[18]

Whether urine biochemical testing, contrast-enhanced ultrasonography, or CT angiography (CTA) can successfully distinguish a pheochromocytoma or adrenocortical carcinoma when this tumor is greater than 1.0 cm but still less than 2.0 cm has yet to be determined, but is an interesting area of investigation. The advantages and disadvantages of various modalities used to distinguish tumor type are shown in **Table 1**.

PRETREATMENT OF ENDOCRINOPATHIES BEFORE SURGERY

For dogs with a cushingoid presentation, the standard recommendation is to pretreat with trilostane to decrease the risk of complications associated with steroid excess, for example, poor wound healing/surgical site infections. Although ideal, this must be offset against the delay in treatment and risk of increase in size of the tumor and/or progression to vascular invasion/thrombus generation. Although an association between Cushing disease and surgical site infection risk in dogs has not been well established in the literature, an association between iatrogenic steroid administration and surgical site infection (SSI) has been reported.[19]

Adrenoceptor Blockade

Dogs with pheochromocytoma should receive appropriate preoperative medical management to block the effects of released catecholamines. The goals of treatment are to normalize blood pressure and heart rate, restore volume depletion, and protect the animal from surgical manipulation-induced catecholamine storm and its consequences on the cardiovascular system. Spontaneous arrest and autoresuscitation during catecholamine crisis has been reported.[20] Hypertension is not a prerequisite for treatment.[21] Phenoxybenzamine, which is an irreversible noncompetitive alpha-adrenoceptor blocker is most commonly used and has been associated with a 35% mortality risk reduction at a dose of 0.6 mg/kg administered orally every 12 hours for 20 days before surgery.[22] Owing to the polymorphic endocrine activity possible with adrenal tumors, the author prefers to use this protocol before any adrenalectomy. For the adrenal tumor that is actively hemorrhaging at the time of diagnosis, where pretreatment is not feasible, phentolamine or sodium nitroprusside can be used intraoperatively to control hypertension and reduce hemorrhage.[21]

Table 1
Preoperative testing to distinguish tumor type

Test	Advantages	Disadvantages
Diameter >2.0 cm on advanced imaging	Highly specific (few false-positives) for malignancy (adenocarcinoma and pheochromocytoma)	Will miss 68% of malignancies (adenocarcinoma and pheochromocytoma) if used in isolation
Fine-needle aspiration cytology	Some reliability for distinguishing cortical tumors from pheochromocytoma	7% complication risk up to and including death; 70% diagnostic yield
Contrast-enhanced ultrasonography	Highly sensitive and specific for distinguishing pheochromocytoma from adrenocortical tumors in a single study	Accuracy may be operator dependent; availability not widespread
Computed tomographic angiogram, triple phase	Contrast uptake and washout patterns appear useful for distinguishing tumor type as well as surgical planning	Sensitivity and specificity not defined; study requires general anesthesia
Urine biochemical testing	Urine vanillylmandelic acid:creatinine ratio highly sensitive and specific	Poor availability

ADRENALECTOMY

The techniques required for successful adrenalectomy vary widely with the presence and extent of vascular invasion, which in turn often correlates with the size and type of tumor. Pheochromocytomas have been associated with a higher risk of vascular invasion.[23] On a sliding scale of increasing technical challenges, adrenalectomies can be categorized as follows: less than or equal to 2.0 cm without vascular invasion (adrenal nodules), greater than 2.0 cm without vascular invasion, greater than 2.0 cm with vascular invasion and prehepatic caval or renal thrombus, greater than 2.0 cm with vascular invasion and hepatic or posthepatic caval thrombus, greater than 2.0 cm with caval wall invasion necessitating partial or complete cavectomy.

Minimally Invasive Techniques

Laparoscopic adrenalectomy has been well reported in 2 case series[24,25] and is typically reserved for adrenal nodules or small adrenal tumors without vascular invasion. Average tumor size was 2.95 and 2.50 cm in these studies, with >85% of tumors left sided. A left-sided tumor is typically easier to access due to a more caudal position, as well as a position lateral to the cava rather than dorsolateral. These studies positioned the patient in lateral or sternal recumbency and used a 3- or 4-port technique (**Fig. 1**). A retroperitoneal single-port approach has also been described in a case series of normal experimental animals.[26] Reported complications in the laparoscopic patient population were minimal, but included splenic laceration during port placement, iatrogenic pneumothorax from Veress needle placement, and capsular rupture of the tumor during manipulation. A more recent case-control study[27] sort to compare laparoscopic versus open adrenalectomy in a patient population recruited over a 15-year period between 1995 and 2020. Enrollment was limited to smaller (3.5 cm diameter), 70% left-sided tumors. Laparoscopic cases were matched on tumor size, histologic type, and laterality to open cases in a 1:2 ratio. Despite valiant attempts at matching, the mean tumor size in the open group was still somewhat larger at 4.6 cm. Reduced incidence of intraoperative hypotension and an average 40-minute reduction in surgical time were identified in the laparoscopic group over the 14 intraoperative and postoperative outcomes examined. Neither the level of surgical experience of the surgeons working with each group nor the average recruitment date for each group were assessed; however, the study did serve to confirm previous

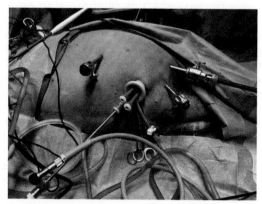

Fig. 1. Port setup for laparoscopic adrenalectomy. (*Image courtesy of* Dr Ameet Singh DACVS.)

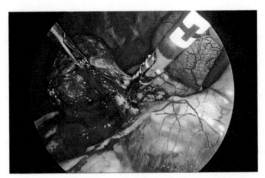

Fig. 2. Laparoscopic adrenal mass. The partially dissected tumor is being grasped and manipulated by the lateral stump of the phrenicoabdominal vein while the medial dissection is competed. (*Image courtesy of* Dr Ameet Singh DACVS.)

findings[28] that with appropriate case selection laparoscopic adrenalectomy can be considered safe. Reported concerns with the laparoscopic technique include increased risk of tumor capsule disruption and inadvertent tumor spillage particularly with larger tumors, and the relative dependence of successful performance of the technique on surgical experience. Recommendations made by a human patient study reviewing 35 years of single-center experience in laparoscopic adrenalectomy included the statement "The choice of laparoscopic vs open approach should depend on the surgeon's experience, regardless of the dimension of the lesion,"[29] emphasizing the importance of this component. **Fig 2** shows a left sided laparoscopic adrenalectomy in progress with an experienced laparoscopic surgeon.

Open Techniques

Techniques to improve surgical exposure

- Positioning patient over bolster at thoracolumbar junction to achieve mild to moderate spinal hyperextension
- Long laparotomy incision
- Neuromuscular blockade
- Exteriorization of the small bowel and spleen

Successful open resection requires full visualization and access to the area in question. Both paracostal, intercostal,[30] and midline laparotomy approaches have been described. An intercostal approach may offer improved access to the right adrenal gland compared with a central midline approach; however, a full abdominal explore is not possible and the approach cannot be readily extended to allow access to the intra-thoracic caudal vena cava if required. When approaching an adrenalectomy via a midline laparotomy, several additional maneuvers may be helpful for improving exposure. Positioning the patient over a sandbag placed at the thoracolumbar (TL) junction to moderately hyperextend the spine can bring the operative site closer to the incision, particularly in deep-chested animals. Wide retraction on the laparotomy incision will be needed, which is facilitated by a long incision and neuromuscular blockade. Neuromuscular blockade and mechanical ventilation also ensures a very regular respiratory pattern, which allows the surgeon to better time their movements to co-ordinate with respiratory motion; this is particularly useful during cavotomy. Exteriorization of the small intestine and wrapping in saline-soaked laparotomy towels creates more working room in the abdominal cavity. For a right adrenalectomy, a duodenal maneuver can be performed using umbilical tape or elastic vessel loops to secure the duodenum temporarily to the sterile drape field on the left side. The hepatic triangular ligaments will typically require transection to allow the caudate hepatic lobe to be manipulated out of the surgical field. Additional assistance from an assistant with a malleable retractor may also be helpful. For a left adrenalectomy, exteriorizing the spleen to the right may help achieve exposure of the area.

The adrenalectomy then typically proceeds in a lateral to medial progression. Pheochromocytomas in particularly are highly vascular and recruit numerous small vessels from the surrounding tumor bed, which will bleed copiously if not respected. Pheochromocytomas may also have generated omental adhesions, which should be ligated or sealed and transected rather than dissected away to minimize capsular disruption. A bipolar vessel sealing device can be very helpful for making the initial lateral incision between the adrenal gland and retroperitoneal tissues and establishing that working plane. The phrenicoabdominal vein will course over the ventral surface of the mass and can be substantially enlarged. Ligation and transection laterally as it leaves the gland can provide a useful vascular stump for further handling and manipulation of the gland. Once the vascular plane is well established, the dissection generally then progresses both dorsally and along the cranial, caudal, and medial planes to separate the mass from the cava and the renal vein. Preoperative CTA can be very helpful to the surgeon in planning both for any venotomies that will be required and having a visual map of the anatomy of the mass, particularly in obese patients in whom the renal vasculature may not be readily visible. When completing the dorsal dissection for a left adrenalectomy, it must be appreciated that the left adrenal gland is often positioned directly ventral to the aorta, thus it may be prudent not to use a vessel sealing device in this area and to proceed patiently. Progressive dissection with small Mixter forceps, followed by bipolar electrocoagulation for small vessels or vessel clips for larger vessels, can be helpful. When the mass is closely associated with the renal vein, multiple additional small veins providing connections between the renal vein and the mass may have been recruited. If the renal vein is to be preserved successfully, these will need to be dissected and coagulated or clipped as distal as possible from their point of origin on the renal vein. For a right-sided adrenalectomy, a segment of the adrenal mass will be located dorsal to the cava and access to this area may be challenging; completing the lateral, cranial, and caudal dissection components first will be necessary. The cava will then generally tolerate some substantial "rolling" to allow this area to be visualized, which can be facilitated with dry cotton-tipped applicators or gentle handling using DeBakey forceps. Once the mass has been isolated in all planes with only the medial origin of the phrenicoabdominal vein from the cava remaining, this can be ligated and transected, assuming that no caval wall invasion has occurred. The point of origin of the left phrenicoabdominal vein on the cava is much closer to the left renal vein than on the right, where there is distinct separation; this can create a greater challenge for the final part of the dissection without renal vein injury.

Open Techniques With Vascular Invasion

As adrenal tumors enlarge, they may progress into the surrounding vasculature; this usually initiates with phrenicoabdominal vein penetration with propagation of tumor thrombus into the vena cava. The tumor thrombus is generally firm and well organized. In more severe cases, the tumor thrombus will ascend into the hepatic cava and eventually into the right atrium.[28] Propagation of tumor thrombus will eventually be followed by tumor invasion into the caval wall, where tumor thrombectomy alone will not be sufficient to achieve mass removal.

The presence of a caval thrombus and its location will make a substantial difference to the planning of the surgical procedure. Occasionally both CTA and/or ultrasonography will not provide an accurate preoperative diagnosis for the presence of thrombus, particularly where there is substantially compression of the cava from tumor bulk. If the presence or absence of caval thrombus cannot be readily confirmed by gentle palpation intraoperatively, the author prefers to use intraoperative ultrasonography for direct interrogation of the caval lumen.

Tumor Thrombectomy Techniques

Generally, the larger and more rostral the tumor thrombus, the more challenging its removal.

When the thrombus is relatively small, removal via phrenicoabdominal venotomy alone may be possible, with no need for caval wall repair.[28] In this technique, Rummel tourniquets are preplaced around the local caval segment in case the venotomy needs to be extended. The cranial tourniquet is placed immediately caudal to the liver. For a right-sided tumor, the caudal tourniquet can typically be placed around the cava between the right phrenicoabdominal and the right renal vein. Depending on the individual's anatomy, if there is insufficient space between the left phrenicoabdominal and left renal vein, for a left-sided tumor a caval tourniquet may be needed caudal to the left renal vein, and on the left and right renal veins if full inflow occlusion into the segment is required. Care is required due to the risk of renal vein injury and subsequent thrombosis. These tourniquets are placed but not tightened. The mass is isolated until only the phrenicoabdominal vein attachment remains. A suture is preplaced around the phrenicoabdominal vein at the point of entry to the cava but not tightened. A venotomy is then started in a longitudinal fashion in the phrenicoabdominal vein as distal as possible to the cava. Once the thrombus can be visualized it is grasped with forceps and pulled from the cava and exteriorized. The phrenicoabdominal vein is then ligated at the point of entry into the caval wall using the preplaced suture. This procedure can be facilitated by the fact that the phrenicoabdominal vein is often considerably dilated and expanded when a tumor thrombus is present.

For a large thrombus that extends into the cava, where the thrombus diameter is expanded such that removal via a venotomy into the phrenicoabdominal vein is not possible, a cavotomy is the next step. The challenge here is achieving good control of hemorrhage such that visualization can be maintained to allow a controlled venotomy to be made and subsequently repaired, while preventing any tourniquets from being tightened onto the thrombus either fracturing it or impeding its removal. Tourniquets can be conceptualized as "inflow" and backflow. The placement of the inflow tourniquets is dictated by whether the tumor is left or right sided, and individual anatomy, as discussed earlier. If the author has concerns about additional injury to a renal vein that has been recently dissected from tourniquet placement and tightening, then occasionally persistent inflow from an unoccluded renal vein into an otherwise occluded caval segment will be tolerated for the cavotomy period. The placement of the backflow tourniquet is dictated by the size of the thrombus and the difficulty level that the surgeon predicts for its removal. For a short thrombus that ends before the hepatic caval segment, the backflow tourniquet can be placed caudal to the liver. For a moderate thrombus that extends into the hepatic caval segment where thrombus diameter is small and ready removal predicted, the tourniquet can still be placed caudal to the liver but will not be tightened until the cavotomy and thrombectomy is complete. For a large thrombus in the intrahepatic caval segment or higher, the laparotomy will need to be extended into a caudal median sternotomy so access to the intrathoracic portion of the caudal vena cava can be achieved and a tourniquet placed

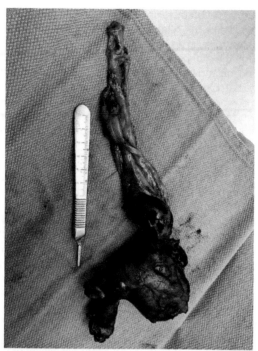

Fig. 3. Rummel tourniquet placement during adrenalectomy for a mass with intrathoracic thrombus extension. Rummels were placed on the intrathoracic cava, the portal vein and hepatic artery (single tourniquet on both), and the suprarenal infraphrenicoabdominal cava.

at this location (**Fig. 3**). In this situation, a Budd-Chiari syndrome with a protein-rich abdominal effusion due to partial occlusion of the hepatic veins may be present preoperatively. Thrombi extending to within the atrium can typically be "milked" back until the thoracic tourniquet can be tightened. Of course the hepatic veins are not amenable to tourniquet placement and empty into the intrahepatic caval segment, so if full backflow occlusion is needed at a large venotomy site then hepatic inflow occlusion will be required; this is achieved by Rummel tourniquet placed on the hepatic artery and portal vein at the epiploic foramen. Examining the level of extension of the thrombus on the CTA and preplanning the tourniquet sites, surgical exposure needed, and order of occlusion and communicating this information to the surgical and anesthesia team is important. The length of the venotomy will also dictate how long the occlusion period needs to be. If the cavotomy is relatively short (<2 cm) then it can be contained within a large tangentially placed Satinsky clamp, allowing release of the tourniquets and partial caval flow while the cavotomy is repaired. If longer, then full occlusion must be maintained while the entire length is closed. Speed is facilitated by preplacing the anchor knot of a continuous line before making the cavotomy incision. If the renal vein has been partially occluded by thrombus, renal venotomy can be performed and the kidney preserved.[31] As the cavotomy is closed, slight release of a tangential clamp, one of the tourniquets, or saline irrigation allows air displacement to prevent air embolus.[32] Median occlusion time for venotomies sutured under full occlusion has been reported at 7.9 minutes in one case series; however, full occlusion times up to 25[32] and even 35[33] minutes were tolerated. Paradoxic bradycardia (reverse Bainbridge reflex) may occur following complete caudal vena cava (CVC) occlusion due to decreased preload.[33] Cavotomies are typically closed longitudinally using a simple continuous line to maximize the retention of caval diameter, although a purse string technique was also described in a single case report.[34] For closure, 5-0 polypropylene can be used, although the author prefers to use 5-0 GORE-TEX vascular suture both due to improved handling and because the needle is sized slightly smaller than the suture diameter, minimizing bleeding from the needle tract holes after tourniquet release. Some bleeding at the moment of release is very common and generally resolves with gentle tamponade and fat graft placement, because fibrin formation seals the tracts. The process of cavotomy planning, tourniquet placement, and execution has been well described in a case report by Ref.[35]

Partial Cavectomy Techniques

When the tumor invades the wall of the vena cava, partial cavectomy and repair or caval ligation may be required. If tumor thrombus propagation has achieved slow and near-complete occlusion of the suprarenal infrahepatic cava, then complete occlusion and resection of this segment may be feasible due to rerouting of blood flow from the renal veins via the azygous vein or vertebral sinuses; this has been described in several case reports,[36,37] and a case series in which experimental animal underwent complete suprarenal infrahepatic caval occlusion over a 2-week period. This study identified extensive formation of collateral vessels between the renal capsule, renal veins, and caudal vena cava to the lumbar veins and vertebral veins and sinuses on subsequent venogram. In this study in 8 dogs, glomerular filtration rate (GFR) underwent a slight but nonstatistically significant decrease.[38] Unfortunately, predicting whether a segmental cavectomy procedure and caval ligation procedure will be either necessary or well tolerated in the individual case before surgery is challenging. When invasion of the caval wall is such that partial cavectomy is required but a caval lumen can be maintained following repair, the procedure can be facilitated by full inflow occlusion into the relevant segment as described earlier. The right-sided adrenal mass shown in **Figs. 4** and **5** was successfully removed without complication with a 6-cm venotomy and partial cavectomy in a 28-kg patient under full inflow and backflow including hepatic inflow occlusion. Fortunately, the caval wall was minimally invaded such that caval diameter could be maintained to approximately 70% of the original dimension. Where caval wall patching is required to maintain diameter, the preparation and use of autogenous small intestinal

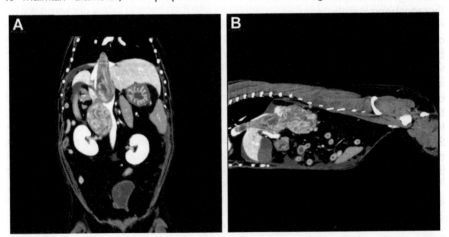

Fig. 4. CTA showing a large right-sided adrenal mass requiring a 6-cm cavotomy and partial cavectomy for successful resection. (*A*)Coronal image, (*B*) sagittal image.

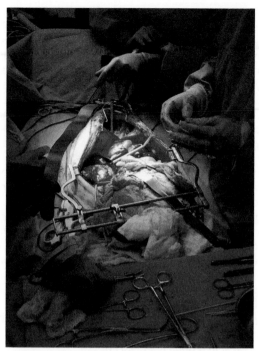

Fig. 5. Adrenal mass in **Fig. 2** following removal; the restriction point of entry into the phenicoabdominal vein and associated invaded caval wall segment can be seen.

submucosa has been described in a series of experimental animals.[39] Use of an autogenous jugular vein graft may also be feasible, although forward planning would be required to harvest the graft before need.

Postoperative Management

There is limited available evidence for optimal postoperative management protocols following adrenalectomy requiring cavotomy. The author uses local blocks (line or thoracoabdominal plexus) in combination with systemic opioids for analgesia. Nonsteroidal anti-inflammatories are avoided in the first 24 hours due to the risk of summation on intraoperative renal injury. Maropitant and pantoprazole are routinely administered preoperatively and maintained while the animal is in hospital. Oxygen supplementation via nasal prongs is routinely provided for 12 hours postoperatively if the patient has atelectasis postanesthesia or if a median sternotomy has been performed. A urinary catheter is placed and urine output monitored closely for the first 12 hours. If the patient has a strongly cushingoid phenotype, unfractionated heparin at a dose of 150 IU/kg is given subcutaneously and followed by a constant rate infusion of 10 IU/kg/h for 24 hours, after which it is tapered and discontinued over 6 to 12 hours. If renal venotomy or extensive renal vein dissection/manipulation has been required, a focal ultrasonography to check renal vein flow 12 hours postoperatively is performed.

PROGNOSIS FOLLOWING ADRENALECTOMY
Short-Term Survival

For small adrenal tumors where removal can be performed without cavotomy (median tumor size = 2.2 cm, n = 51 dogs), perioperative mortality has been reported at 8%

with 83.3% 1-year and 76.1% 2-year survival rates (Cavalcanti 2020). An additional 24% of dogs experienced a minor or major postoperative complication, including hypoadrenocorticism, regurgitation and aspiration pneumonia, acute kidney injury, pancreatitis, and hypertension or hypotension; 53% of dogs experienced major or minor intraoperative complications, including hemorrhage, hypertension or hypotension, bradycardia, tachycardia, regurgitation, and capsular rupture of the tumor.

In a case series of larger adrenal tumors wherein cavotomy was required (median tumor size 2.6 cm, n = 45 dogs) perioperative mortality was 24% and median survival time was 547 days (95% confidence interval 146–710).[40] The reasons for the perioperative deaths were not reported, but the presence of thrombus extending into the intrathoracic cava was associated with a greater risk of death. An additional 31% experienced a postoperative complication including pancreatitis, persistent bleeding, renal failure, respiratory crisis due to acute respiratory distress syndrome or aspiration pneumonia, and acute kidney injury.

Outcome following bilateral adrenalectomy (n = 9) has also been reported (Oblak 2016). These dogs received intraoperative steroid supplementation with dexamethasone and desoxycorticosterone pivalate. Outcomes in this small series were similar to those reported in a unilateral adrenalectomy population: 1 dog died postoperatively and 3 additional dogs experienced perioperative complications. Median survival time was 525 days, and long-term management of the iatrogenic hypoadrenocorticism was reported as straightforward.

Prognosis following emergency adrenalectomy performed for acute paraneoplastic adrenal hemorrhage seems poorer than for elective adrenalectomy, with a perioperative mortality risk of 50% in 8 dogs (Lang 2011).

Although hypercoagulability secondary to hypercortisolism is a well-cited concern, respiratory crisis due to pulmonary thromboembolism was not a notable reported complication in the studies cited, although some instances of sudden death due to cardiac arrest, which could be due to an embolic event, were reported.

Long-Term Survival

The metastatic risk for adrenal tumors following adrenalectomy is not well established due to the absence of long-term posttreatment necropsy studies, but may be higher for pheochromocytomas than adrenocortical carcinomas, with both local recurrence at the original tumor site and metastasis to other organs reported. In a population of dogs that required cavotomy for adrenal tumor removal, imaging findings consistent with metastasis were reported in 5 of 45 (11%) dogs with a median survival of 547 postoperative days.[40] A necropsy study evaluating dogs with untreated pheochromocytoma identified metastatic lesions in 20% of animals at the time of death or euthanasia (Barthez 1997). In 7 dogs that underwent adrenalectomy for pheochromocytoma and had long-term follow-up, diffuse metastasis to regional lymph nodes, spleen, liver, and lung was identified 3 years postoperatively in 1 dog (Barthez 1997). In another case series a dog undergoing adrenalectomy for adrenocortical carcinoma developed pulmonary metastasis at an unspecified time after surgery (Lang 2011). In 50 dogs with adrenocortical tumors that underwent adrenalectomy, recurrence of clinical signs of hyperadrenocorticism, which may have been due to local recurrence or metastasis or contralateral disease, occurred in 38% with a median survival of 507 days (Sanders 2019).

Histopathological Prognosis

Histopathological differentiation of adrenocortical adenoma from adenocarcinoma can be challenging and is likely to impact both prognosis and the long-term monitoring protocol for the patient. A scoring system based on the histopathological features of these tumors has been developed, with the goal of improving consistency in differentiation of these tumor types and improving prognosis; however, the score has yet to be validated on an independent population (Sanders 2019).

SUMMARY

Improvements in early diagnosis with many tumors now being identified on advanced imaging for other reasons and before the development of any clinical signs, together with improvements in preoperative treatment, anesthetic management, and surgical familiarity with the multiple techniques available for the specific challenges of any individual adrenalectomy have all contributed to an improved prognosis for these tumors over the last decade. A recent report on extended survival times following stereotactic radiation for the treatment of adrenal tumors showing vascular invasion may offer another treatment option for cases with advanced disease (Dolera 2016) if results are repeatable. Additional avenues for improving care may be available in simulator training to accelerate the learning curve for management of vascular invasion in inexperienced surgeons, and evidence-based definitions of appropriate case selection for minimally invasive techniques.

DISCLOSURE

The author has nothing to disclose

REFERENCES

1. Cook AK, Spaulding KA, Edwards JF. Clinical findings in dogs with incidental adrenal gland lesions determined by ultrasonography: 151 cases (2007-2010). J Am Vet Med Assoc 2014;244:1181–5.
2. Melián C, Pérez-López L, Saavedra P, et al. Vet Rec 2020. https://doi.org/10.1002/VETR.80. in press.
3. Pagani E, Tursi M, Lorenzi C, et al. Ultrasonographic features of adrenal gland lesions in dogs can aid in diagnosis. BMC Vet Res 2016;12. https://doi.org/10.1186/S12917-016-0895-1.
4. Bertazzolo W, Didier M, Gelain ME, et al. Accuracy of cytology in distinguishing adrenocortical tumors from pheochromocytoma in companion animals. Vet Clin Pathol 2014;43:453–9.
5. Pey P, Diana A, Rossi F, et al. Safety of percutaneous ultrasound-guided fine-needle aspiration of adrenal lesions in dogs: Perception of the procedure by radiologists and presentation of 50 cases. J Vet Intern Med 2020;34:626–35.
6. Sumner JA, Lacorcia L, Rose AM, et al. Clinical safety of percutaneous ultrasound-guided fine-needle aspiration of adrenal gland lesions in 19 dogs. J Small Anim Pract 2018;59:357–63.
7. Lee S, Lee A, Chai SH, et al. Ectopic Cushing's syndrome associated with a pheochromocytoma in a dog: a case report. BMC Vet Res 2020;16. https://doi.org/10.1186/S12917-020-2244-7.
8. Baek Y, Ang M, Park J. Canine adrenocorticotropic hormone-producing sinusoidal neuroendocrine tumor associated with Cushing's disease. J Vet Med Sci 2019;81(12):1863–7.
9. Hylands R. Veterinary diagnostic imaging. Malignant pheochromocytoma of the left adrenal gland invading the caudal vena cava, accompanied by a cortisol

secreting adrenocortical carcinoma of the right adrenal gland. Can Vet J 2005; 46(12):1156–8.

10. Gójska-Zygner O, Lechowski R, Zygner W. Functioning unilateral adrenocortical carcinoma in a dog. Can Vet J 2012;53(6):623–5.

11. Cook. Suspected bilateral adrenal gland tumour causing primary Addison's disease in a dog. Tierarztl Prax Ausg K Kleintiere Heimtiere 2020;48(2):132–8.

12. Merino-Gutierrez V, Feo-Bernabé L, Clemente-Vicario F, et al. Addison's Disease Secondary to Bilateral Adrenal Gland Metastatic Mammary Carcinoma in a Dog. J Am Anim Hosp Assoc. Mar/Apr 2020;56(2):e56203.

13. Cavalcanti JVJ, Skinner OT, Mayhew PD, et al. Outcome in dogs undergoing adrenalectomy for small adrenal gland tumours without vascular invasion. Vet Comp Oncol 2020;18(4):599–606.

14. Nagumo T, Ishigaki K, Yoshida O, et al. Utility of contrast-enhanced ultrasound in differential diagnosis of adrenal tumors in dogs. J Vet Med Sci 2020;82: 1594–601.

15. Yoshida O, Kutara K, Seki M, et al. Preoperative Differential Diagnosis of Canine Adrenal Tumors Using Triple-Phase Helical Computed Tomography. Vet Surg 2016;45:427–35.

16. Soler Arias EA, Trigo RH, Miceli DD, et al. Urinary vanillylmandelic acid:creatinine ratio in dogs with pheochromocytoma. Domest Anim Endocrinol 2021;74. https:// doi.org/10.1016/J.DOMANIEND.2020.106559.

17. Salesov E, Boretti FS, Sieber-Ruckstuhl NS, et al. Urinary and plasma catecholamines and metanephrines in dogs with pheochromocytoma, hypercortisolism, nonadrenal disease and in healthy dogs. J Vet Intern Med 2015;29:597–602.

18. Sasaki N, Ikenaka Y, Inoue Y, et al. Urinary free metanephrines measurement in dogs with adrenal gland diseases using a new simple liquid chromatography tandem mass spectrometry method. J Vet Med Sci 2021;83:648–55.

19. Espinel-Rupérez J, Martín-Ríos MD, Salazar V, et al. Incidence of surgical site infection in dogs undergoing soft tissue surgery: risk factors and economic impact. Vet Rec Open 2019;6. https://doi.org/10.1136/VETRECO-2017-000233.

20. Kato MT, Mallard JM. Autoresuscitation and pheochromocytoma multisystem crisis in a dog. J Vet Emerg Crit Care (San Antonio) 2021;31:525–30.

21. Pacak K. Preoperative management of the pheochromocytoma patient. J Clin Endocrinol Metab 2007;92:4069–79.

22. Herrera MA, Mehl ML, Kass PH, et al. Predictive factors and the effect of phenoxybenzamine on outcome in dogs undergoing adrenalectomy for pheochromocytoma. J Vet Intern Med 2008;22:1333–9.

23. Gregori T, Mantis P, Benigni L, et al. Comparison of computed tomographic and pathologic findings in 17 dogs with primary adrenal neoplasia. Vet Radiol Ultrasound 2015;56:153–9.

24. Naan EC, Kirpensteijn J, Dupré GP, et al. Innovative approach to laparoscopic adrenalectomy for treatment of unilateral adrenal gland tumors in dogs. Vet Surg 2013;42:710–5.

25. Pitt KA, Mayhew PD, Steffey MA, et al. Laparoscopic Adrenalectomy for Removal of Unilateral Noninvasive Pheochromocytomas in 10 Dogs. Vet Surg 2016;45: O70–6.

26. Ko J, Jeong J, Lee S, et al. Feasibility of single-port retroperitoneoscopic adrenalectomy in dogs. Vet Surg 2018;47:O75–83.

27. Taylor CJ, Monnet E. A comparison of outcomes between laparoscopic and open adrenalectomies in dogs. Vet Surg 2021;50(Suppl 1):O99–107.

28. Mayhew PD, Culp WTN, Hunt GB, et al. Comparison of perioperative morbidity and mortality rates in dogs with noninvasive adrenocortical masses undergoing laparoscopic versus open adrenalectomy. J Am Vet Med Assoc 2014;245: 1028–35.
29. Battistella E, Ferrari S, Pomba L, et al. Adrenal surgery: Review of 35 years experience in a single centre. Surg Oncol 2021;37. https://doi.org/10.1016/J. SURONC.2021.101554.
30. Andrade N, Rivas LR, Milovancev M, et al. Intercostal approach for right adrenalectomy in dogs. Vet Surg 2014;43:99–104.
31. Chiti LE, Mayhew PD, Massari F. Renal venotomy for thrombectomy and kidney preservation in dogs with adrenal tumors and renal vein invasion. Vet Surg 2021;50:872–9.
32. Knight RC, Lamb CR, Brockman DJ, et al. Variations in surgical technique for adrenalectomy with caudal vena cava venotomy in 19 dogs. Vet Surg 2019;48: 751–9.
33. Davis J, Raisis AL, Haitjema H, et al. Paradoxical bradycardia during surgical caudal vena cava occlusion in an anesthetized dog. J Vet Emerg Crit Care (San Antonio) 2017;27:243–9.
34. de Andrade CR, Barboza WM, Silva Lessa DF, et al. Acta Sci Vet 2020. https://doi. org/10.22456/1679-9216.100113. in press.
35. Lipscomb VJ. Surgical management of an adrenal gland tumor that had extended into the thoracic portion of the caudal vena cava in a dog. J Am Vet Med Assoc 2019;254:1309–15.
36. Guillaumot PJ, Heripret D, Bouvy BM, et al. 49-month survival following caval venectomy without nephrectomy in a dog with a pheochromocytoma. J Am Anim Hosp Assoc 2012;48:352–8.
37. Louvet A, Lazard P, Denis B. Phaeochromocytoma treated by en bloc resection including the suprarenal caudal vena cava in a dog. J Small Anim Pract 2005; 46:591–6.
38. Peacock JT, Fossum TW, Bahr AM, et al. Evaluation of gradual occlusion of the caudal vena cava in clinically normal dogs. Am J Vet Res 2003;64:1347–53.
39. Lantz GC, Badylak SF, Coffey AC, et al. Small intestinal submucosa as a superior vena cava graft in the dog. J Surg Res 1992;53:175–81.
40. Mayhew PD, Culp WTN, Balsa IM, et al. Phrenicoabdominal venotomy for tumor thrombectomy in dogs with adrenal neoplasia and suspected vena caval invasion. Vet Surg 2018;47:227–35.

Current Concepts in Head and Neck Surgery

Judith Bertran, DVM, MSc[a,b],*, Alexander C.S. Thomson, DVM[c]

KEYWORDS

- Maxillectomy • Mandibulectomy • Oral surgery • Oncology • Dental lymphogram

KEY POINTS

- Complete staging for oral tumors and understanding the biological behavior of the tumor is essential for the decision-making therapeutic plan.
- Oral surgical oncology principles are extremely important to maximize success and achieve adequate prognosis in the first surgical tumor removal attempt.
- A high (43.8%) false-negative rate of aspirated lymph nodes is detected in histopathology in dogs with oral malignant melanoma
- Bone regeneration and internal fixation after mandibulectomy or maxillectomy is not necessary; however, several emerging techniques have achieved successful outcomes and may be alternative options for some owners.
- Cosmetic and functional outcomes after aggressive oral tumor surgical excisions are acceptable by most of the owners and preserve patient's good quality of life.

INTRODUCTION

Oral cavity tumors and tumorlike lesions are detected commonly during routine clinical examination in dogs and cats. Oral tumorlike lesions may be benign or malignant, but hyperplastic and inflammatory lesions may clinically masquerade neoplasia.[1] Historically, oral malignant neoplasms represented approximately 6% to 7% of all canine cancers, and 3% of all feline cancers.[2] A recent demographic study showed that the incidence of oral tumors is considerably higher than previously reported, and about 53.6% and 58.1% were classified as malignant in dogs and cats, respectively.[3] The most common oral malignancies in dogs are melanomas (**Fig. 1**), squamous cell carcinomas (SCC), fibrosarcomas, and osteosarcomas.[1] In cats, 69% of malignant oral tumors are SCC and 18% are fibrosarcomas.[1,4] Other

[a] Surgical Oncology, Small Animal Clinical Sciences, University of Florida, Gainesville, FL, USA;
[b] Veterinary Clinical Sciences, University of Florida, 2015 Southwest 16th Avenue, Gainesville 32608, FL, USA; [c] City University of Hong Kong Veterinary Medical Centre, 202 Yee Kuk Street, Sham Shui Po, Kowloon, HK
* Corresponding author. Veterinary Clinical Sciences, University of Florida, 2015 Southwest 16th Avenue, Gainesville, FL 32608.
E-mail address: Bertran.judith@ufl.edu

Vet Clin Small Anim 52 (2022) 489–512
https://doi.org/10.1016/j.cvsm.2021.12.006
0195-5616/22/© 2021 Elsevier Inc. All rights reserved.

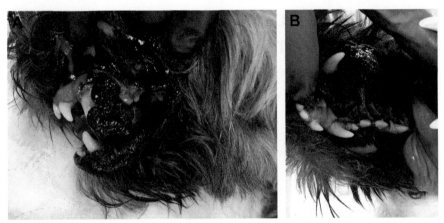

Fig. 1. Left maxillary oral malignant melanoma in a dog (*A*). Notice how the tumor extends across the rostral aspect of the hard palate (*B*). This illustrates the importance of a complete, under sedation/anesthesia oral examination.

oral tumors that can occur are acanthomatous ameloblastoma (**Fig. 2**) and peripheral odontogenic fibromas. Infectious and inflammatory lesions and nonneoplastic growths such as gingival hyperplasia may be mistaken for neoplastic lesions. Despite their different nature, these lesions appear similar macroscopically, and therefore their clinical classification is difficult or impossible without cytologic or histopathological analysis. Oral tumors often go unnoticed by the pet's owner until they reach an advanced stage of the disease. Understanding the tumor's biological behavior is essential to formulate a diagnostic and therapeutic plan, and to provide necessary information to the client.

CLINICAL STAGING

Accurate assessment of the primary tumor and the stage of the disease is crucial, and it requires a systematic approach using the universally recognized TNM system.[5] This system evaluates the tumor, the regional lymph nodes (LNs), and other distant organs targeted by the metastatic potential of the tumor.

1. *Tumor:* Complete inspection and evaluation of the tumor often require sedation. Assessment of size, location, evidence of necrosis, ulceration, pain, bone involvement, and abnormal mobility of the teeth is of paramount importance. Diagnostic imaging of the oral cavity will help determine the extension of the tumor's local soft tissue and bone invasion. Ultimately, cytologic and/or histopathological diagnosis of the tumor is essential to comprehend the biology of the tumor.
2. *Lymph node:* LN evaluation is an important part of the staging process for oral neoplasia in human and veterinary patients and is an important predictor of prognosis in many tumor types. Metastasis to the LNs may also indicate the potential for distant metastasis.[6] It has been shown in veterinary patients that palpation and cytology of the metastatic LNs lack sensitivity and specificity.[7] Nonetheless, evaluation of LNs is still an essential part of the TNM staging classification. However, because head and neck lymphatic drainage is abundant, extremely convoluted, and unpredictable, selection of the LNs that drain the tumor's anatomic area (also known as the sentinel LN [SLN]) is extremely important for accuracy of the

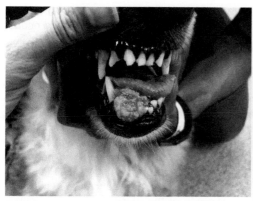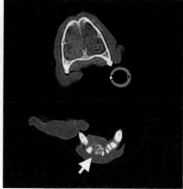

Fig. 2. Acanthomatous ameloblastoma of the right rostral mandible (*A*) and CT transverse image showing the local bone invasion of this tumor (*B*).

staging process and to target nodal dissection if indicated. Therefore, methods for diagnostic imaging and intraoperative detection of SLNs are emerging in veterinary surgical oncology and should be implemented when available.[8]

3. *Distant metastasis:* Thoracic radiographs for the detection of pulmonary metastasis should be obtained for any dog with a suspected oral tumor. Up to 41% of dogs diagnosed with oral malignant melanoma (OMM) can have pulmonary metastasis by the time of diagnosis.[9] Although the yield of this test is generally low,[10] the presence of visible pulmonary metastasis on plain radiographs indicates a poor prognosis. Computed tomography (CT) is significantly more sensitive than thoracic radiography to detect soft tissue nodules in the lungs and can be paired with CT imaging of the head for surgical planning.[11]

DIAGNOSTIC IMAGING FOR ORAL TUMORS

Investigating the local extent of tumor invasion is important for determining first-line therapy options. Because bone must lose a significant proportion of its mineral before it acquires lytic radiographic appearance, plain radiographs tend to underestimate the extent of bone destruction. In addition, plain radiography gives poor representation of the degree of involvement of normal and abnormal soft tissues. Dental radiographs are commonly used in maxillofacial surgery and dental practices; they are useful for identifying mass-associated tooth destruction and to assess periodontal ligament tumors, like fibromatous epulis.[12,13] Dental radiographs may be adequate and sufficient for small rostrally located masses. CT provides a comprehensive and accurate assessment of both bone and soft tissue margins. In addition, CT is particularly valuable for assessment of tumor sizes and locations that may make complete surgical resection difficult (eg, caudal maxilla and mandible, tumors that invade the nasal cavity or the periorbital region, and tumors that grow beyond midline).[13]

BIOPSY VERSUS CYTOLOGY

Oral malignancies have similar local invasive behavior but different metastatic potential. Therefore, the histologic type influences the long-term survival but minimally affects surgical planning. Nonetheless, preoperative cytology or biopsy is strongly advised and has several advantages for the client and the clinician: to discriminate benign versus malignant lesions, to plan diagnostic tests for tumor staging, to obtain accurate prognosis before considering treatment, to decide on the extent of the treatment (conservative versus aggressive), and to investigate tumor responses to neoadjuvant or adjuvant treatments.

Fine-needle aspiration (FNA) and cytology has shown to carry high sensitivities and moderate specificities for neoplastic oral lesions.[14] This study showed that fine-needle insertion (needle tissue penetration without aspirating with a syringe) is superior due to preservation of intact cells when compared with FNA. However, hypocellularity, hemodilution, inflammation, and necrosis are known factors to affect cytologic analysis. In addition, masses with high percentage of stroma (like peripheral odontogenic fibroma and gingival fibroepithelial hyperplasia) may prevent adequate cytology sampling. Because most animals will require some type of tranquilization to perform a thorough oral examination and obtain either type of sample from an intraoral location, some clinicians prefer to perform a biopsy to maximize the chances of achieving a diagnosis during the sedation period.[15] The site of the biopsy should be planned such that it falls within the boundaries of the tissue to be excised once the diagnosis is made to maintain the tumor margins for surgical planning.[16] Similarly, macroscopically normal tissue on the margin of the tumor should not necessarily be included in an incisional biopsy because this may violate previously unopened tissue planes.[17] Obtaining multiple deep biopsies from different parts of the lesion is sometimes necessary.[18] In selected cases (small tumors or pedunculated masses) an excisional biopsy may be indicated. The results from histopathology should be compared with the clinical findings, and if they are not found to be compatible with the clinical picture further discussion with the pathologist is warranted to decide and select the most appropriate therapeutic plan.

LYMPH NODE STAGING AND CONTROVERSIES

Metastasis to LNs is a negative prognostic factor in oral cancers in humans and dogs.[19,20] Evaluation of regional LNs or SLNs is necessary for staging oral cancers because results can provide prognostic information and early detection of nodal metastasis can impact survival.[9,20] Moreover, excision of the metastatic LNs has a therapeutic benefit.[21] Equivalent data are not available in the dog or the cat; however, the excision of metastatic LNs in nonoral cancers has documented similar benefits in disease-free intervals and overall survival.[22]

As previously stated, LN size and cytology lack sensitivity and specificity for metastatic detection in solid tumors of the head.[7,23–25] Lymphatic drainage of the head and neck involves multiple lymph centers, with individual variation reported; however, the main sites are the parotid, the mandibular (lateral and medial), and the retropharyngeal LNs.[26] In addition, bilateral and overlapping drainage pathways have been identified in the dog's head with metastasis occurring to the contralateral LNs in 62% of cases.[27]

Nonselective extirpation of the regional LNs has been used in humans and dogs; although the therapeutic benefit of this approach is unknown, it may provide valuable staging information. A technique for extirpation of bilateral mandibular and retropharyngeal LNs using a single cervical incision has been reported.[28] In addition, another technique allows for ipsilateral removal of the parotid, mandibular, and retropharyngeal lymph centers.[29] In humans, however, selective SLN mapping is commonly accepted as the gold standard for LN dissection and has been associated with decreased surgical time, decreased complication rate, and similar prognostic benefits.[30] Nonetheless, with the complexity of the head and neck lymphatics and the biologically aggressive behavior of tumors such as melanoma, risks of false-negative SLNs is still a limitation.[31] Indirect computed lymphography (**Fig. 3**A) and

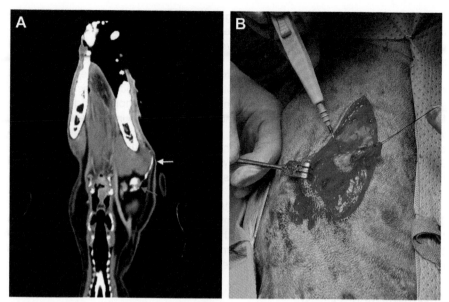

Fig. 3. CT lymphography (CTL) of a dog with right maxillary OMM (*A*). A lymphatic efferent vessel (*white arrow*) is entering the lateral right submandibular lymph node (*blue arrow*). Intraoperative picture of the sentinel lymph node detected via a combination of CTL and methylene blue (*B*).

intraoperative use of a variety of dyes (methylene blue, **Fig. 3**B) and near-infrared technology (indocyanine green) are currently in use and under investigation.[32] There is an emergent need for novel SLN visualization techniques that can help easier identification of SLNs reducing the amount of false-negative SLNs associated with head and neck tumors. Failure to identify sites of LN metastasis may result in less aggressive treatment than is warranted by the disease process and a decreased survival time.

DECISION MAKING

The therapeutic plan is made after clinical staging and tumor type identification. A team approach involving a surgical oncologist, a dentist, a radiation oncologist, and a medical oncologist is ideal. Surgical excision of oral tumors remains the gold standard treatment. Generally, wide surgical excision is required to appropriately treat malignant tumors of the oral cavity, whereas marginal excision including the affected tooth and the periodontal ligament may be sufficient for some benign tumors. When surgical options are limited, local treatment with radiation therapy (RT) should be considered as a definitive intent or palliative option. In selected cases, preoperative RT may be indicated for tumor size reduction. Adjuvant RT should be discussed and anticipated if the size or location of the tumor makes complete surgical excision unlikely.

PRINCIPLES OF ORAL SURGERY

Surgical excision is the most commonly used modality for treatment of oral tumors. A thorough knowledge of the regional anatomy (neurovascular bundles, muscular attachments, options for local flaps, and so forth) is necessary for a successful surgical outcome. Presurgical biopsy site planning allows the surgeon to excise the biopsy tract en bloc with the tumor and the desired tissue margins during the definitive surgery. Extensive anatomic descriptions have been published and should be reviewed before any maxillofacial surgery.[15,17]

Except for peripheral odontogenic fibroma, most tumors involving the mandible and maxilla have some underlying bone involvement, and surgical resection of these should include bony margins to increase the likelihood of complete surgical excision. Margins required for resection of oral tumors have not been investigated; however, when possible, 2- to 3-cm margins for malignant tumors are recommended to decrease recurrence rates.[33] Depending on the size and location of some oral tumors, 2 to 3 cm may not be possible; therefore whenever possible 1 cm of grossly normal tissue beyond the visible tumor or previously determined by imaging may be acceptable for malignant tumors.

Surgical principles of oral surgery need to be considered during these procedures. The oral cavity is a remarkable environment in which effective healing occurs despite the several local factors that could disturb the wound (**Table 1**). However, it is essential that surgeons have an improved understanding of these challenges to help address issues that can lead to poor oral wound healing.

ANESTHETIC MANAGEMENT

Anesthetic preparation is critical to mitigate risk associated with surgeries of the head. Blood products and various airway management strategies should be readily available

Craniofacial pathology can render normograde intubation difficult or impossible. Supplies for guided intubation and tracheostomy should be available throughout the anesthetic and recovery periods. Care should be taken not to embolize friable tissue or foreign material into the airway. The pharynx should be inspected before extubation; clotted blood or other material can cause postoperative airway obstruction.

A balanced anesthetic protocol should be used whenever possible. Nerve blocks reduce systemic anesthetic requirements and are associated with improved postoperative analgesia.[39–42]

Regional Anesthetic Techniques

Selection of a technique is predicated on the individual procedure and anatomy. Intraneural and intravascular injections should be avoided, and the needle should not pass through diseased tissue (**Fig. 5**).

Mixing local anesthetics has been suggested.[43,44] However, this alters the pH and concentration of each drug, reducing the duration of blockade without appreciably improving the onset time.[45,46]

Maxillary Techniques

The maxillary nerve can be blocked in the pterygopalatine fossa,[47–49] desensitizing the entire maxilla and its associated soft tissue structures. The palate may also be desensitized due to blockade of the pterygopalatine nerve.

A Quincke needle is introduced by a maxillary tuberosity approach, in which the needle is inserted perpendicularly to the hard palate caudal to the last molar, or a transcutaneous subzygomatic approach, in which the needle is inserted perpendicular to the skin ventral to the rostral zygomatic arch and cranial to the mandibular coronoid process. The bevel is directed rostrally toward the pterygopalatine fossa; the depth depends on the size of the patient. Recommended injection volume is 0.25 mL for a cat or up to 0.5 mL for a large dog.[47]

Table 1
Local factors affecting wound healing

	Key points
Local infection	• Incidence of local infection is low due to excellent blood supply • Infection maintains wound in an inflammatory state resulting in dehiscence and fistulation • "Clean-contaminated" procedure: prophylactic antibiotics (ie, clindamycin, amoxicillin-clavulanic acid every 90 min during anesthesia[34]). Definitely consider if systemic disease, immunosuppression, radiation treatment, etc.
Thermal damage	• Avoid excessive monopolar use in mucosa/submucosa—associated with delayed healing[35] • Mucosal layer ultimately responsible for epithelialization—protective function • Frequent irrigation of the saw blade or high speed burr during bone cutting to avoid bone necrosis and maintain the blood supply
Sutures	• Tissue reactivity may enhance inflammatory response • Polydioxanone and polyglyconate are preferred absorbable sutures—low tissue reactivity and microbial adherence[36] • Other braided sutures (potentially softer and more secure knots) are contraindicated due to increased surface area and likelihood of infection
Tension at incision	• Important principle to avoid wound breakdown—mucosal apposition without tension • Incision challenges; tension from tongue motion, swallowing patterns, masticatory functions • Suturing tricks: appositional pattern, interrupted/cruciate/horizontal patterns preferred[37] • Two- or 3-layer closure whenever possible using tissues with better holding properties than mucosa (submucosa, subcutaneous, muscular, mucoperiosteum) **Fig. 4** • Mobilize buccal mucosal flaps to where final incision lays over thicker muscle, submucosal or bone tissue
Nerve damage	• Causes loss of sensation potentially perpetuating self-trauma • Dysfunction in the form of neuropathic pain with or without hypoesthesia of the innervated area has been detected in people[38]

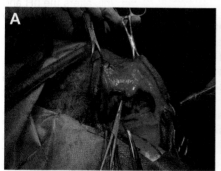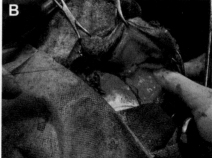

Fig. 4. Closure of a bilateral rostral maxillectomy using a 3-layer closure. The deeper sutures are placed to ensure good placement onto the muscular layer (*A*). Subcutaneous layer closure with simple interrupted sutures (*B*) before mucosal layer closure.

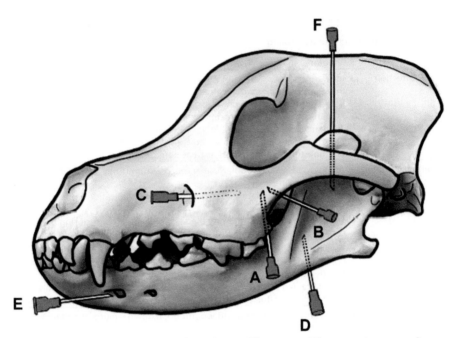

Fig. 5. Maxillary tuberosity approach to the maxillary nerve (A); transcutaneous subzygomatic approach to the maxillary nerve (B); infraorbital approach to the maxillary nerve (C); extraoral approach to the inferior alveolar nerve (D); approach to the middle mental nerve (E); approach to the trigeminal nerve (F).

Alternatively, a catheter can be fed caudally through the infraorbital canal.[50–52] This technique reduces the risk of damage to retrobulbar structures and resulted in higher success than a transcutaneous approach in both dogs and cats.[50,51]

The maxilla rostral to the third premolar can be anesthetized with an infraorbital nerve block. A needle is positioned over the foramen under direct palpation, with the bevel facing medially. The same volume of local anesthetic is used as for the maxillary nerve block.[47]

Mandibular Techniques

Inferior alveolar nerve block results in desensitization of the mandible, mandibular teeth, gingiva, and associated soft tissue structures. The mandibular foramen and neurovascular bundle can be palpated intraorally on the medial ventral ramus. A Quincke needle is introduced either intraorally or percutaneously and advanced beneath the mucosa until the tip is palpated directly over the foramen. The recommended injection volume is 0.15 to 0.6 mL, depending on the size of the patient.[47] Injection of too much volume may cause blockade of the lingual nerve, tongue desensitization, and potential self-inflicted trauma.[53]

The rostral buccal gingiva or lower lip can be anesthetized by blocking the middle mental nerve. However, analgesia of the rostral mandible may be ineffective, so inferior alveolar nerve block should be considered for more invasive procedures.[54]

Trigeminal Nerve Block

Ultrasound-guided trigeminal nerve block has been reported in a dog undergoing exenteration, caudal maxillectomy, and zygomatic arch resection.[55,56] A Quincke spinal needle is introduced in-plane to the ultrasound transducer caudal to the orbital ligament and advanced ventrally, where the branches of the trigeminal nerve and the maxillary artery can be seen overlying the sphenoid bone.[56] The volume delivered is calculated as 0.1 mL/cm from the cranium length, measured from the inion (ridge felt ventral to the external occipital protuberance) to the nasion (indentation between forehead and nose).[55]

SURGICAL TECHNIQUES: AN UPDATE

Patient preparation and aseptic techniques for oral surgery are described elsewhere and are beyond the scope of this article.[17] In this article we cover the most updated techniques; therefore standard surgical textbooks can be consulted by the reader for step-by-step procedures.[17,57,58] Generally speaking, the surgical dose for an oral tumor should be decided based on preoperative advanced imaging, tumor biological behavior, tumor location, and tumor size. In addition, clients should be thoroughly educated about postoperative care and esthetics, survival times, risks, and costs in advance of surgery.

Removing Tooth Roots: Is There a Debate?

Often the osteotomies fall across a tooth root during mandibulectomy and maxillectomy. Pulpal tissue is sensitive, and dogs have a propensity to develop periodontitis and periapical lesions. Irreversible pulpitis, necrosis, and pain resulting from exposure of the tooth root can occur, leading most dentists to recommend removing the exposed tooth roots. Additionally, intact alveoli removal is recommended because many tumors like to infiltrate the periodontal ligament space. Dental elevators, a high-speed bur, or piezoelectric equipment can be used with minimal added surgical time (**Fig. 6**). Conversely, others may leave the tooth roots in situ as long as they do not present signs of disease. In a review of the literature, it was seen that up to 84% of humans with retained tooth fragments observed in radiographs did not have any associated symptoms.[59] Although there are no clear data on this controversial topic, given the possibility of chronic discomfort and the chances of potential complications (16% in humans),[59] the decision would fall in favor of removing the exposed tooth roots as long as the patient is doing well under anesthesia.

Updates in Mandibulectomy Techniques

Anatomically, the mandibular canal is an important oncological consideration and extends along the body of the mandible until reaching the mandibular foramen. Tumors involving the mandibular body can extend along the mandibular canal, thus the caudal margins of the excision should be taken caudal to the mandibular foramen to minimize the risk of incomplete tumor excision.

A mandibulectomy is the en bloc excision of a mandible (total mandibulectomy), or part of one (partial mandibulectomy) or part of both mandibles (rostral mandibulectomy), bearing an oral tumor. Mandibulectomy should be considered for local control of mandibular neoplasms.

Rim excision: A rim excision on the mandible is defined as a partial segmental excision that removes the occlusal part of the mandible but leaves a strong ventral border intact.[60] This is an effective oncologic procedure that may provide local cancer control comparable with segmental mandibulectomy in certain cases. This procedure is indicated for marginal excision of benign tumors or wide excision of small malignant tumors that are not invading beyond the alveolar margin.[61] Malignant nonodontogenic tumors (fibrosarcoma, OMM, SCC, and other tumors) should be treated with wider

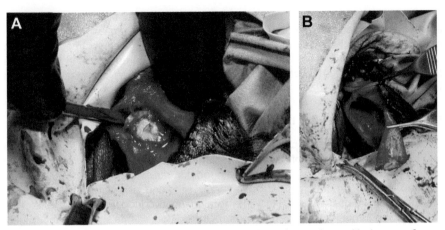

Fig. 6. Lower canine tooth root removal after a unilateral rostral mandibulectomy for an oral plasmacytoma (*A, B*). (Pictures courtesy of Dr Don Hoover.)

margins and are contraindicated for this technique (**Fig. 7**). This procedure has the main advantages of superior postoperative function, absence of mandibular drift, maintenance of normal tongue carriage, elimination of traumatic malocclusion, and preservation of cosmetics. In addition, this technique is versatile and can be performed in the rostral mandible, in the caudal aspect of the mandibular ramus, and in the maxilla in dogs.[62] Because the current veterinary literature does not provide a uniform opinion regarding the surgical dose needed to obtain cancer-free margins, this technique may seem attractive to some veterinarians as a simple and less aggressive procedure. However, it is of paramount importance to consider tumor biology, tumor extension, surgical oncology principles, and anatomic constraints (**Box 1**).

Postoperative iatrogenic fractures have been seen in 15% of people undergoing this procedure, likely due to decreased blood supply, excessive periosteal stripping, and wound dehiscence. In dogs, although literature is sparse in relation to this technique, 1 of 13 dogs had a subclinical fracture after crescentic osteotomy rim resection for acanthomatous ameloblastoma.[60] Although a biomechanical study in the dog shows no differences between curvilinear and right-angled osteotomy,[63] it seems that the curvilinear cut resists higher occlusal forces in humans.[64] Some important oncological considerations need to be made in view of using this technique. Rim excision can be performed with a pneumatic bur, a semicircular saw blade, or piezoelectric technology

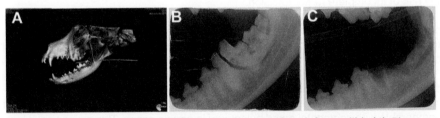

Fig. 7. CT reconstruction of a dog with previous fibroma of the left mandible (*A*). Rim resection dental pictures of the marked bone cut (*B*) and after removing the tumor with the left 3 molars with additional tooth root removal of M1 (*C*). (*Pictures courtesy* of Dr Cindy Eward.)

Box 1
Oncological considerations for rim excision: contraindications

Gross periodontal ligament involvement in the tumor burden

Tumor is involving the mandibular canal

Small dogs with tumors involving the first molar[62]

for different types of osteotomies.[60,65] One needs to consider that adequate surgical margin assessment may not be feasible when using the bur because further bone removal may be performed after tumor excision.[66] When considering where to locate the most ventral point of the osteotomy, it is recommended to consider 40% of the total height of the mandibular body to avoid entering the mandibular canal.[63] Osteotomies measuring greater than 50% of the dorsal mandibular body risk entering the canal and lacerating the neurovascular bundle, weakening the remaining fragments and compromising the vitality of the dental structures. However, the surgical margin should not be dictated by those limitations, and decision making of the surgical technique should be performed with the goal of curative intent. Although rim excision is a promising technique for treatment of minimally invasive odontogenic oncological surgery, appropriate case selection is key for decision making to use this technique.

Symphyseal-sparing rostral mandibulectomy: This procedure is indicated for dogs with neoplasms located at or near the mandibular incisor and canine teeth. The goal remains to remove a minimum of 1 cm margin of grossly normal tissue while preserving some portion of the symphysis. A symphyseal-sparing technique should prevent mobility of the mandibles and allow for an optimal occlusion, aiding preservation of function and cosmesis. Knowledge of the regional anatomy of the caudal mandibular symphysis and the mental foramen in relation to the first premolar teeth is important to serve as guideline for symphysis preservation. Ostectomies performed during this procedure will be at or immediately rostral to the middle mental foramen. The reconstruction of the lip should be previously planned accounting for the soft tissue margins that need to be excised and with the goal of achieving mucosal apposition, coverage of the excised bone, and support for food and saliva[67] (**Fig. 8**).

Rostral bilateral mandibulectomy: More extensive rostral mandibulectomies are indicated for dogs with malignant tumors or benign acanthomatous ameloblastoma rostral to the first premolar tooth and across the mandibular symphysis. The extent of the excision can be as far caudal as the fourth premolar; however, greater difficulty prehending food can occur. For this reason, immediate or delayed reconstruction techniques with preoperative 3D printing, titanium locking plates, and regenerative materials have been described with good outcomes.[68] Despite this, outcomes after bilateral rostral mandibulectomy are well accepted and reconstruction of the area is generally considered unnecessary (**Fig. 9**). Cheiloplasty for the excision of the redundant lower lip tissue is usually necessary and determined during the initial planned incision depending on tumor location. The main considerations should be a tension-free closure to avoid any dehiscence and to close the lip margin higher than the alveolar margin to avoid excessive drooling. The reconstruction of the lower lip is better assessed when the patient is on sternal recumbency compared with dorsal recumbency.

Subtotal mandibulectomy: This technique is indicated for rostral to midmandible tumors invading into the medullary cavity or mandibular canal (**Fig. 10**). In the past, the

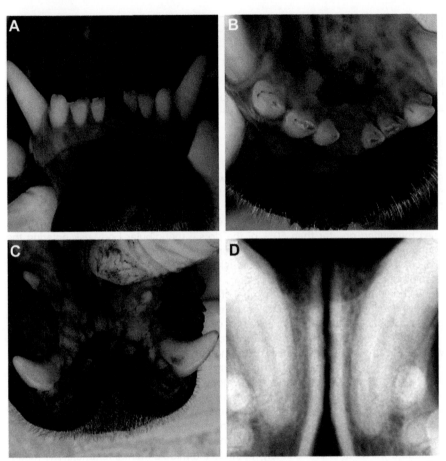

Fig. 8. Photographs before (*A*, *B*) and after (*C*) a bilateral rostral mandibulectomy in dog with an acanthomatous ameloblastoma. Surgical margins of 2 cm were achieved by en bloc resection of the mandibular incisors and associated alveolar bone. The postoperative intraoral radiograph shows preservation of the mandibular symphysis (*D*). (*Picture courtesy of* Dr Christopher Smithson.)

caudal osteotomy for subtotal mandibulectomy was positioned immediately rostral to the cranial attachment of the masseter muscle, just caudal to the third molar.[58] However, an important oncological observation is that the entire mandibular canal is not fully excised. Therefore, a surgical technique that allows an en bloc excision of the mandibular canal without the more technically demanding disarticulation of the temporomandibular joint (TMJ) has been recently described.[69] The extended subtotal mandibulectomy is intended to remove the mandibular canal entirely, while retaining the coronoid and the condylar processes. Patients are placed in dorsal recumbency, and an intraoral approach is used to expose the bone, from symphysis to caudal mental foramen. The symphysis is incised with an oscillating saw or an osteotome, and the hemimandible is gently retracted laterally to identify the mandibular foramen and ligate the inferior alveolar artery and vein. After this, the caudal osteotomy is performed assuring to excise the mandibular foramen and the angular process.[69] Based on 3 cases, mandibular drift and tongue protrusion were the only complications described.

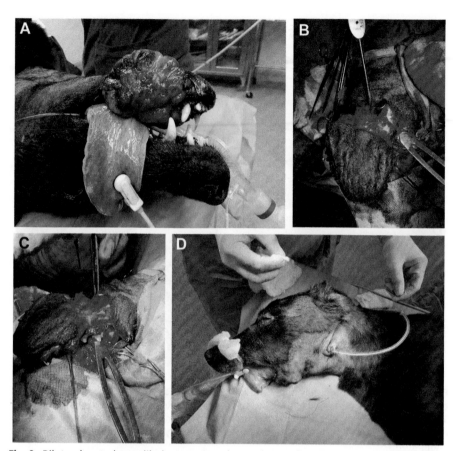

Fig. 9. Bilateral rostral mandibulectomy in a dog with a grade II fibrosarcoma of the rostral to left mandible (*A*). An intraoral and ventral excision were performed with surgical margins marked at 3 cm from the tumor edges (*B* and *C*). An esophagostomy tube was placed for post-operative nutrition support (*D*). (*Courtesy of* Dr Carlos Souza.)

Total and caudal mandibulectomy: These techniques are indicated for malignant tumors that invade the rostral, mid, and/or caudal mandible (**Fig. 11**). The patient is usually positioned in lateral recumbency. The dissection is similar to the extended subtotal mandibulectomy, but it is continued further caudally including incising insertions of the masseter (ventrolateral), the pterygoid (caudomedial), and the digastricus (caudoventral) muscles. Depending on the location of the tumor, the masseter muscle is included in the oncological margins or elevated from the masseter fossa. Thereafter the TMJ is incised and the hemimandible is luxated laterally exposing the temporalis muscle insertion at the coronoid process of the mandibular ramus, which will be dissected off. Recently, a novel ventral approach has been described for a total unilateral mandibulectomy or a caudal mandibulectomy.[70] This approach claims to be advantageous in regard to the ease of the procedure, allowing a direct visualization of the inferior alveolar artery and TMJ, and provides access to locoregional LNs without the need to reposition the patient. Furthermore, the ostectomy of the zygomatic arch to access the mandibular vertical ramus may not be needed, hence decreasing the potential morbidity. Complications reported with this technique seem to be comparable to the standard approach for total mandibulectomy including

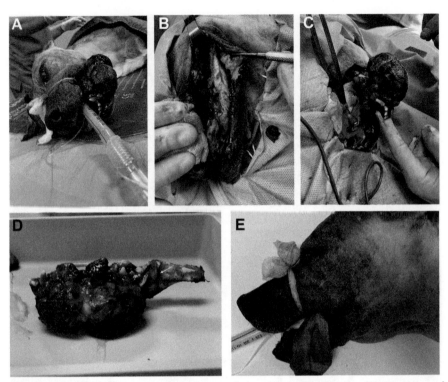

Fig. 10. Dog with a biologically high histologically low-grade fibrosarcoma (*A*). Dissection of the soft tissues down to bone at the surgical margins (*B*). Rostral mandibular osteotomy (*C*). Specimen after the caudal osteotomy, just dorsal to the mandibular foramen (*D, white arrow*). Cosmetic aspect of the dog immediately after surgery (*E*). (*Picture courtesy* of Dr Brian Trumpatori.)

hemorrhage, ventral edema, and sublingual swelling. Although those techniques have never been compared, the ventral approach was perceived as superior for en bloc resection of a hemimandible due to the aforementioned advantages,[70] making this technique a potential alternative for caudal and unilateral mandibulectomy in dogs.

Segmental mandibulectomy: This technique is indicated for animals that have low-grade malignant tumor or locally invasive benign tumors located in the mid mandibular body, and the desired surgical margins exceed the limit of the more conservative rim excision procedure. Segmental mandibulectomy is contraindicated for malignant tumors other than SCC.[58] Regenerative techniques combined with immediate rigid fixation have also been successful with the goal of achieving appropriate occlusion immediately after surgery and a rapid return to normal function.[68] In that case series, bone regeneration filling up the mandibular defect was seen as soon as 4 weeks after surgery and appeared fully healed by 3 months, however, with decreased bone density and porosity compared with the contralateral site.[68] Nonetheless, cosmetic and functional outcome is acceptable after segmental mandibulectomy, making reconstruction of the defect a potential alternative.

Mandibulectomy Complications

Intraoperative complications are uncommon during mandibulectomy; however, blood loss and hypotension can occur with more extensive surgeries.[58] A recent study found

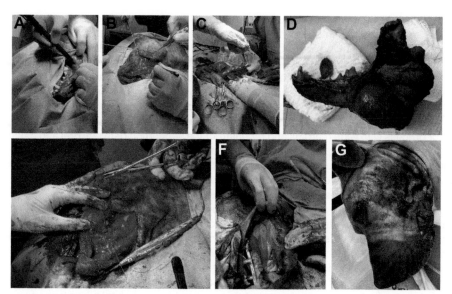

Fig. 11. Total left mandibulectomy for a mandibular osteosarcoma in a dog. The soft tissue margins are marked including the biopsy tract (*A*). The mandibulectomy was performed using the ventral approach (*B*). After the rostral mandibular osteotomy, the hemimandible is gently manipulated laterally to allow dissection of the remaining soft tissue attachments (*C*). Hemimandible specimen with the tumor (*D*). Reconstruction of the oral mucosa through the ventral approach (*E*). Intraoral reconstruction (*F*). Final cosmetic appearance (*G*). (*Courtesy of* Dr Janis Lapsley and Andrea Erickson.)

that 38% of patients were affected by more than one complication after mandibulectomy, with 26% being considered major.[71] The most common were mandibular drift and malocclusion (14% of dogs).[71]

- Malocclusion can result in difficulty eating and drinking, prehension, and pain of the contralateral TMJ.
- Mandibular drift is the phenomenon by which the mandible shifts to the side of the ostectomy due to disruption of the mandibular symphysis. This complication is eliminated with reconstructive or symphysis-sparing techniques, thus permitting normal TMJ mechanics and articulation. Elastic training is a viable option for preventing mandibular drift but requires good client compliance, and only 50% of the cases may benefit.[72]
- Others: Incisional dehiscence, ranula formation, increased salivation, and pain.

Updates in Maxillectomy Techniques

Maxillary surgery is complex and requires excellent knowledge of the regional anatomy, not only the bones of the maxilla (frontal, nasal maxillary, incisive, and pterygoid) but also the detailed appreciation of the 3D relationship of the bones and different structures of the skull.[17] It is strongly recommended to have an appropriate skull for surgical planning as well as for intraoperative review during surgery. It is essential to understand the vascular anatomy of the maxilla, mandible, and orbit because of the risk of hemorrhage and hypotension. For rostral maxillectomies, the major palatine and sphenopalatine arteries are of importance, and the maxillary and infraorbital arteries for the caudal maxillectomies. Owing to the proximity to the surgical area of this network of large blood vessels, it is strongly recommended to blood type and cross-match the patients and have accessibility to blood transfusion products. In the event of major blood loss additional techniques to decrease blood loss such as maxillary or carotid artery ligation can be considered.

Maxillectomy refers to the en bloc excision of a tumor involving parts of the incisive, palatine, lacrimal, zygomatic, frontal, and/or vomer bones in addition to the maxilla.[58] As with the mandible, depending on the area removed, the nomenclature of the maxillectomy varies. General goals of maxillectomies are to achieve local control of the tumor process with wide margins and reconstruct the separation between oral and nasal cavity. Most of these maxillectomy procedures, especially the rostral and caudal maxillectomies, are considered advanced oral surgery, and initial attempts are best used with an experienced mentor or colleagues help.

Incisivectomy and rostral maxillectomy: This technique is indicated for small malignant or benign tumors affecting the incisor bone (**Fig. 12**). Larger lesions extending more caudally are treated with rostral maxillectomy but may also require a nasal planectomy. The patient is positioned in dorsal to allow better visualization of the oral cavity for reconstruction and suturing. For the osteotomy, a high-speed bur, oscillating sagittal bone saw, or piezoelectric equipment is recommended over an osteotome to avoid bone fractures or soft tissue injuries. Usually, the turbinates are cut sharply with the osteotomy of the palatine bone and removed en bloc to maintain the planned surgical margins. The final wound bed should be free of sharp bone fragments. The formation of a vestibular mucosal-submucosal flap from both lips to reconstruct the wound is started from the maxillectomy site and working toward the lip margin. Bone tunnels can be used to anchor areas of the flap submucosa to the palatine bone on midline. Final wound closure initiated at midline is carried rostrally and buccally in a simple interrupted pattern, creating a T-shaped closure.[73] A nasal cantilever suture technique is used to repair a functional or/and cosmetic ventral drop of the muzzle (see **Fig. 12D**).

Caudal maxillectomy: This technique can be perform via 2 approaches: intraoral (for tumors located along the alveolar margins of the mid to caudal maxilla) or combined dorsolateral and intraoral (for tumors of the mid-to-caudal maxilla that extend dorsolaterally and caudally into the inferior orbit)[74] (**Fig. 13**). The latter improves exposure and increases the ability to achieving clean surgical margins. Hemorrhage is the most common intraoperative complication reported during these procedures because maxillary artery ligation is not performed until completion of all osteotomies allowing tumor-bearing bone mobilization. A clinical study demonstrated that preligation of the maxillary artery decreases the probability of intraoperative hemorrhage and hypotension.[75] For that, the animal is placed in lateral recumbency with the affected side up. If the animal requires an enucleation, the maxillary artery is identified caudal to the entrance into the infraorbital canal (maxillary foramen) within the orbit. If no enucleation is needed, the skin incision made for the combined approach is extended caudally over the zygomatic arch. The masseter muscle and the periosteum are dissected off the ventral aspect of the zygomatic arch and the ostectomy is performed. Through the defect the maxillary artery can be exposed by retracting the eye dorsocaudally.[75] The remainder of the procedure is performed as previously described.[74]

Bilateral caudal maxillectomy: This technique is indicated for surgical resection of caudal maxillary tumors that abut or cross the palatal midline. It is not uncommon that these tumors get diagnosed when they are already large, likely because of the difficulty for the owners to notice lesions in the caudal aspect of the oral cavity. Therefore, they often present significant challenges for surgical resection, especially if the

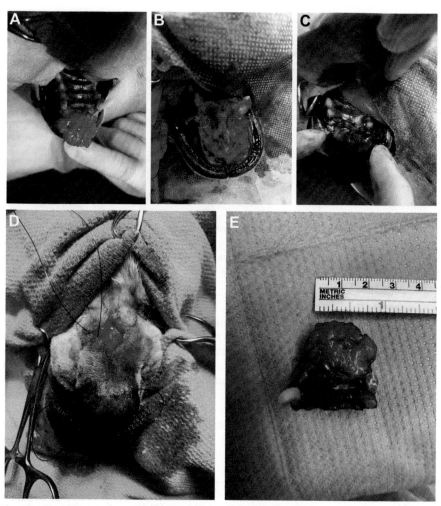

Fig. 12. Acanthomatous ameloblastoma of the maxillary incisors in a dog (*A*). Rostral maxillectomy with 1-cm surgical margins was performed (*B*). Reconstruction of the defect was made with buccal mucosa from the upper lips (*C*). A nasal cantilever technique is performed after the rostral maxillectomy (*D*). Tumor-bearing specimen (*E*). (*Courtesy of* Dr Elizabeth Maxwell.)

tumor crosses midline. A recent case series described the technique and demonstrated feasibility and success of this procedure.[76] Briefly, with the dog in dorsal recumbency and the pharyngeal area packed with sponges, the surgical margins are marked on the mucosal surface. Bilateral buccal mucosal incisions are made, dissecting down to the bone at the marked level to include the left infraorbital foramen and last molar caudally, to the second premolar rostrally. Depending on the case, part of the orbital bone can be included on the osteotomy plan. The osteotomies are performed in the following order to minimize hemorrhage: (1) dorsolateral (bilaterally); (2) caudal, across the palatine bone; (3) rostral (bilateral). After the tumor-bearing tissue is removed, buccal mucosal flaps are elevated bilaterally in preparation for closure, trying to preserve the *angularis oris* vessels bilaterally if possible. After suturing the

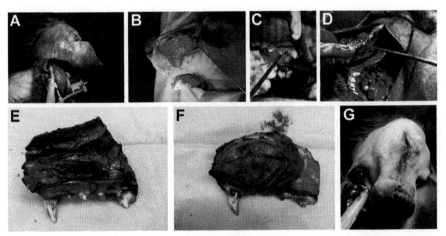

Fig. 13. Right maxillary osteosarcoma in a dog (*A*). Combined dorsolateral (*B*) and intraoral approach to a right maxillary (*C, D*). The resected en bloc segment's surgical margins are inked and submitted for histopathology analysis (*E, F*). Cosmetic aspect of the patient immediately after surgery (*G*).

buccal mucosa flaps to the soft palate (caudally), to themselves (medially) and to the hard palate mucoperiosteum (rostrally), an esophagostomy tube is placed for 14 days to bypass the oral cavity.[76] The only intraoperative complications documented were hemorrhage and secondary hypotension. Although blood transfusion products are usually enough to correct acute hypotension, temporary carotid artery ligation should be considered. Postoperative complications were facial swelling, epistaxis, subcutaneous emphysema, and dehiscence (oronasal fistulation). All the complications were self-limiting except the wound dehiscence, which had to be revised with an *angularis oris* flap in both dogs.

Maxillectomy Complications

Complications from maxillectomy are usually more prevalent than with mandibulectomy. More than one complication has been seen in 36.1% patients that underwent maxillectomy.[71] When compared with mandibulectomy, maxillectomy was associated with higher risk of hemorrhage and oronasal fistula.

- Bleeding is the most common intraoperative complication (53.4%) for which 43% of these patients will receive intraoperative blood transfusion.[77] Dogs treated with the combined dorsolateral/intraoral approach were more likely to have excessive bleeding (83%) than only using intraoral approach (54%).
- Wound dehiscence is a major complication of maxillary surgery, with 33% reported in maxillectomies caudal to the second premolar.[78] A more recent large case series only detected an 11% rate of oronasal fistula formation.[77] In addition, other factors like RT or chemotherapy increase the odds of incisional dehiscence or oral fistula formation.[71] Generally, repair of oronasal fistulas is required if they are causing clinical signs (regurgitation, nausea, rhinitis, and so forth). Several methods have been used to correct these defects, including both single- and double-layer mucoperiosteal flaps, *angularis oris* axial pattern flap, use of synthetic[79] or natural tissue (ie, auricular cartilage) regeneration material, and placement of permanent or removable obturator.[76,79–81] The success of those

methods is variable, and decision making usually depends on available viable tissue, surgeon's experience, and patient factors.

- Others: epistaxis, excessive facial swelling, difficulty eating, ulcer formation secondary to teeth trauma, and infection.

Postoperative Care

Pain management depends on the extent of the surgery and varies between patients. Multimodal analgesia allows dose and side effects reduction. For the first 24 to 48 hours after surgery, a combination of a mu-agonist opioid and nonsteroidal anti-inflammatory is usually sufficient.

If additional analgesia is required, ketamine or lidocaine infusions are excellent choices. Moreover, intravenous fluid therapy is continued until normal oral intake is established. Nutritional support with a feeding tube should be considered if the animal is not eating and drinking adequately within 3 days, which is unusual.[18] To prevent disruption of intraoral incisions cats and dogs should only be fed soft canned food and prevented from chewing or playing on any toys for 4 to 6 weeks. An Elizabethan collar should be worn at all times to avoid self-trauma.

Outcome, Cosmetics, and Function

The cosmetic appearance of cats and dogs undergoing mandibulectomy and maxillectomy is usually considered good to excellent by the owners (85% satisfaction).[82] Thorough discussion, including the use of preoperative and postoperative images of the appropriate procedure, with the owner is key to meet owner satisfaction and acceptance. Eating difficulties are uncommon following most of these procedures. Some patients undergoing mandibulectomy may require initial assistance in feeding due to the malocclusion of the rostral aspect of the oral cavity and loss of prehension ability. However, most of these patients adapt to unassisted eating in 2 to 3 weeks. Supplemental feeding may be required for cats following complex maxillectomy procedures.

SUMMARY

The prognosis for dogs undergoing surgical resection of malignant orofacial tumors has improved steadily over the years. This improvement is likely due to a combination of important factors that have been discussed in this article.

Factors to consider before recommending surgical removal:

- Oral examination findings
- Diagnostic imaging results
- Histopathologic (or cytologic) diagnosis
- Understand the tumor biological behavior
- Recommend surgical margins based on tumor type and biology
- Determine the intent of surgery (definitive vs palliative)
- Apply oral surgery principles
- Owner preparation and set expectations
- Understand regional anatomy, techniques available, and complications
- Availability of local tissues for surgical closure
- Determine neoadjuvant or adjuvant therapies
- Accept and prepare for complications

Generally, dogs and cats tolerate orofacial surgery extremely well. Surgeons have become more experienced and more aggressive in treating those tumors. Accepting and treating postoperative complications is also an intrinsic part of the comprehensive treatment of orofacial tumors; however, preventive actions to avoid complications should be taken and planned surgeries with preoperative biopsies are recommended.

CLINICS CARE POINTS

- Know the biological behavior of the tumor
- Take an intra-oral biopsy to obtain histopathological tumor information
- Lymph node mapping techniques allow sentinel lymph node detection
- Advanced imaging, like CT scan is very useful for staging the tumors and aid with surgical planning.
- Surgical doses should be planned for each tumor depending on biological behavior

DISCLOSURE

The authors have nothing to disclose.

REFERENCES

1. Mikiewicz M, Paździor-Czapula K, Gesek M, et al. Canine and Feline Oral Cavity Tumours and Tumour-like Lesions: a Retrospective Study of 486 Cases (2015-2017). J Comp Pathol 2019;172:80–7.
2. Liptak JM, Withrow S. Oral tumors. In: Withrow SJ, editor. Small animal clinical oncology. St. Louis (MO): Elsevier Saunders; 2013. p. 381.
3. Cray M, Selmic LE, Ruple A. Demographics of dogs and cats with oral tumors presenting to teaching hospitals: 1996-2017. J Vet Sci 2020;21(5):e70.
4. Cotter SM. Oral pharyngeal neoplasms in the cat. J Am Anim Hosp Assoc 1981; 17(6):917–20.
5. Owen LN. TNM classification of tumours in domestic animals. Geneva (Switzerland): World Health Organization; 1980.
6. Atherton MJ, Morris JS, McDermott MR, et al. Cancer immunology and canine malignant melanoma: a comparative review. Vet Immunol Immunopathol 2016; 169:15–26.
7. Williams LE, Packer RA. Association between lymph node size and metastasis in dogs with oral malignant melanoma: 100 cases (1987-2001). J Am Vet Med Assoc 2003;222(9):1234–6.
8. Beer P, Pozzi A, Rohrer Bley C, et al. The role of sentinel lymph node mapping in small animal veterinary medicine: a comparison with current approaches in human medicine. Vet Comp Oncol 2018;16(2):178–87.
9. Grimes JA, Mestrinho LA, Berg J, et al. Histologic evaluation of mandibular and medial retropharyngeal lymph nodes during staging of oral malignant melanoma and squamous cell carcinoma in dogs. J Am Vet Med Assoc 2019;254(8):938–43.
10. Armbrust LJ, Biller DS, Bamford A, et al. Comparison of three-view thoracic radiography and computed tomography for detection of pulmonary nodules in dogs with neoplasia. J Am Vet Med Assoc 2012;240(9):1088–94.
11. Nemanic S, London CA, Wisner ER. Comparison of thoracic radiographs and single breath-hold helical CT for detection of pulmonary nodules in dogs with metastatic neoplasia. J Vet Intern Med 2006;20(3):508–15.
12. Nemec A, Arzi B, Murphy B, et al. Prevalence and types of tooth resorption in dogs with oral tumors. Am J Vet Res 2012;73(7):1057–66.

13. Amory JT, Reetz JA, Sánchez MD, et al. Computed tomographic characteristics of odontogenic neoplasms in dogs. Vet Radiol Ultrasound 2014;55(2):147–58.

14. Bonfanti U, Bertazzolo W, Gracis M, et al. Diagnostic value of cytological analysis of tumours and tumour-like lesions of the oral cavity in dogs and cats: a prospective study on 114 cases. Vet J 2015;205(2):322–7.

15. Liptak JM, Lascelles Dx. Oral Tumors. In: Veterinary surgical oncology. 1st edition. West Sussex (UK): Wiley-Blackwell; 2012. p. 119–77.

16. Lommer MJ. Oral inflammation in small animals. Vet Clin North Am Small Anim Pract 2013;43(3):555–71.

17. Verstraete FJ. Mandibulectomy and maxillectomy. Vet Clin North Am Small Anim Pract 2005;35(4):1009–39.

18. Margaret C. McEntee. Clinical behavior of nonodontogenic tumors. In: Verstraete FJM, Lommer MJ, editors. Oral and maxillofacial surgery in dogs and cats. St Louis (MO): W.B. Saunders; 2012. p. 387–402.

19. Kowalski LP, Bagietto R, Lara JR, et al. Prognostic significance of the distribution of neck node metastasis from oral carcinoma. Head Neck 2000;22(3):207–14.

20. Tuohy JL, Selmic LE, Worley DR, et al. Outcome following curative-intent surgery for oral melanoma in dogs: 70 cases (1998–2011). J Am Vet Med Assoc 2014; 245:1266–73.

21. Morton DL, Thompson JF, Cochran AJ, et al. Final trial report of sentinel-node biopsy versus nodal observation in melanoma. N Engl J Med 2014;370:599–609.

22. Mendez SE, Drobatz KJ, Duda LE, et al. Treating the locoregional lymph nodes with radiation and/or surgery significantly improves outcome in dogs with high-grade mast cell tumours. Vet Comp Oncol 2020;18(2):239–46.

23. Herring ES, Smith MM, Robertson JL. Lymph node staging of oral and maxillofacial neoplasms in 31 dogs and cats. J Vet Dent 2002;19(3):122–6.

24. Grimes JA, Matz BM, Christopherson PW, et al. Agreement between cytology and histopathology for regional lymph node metastasis in dogs with melanocytic neoplasms. Vet Pathol 2017;54(4):579–87.

25. Boston SE, Lu X, Culp WT, et al. Efficacy of systemic adjuvant therapies administered to dogs after excision of oral malignant melanomas: 151 cases (2001-2012). J Am Vet Med Assoc 2014;245(4):401–7.

26. Odenweller PH, Smith MM, Taney KG. Validation of regional lymph node excisional biopsy for staging oral and maxillofacial malignant neoplasms in 97 dogs and 10 cats (2006-2016). J Vet Dent 2019;36(2):97–103.

27. Skinner OT, Boston SE, Souza CHM. Patterns of lymph node metastasis identified following bilateral mandibular and medial retropharyngeal lymphadenectomy in 31 dogs with malignancies of the head. Vet Comp Oncol 2017;15(3):881–9.

28. Green K, Boston SE. Bilateral removal of the mandibular and medial retropharyngeal lymph nodes through a single ventral midline incision for staging of head and neck cancers in dogs: a description of surgical technique. Vet Comp Oncol 2017;15(1):208–14.

29. Smith MM. Surgical approach for lymph node staging of oral and maxillofacial neoplasms in dogs. J Am Anim Hosp Assoc 1995;31(6):514–8.

30. Rahimi-Nedjat RK, Al-Nawas B, Tuettenberg A, et al. Sentinel lymph node biopsy in malignant melanoma of the head and neck. J Craniomaxillofac Surg 2018; 46(6):1027–31.

31. Madu MF, Wouters MW, van Akkooi AC. Sentinel node biopsy in melanoma: current controversies addressed. Eur J Surg Oncol 2017;43(3):517–33.

32. Wan J, Oblak ML, Ram A, et al. Determining agreement between preoperative computed tomography lymphography and indocyanine green near infrared

fluorescence intraoperative imaging for sentinel lymph node mapping in dogs with oral tumours. Vet Comp Oncol 2021;19(2):295–303.

33. Syrcle JA, Bonczynski JJ, Monette S, et al. Retrospective evaluation of lingual tumors in 42 dogs: 1999-2005. J Am Anim Hosp Assoc 2008;44(6):308–19.

34. Peterson LJ. Principles of antibiotic therapy. In: Topazian RG, Goldberg MH, editors. Oral and maxillofacial infections. 3rd edition. Philadelphia (PA): WB Saunders; 1994. p. 160–97.

35. Liboon J, Funkhouser W, Terris DJ. A comparison of mucosal incisions made by scalpel, CO2 laser, electrocautery, and constant-voltage electrocautery. Otolaryngol Head Neck Surg 1997;116(3):379–85.

36. Dragovic M, Pejovic M, Stepic J, et al. Comparison of four different suture materials in respect to oral wound healing, microbial colonization, tissue reaction and clinical features-randomized clinical study. Clin Oral Investig 2020;24(4):1527–41.

37. Davis B, Smith KD. Oral Surgery suturing. In: StatPearls. Treasure Island (FL): StatPearls Publishing; 2021.

38. Politis C, Schoenaers J, Jacobs R, et al. Wound healing problems in the mouth. Front Physiol 2016;7:507.

39. Kalamaras AB, Aarnes TK, Moore SA, et al. Effects of perioperative saphenous and sciatic nerve blocks, lumbosacral epidural or morphine–lidocaine–ketamine infusion on postoperative pain and sedation in dogs undergoing tibial plateau leveling osteotomy. Vet Anaesth Analgesia 2021;48(3):415–21.

40. Tavakoli A, Tazik ME, Abbasi A. Comparison of production of pain and oxidative stress after induction of local nerve block or use of NSAIDs following painful dental procedures in dogs. Iranian J Vet Surg 2021;16(1):29–33.

41. Romano M, Portela DA, Breghi G, et al. Stress-related biomarkers in dogs administered regional anaesthesia or fentanyl for analgesia during stifle surgery. Vet Anaesth Analgesia 2016;43(1):44–54.

42. Bellows J, Berg ML, Dennis S, et al. 2019 AAHA Dental Care Guidelines for Dogs and Cats*. J Am Anim Hosp Assoc 2019;55(2):49–69.

43. Pascoe PJ, Chohan AS. Comparison of the efficacy and duration of desensitization of oral structures following injection of various volumes of a lidocaine-bupivacaine mixture via an infraorbital approach in dogs. Am J Vet Res 2020;81(6):463–70.

44. Caniglia AM, Driessen B, Puerto DA, et al. Intraoperative antinociception and postoperative analgesia following epidural anesthesia versus femoral and sciatic nerve blockade in dogs undergoing stifle joint surgery. J Am Vet Med Assoc 2012;241(12):1605–12.

45. Sepehripour S, Dheansa BS. Is there an advantage in onset of action with mixing lignocaine and bupivacaine? J Plast Reconstr Aesthet Surg 2017;70(12):1782.

46. Ribotsky BM, Berkowitz KD, Montague JR. Local anesthetics. Is there an advantage to mixing solutions? J Am Podiatr Med Assoc 1996;86(10):487–91.

47. Otero PE, Portela DA. Nerve blocks of the upper jaw. In: Manual of small animal regional anesthesia. 2nd edition. Inter-Medica; 2019. p. 319–25.

48. Gracis M. The oral cavity. In: Campoy L, Read MR, editors. Small animal regional anesthesia and analgesia. Oxford (UK): John Wiley & Sons, Inc.; 2013. p. 119–39.

49. Loughran CM, Raisis AL, Haitjema G, et al. Unilateral retrobulbar hematoma following maxillary nerve block in a dog. J Vet Emerg Crit Care 2016;26(6):815–8.

50. Shilo-Benjamini Y, Letz S, Peery D, et al. Comparison of three regional anaesthetic techniques for infraorbital or maxillary nerve block in cats: a cadaveric study. J Feline Med Surg 2021.

51. Viscasillas J, Seymour CJ, Brodbelt DC. A cadaver study comparing two approaches for performing maxillary nerve block in dogs. Vet Anaesthes Analg 2013;40(2):212–9.

52. Fizzano KM, Claude AK, Kuo L-H, et al. Evaluation of a modified infraorbital approach for a maxillary nerve block for rhinoscopy with nasal biopsy of dogs. Am Vet Res 2017;78(9):1025–35.

53. Chau AYK. Tongue lacerations in a geriatric dog after bilateral inferior alveolar nerve blocks with bupivacaine. Vet Rec Case Rep 2017;5(3).

54. Krug W, Losey J. Area of desensitization following mental nerve block in dogs. J Vet Dent 2011;28(3):146–50.

55. Viscasillas J, ter Haar G. Ultrasound guided trigeminal nerve block as local anaesthetic technique for exenteration and excision of the zygomatic arch with partial caudal maxillectomy in a dog. Vet Anaesth Analgesia 2017;44(3).

56. Otero PE, Portela DA. Block of the trigeminal nerve via a temporal approach. In: Manual of small animal regional anesthesia. 2nd edition. Inter-Medica; 2019. p. 338–41.

57. Berg J. In: Johnson SA, Tobias KM, editors. Mandibulectomy and maxillectomy. 2nd edition. Elsevier; 2018. p. 1663.

58. Kudnig ST, Séguin B. Veterinary surgical oncology. 2nd edition. West Susex (UK): Wiley-Blackwell; 2016.

59. Nayyar J, Clarke M, O'Sullivan M, et al. Fractured root tips during dental extractions and retained root fragments. A clinical dilemma? Br Dent J 2015;218(5): 285–90.

60. Arzi B, Verstraete FJ. Mandibular rim excision in seven dogs. Vet Surg 2010; 39(2):226–31.

61. Brown JS, Kalavrezos N, D'Souza J, et al. Factors that influence the method of mandibular resection in the management of oral squamous cell carcinoma. Br J Oral Maxillofac Surg 2002;40:275–84.

62. Gioso MA, Shofer F, Barros PS, et al. Mandible and mandibular first molar tooth measurements in dogs: relationship of radiographic height to body weight. J Vet Dent 2001;18(2):65–8.

63. Linden D, Matz BM, Farag R, et al. Biomechanical comparison of two ostectomy configurations for partial mandibulectomy. Vet Comp Orthop Traumatol 2017; 30(1):15–9.

64. Melugin MB, Oyen OJ, Indresano AT. The effect of rim mandibulectomy configuration and residual segment size on postoperative fracture risk: an in vitro study. J Oral Maxillofac Surg 2001;59(4):409–13.

65. Fujiwara S, Kato S, Bengazi F, et al. Healing at implants installed in osteotomies prepared either with a piezoelectric device or drills: an experimental study in dogs. Oral Maxillofac Surg 2021;25(1):65–73.

66. Murray RL, Aitken ML, Gottfried SD. The use of rim excision as a treatment for canine acanthomatous ameloblastoma. J Am Anim Hosp Assoc 2010;46:91–6.

67. Smithson CW, Taney K. Symphyseal sparing rostral mandibulectomy. J Vet Dent 2009;26(4):264–9.

68. Arzi B, Cissell DD, Pollard RE, et al. Regenerative Approach to Bilateral Rostral Mandibular Reconstruction in a Case Series of Dogs. Front Vet Sci 2015;2:4.

69. Fiani N, Peralta S. Extended Subtotal Mandibulectomy for the treatment of oral tumors invading the mandibular canal in dogs-a novel surgical technique. Front Vet Sci 2019;6:339.

70. de Mello Souza CH, Bacon N, Boston S, et al. Ventral mandibulectomy for removal of oral tumours in the dog: Surgical technique and results in 19 cases. Vet Comp Oncol 2019;17(3):271–5.

71. Cray M, Selmic LE, Kindra C, et al. Analysis of risk factors associated with complications following mandibulectomy and maxillectomy in dogs. J Am Vet Med Assoc 2021;259(3):265–74.

72. Bar-Am Y, Verstraete FJ. Elastic training for the prevention of mandibular drift following mandibulectomy in dogs: 18 cases (2005-2008). Vet Surg 2010;39(5): 574–80.

73. Gingerich W, Stepaniuk KS. Bilateral rostral maxillectomy in the dog. J Vet Dent 2013;30(2):125–30.

74. Lascelles BD, Thomson MJ, Dernell WS, et al. Combined dorsolateral and intraoral approach for the resection of tumors of the maxilla in the dog. J Am Anim Hosp Assoc 2003;39(3):294–305.

75. Carroll KA, Mathews KG. Ligation of the maxillary artery prior to caudal maxillectomy in the dog-a description of the technique, retrospective evaluation of blood loss, and cadaveric evaluation of maxillary artery anatomy. Front Vet Sci 2020;7: 588–945.

76. Tuohy JL, Worley DR, Wustefeld-Janssens BG, et al. Bilateral caudal maxillectomy for resection of tumors crossing palatal midline and use of the angularis oris axial pattern flap for primary closure or dehiscence repair in two dogs. Vet Surg 2019;48(8):1490–9.

77. MacLellan RH, Rawlinson JE, Rao S, et al. Intraoperative and postoperative complications of partial maxillectomy for the treatment of oral tumors in dogs. J Am Vet Med Assoc 2018;252(12):1538–47.

78. Schwarz PD, Withrow SJ, Curtis CR, et al. Partial maxillary resection as a treatment for oral cancer in 61 dogs. J Am Anim Hosp Assoc 1991;27:617–24.

79. Martin SA, Kirby BM. Incorporation of a polydioxanone absorbable plate in the successful repair of an iatrogenic oronasal fistula in a dog. J Am Vet Med Assoc 2019;254(9):1094–8.

80. Lorrain RP, Legendre LF. Oronasal fistula repair using auricular cartilage. J Vet Dent 2012;29(3):172–5.

81. Cavanaugh RP, Farese JP, Bacon NJ, et al. Oronasal fistula repair utilizing a temporalis muscle flap in a dog with severe trismus. J Am Anim Hosp Assoc 2011; 47(6):447–54.

82. Fox LE, Geoghegan SL, Davis LH, et al. Owner satisfaction with partial mandibulectomy or maxillectomy for treatment of oral tumors in 27 dogs. J Am Anim Hosp Assoc 1997;33(1):25–31.

Updates in Laparoscopy

Nicole J. Buote, DVM, DACVS-SA

KEYWORDS

- Laparoscopy • Near-infrared fluorescence • 3D printing • Retroperitoneal access
- Robotics • Barbed suture • NOTES • Laparoscopic nephrectomy

KEY POINTS

- Retroperitoneal access for laparoscopic adrenalectomy has inherent advantages such as the lack of retraction of intra-abdominal organs needed for dissection which may lead to decreased operative times and fewer ports needed.
- Near-infrared fluorescence (NIRF) imaging is an exciting new diagnostic technology available to veterinary medicine. The applications of this low-energy technology have been investigated for biliary, oncologic, thoracic duct, and lymph node mapping but no standardized doses or protocols have been established as of yet.
- Barbed suture is a significant positive addition to the minimally invasive surgeon and studies show its use reduces surgery time, allows for consistent tension along the suture line, and removes the need for intracorporeal knot-tying.
- 3D printed laparoscopic ports may allow patient-specific port creation leading to additional availability of MIS procedures for our small animal population.
- Robotics use in veterinary medicine for clinical patients is being investigated after decades of experimental use for human surgical models.

INTRODUCTION

The popularity and use of minimally invasive surgery (MIS) in veterinary medicine have increased exponentially over the past few decades. More procedures have become possible because of video-assisted or completely laparoscopic techniques which allow our patients to benefit from less tissue trauma and reduced infection rates.[1–3] The desire to improve patient postoperative comfort and decrease the time until return to normal activity are the main driving forces behind MIS in veterinary medicine. As we are able to add more versatility to these procedures and use new technologies that make them easier or more effective, we can bring these surgeries to more patients.

Randomized controlled trials between traditional open and MIS surgeries looking at postoperative outcomes are uncommon, and most reports are case series or experimental studies, but these are necessary steps in gaining experience and acceptance in the veterinary field. Over the past few years, new access techniques

Department of Clinical Sciences, Small Animal Surgery Soft Tissue Section, Cornell University School of Veterinary Medicine, 930 Campus Road, Ithaca, NY 14853, USA
E-mail address: njb235@cornell.edu

Vet Clin Small Anim 52 (2022) 513–529
https://doi.org/10.1016/j.cvsm.2021.12.007
0195-5616/22/© 2021 Elsevier Inc. All rights reserved.

(retroperitoneal, 3D printed ports) and diagnostic techniques (near-infrared fluorescence) have been investigated as well as continued work on advanced procedures (robotics) which will be discussed in this chapter.

Updates in laparoscopy

Retroperitoneal access

MIS begins, like any surgery, with an incision. The goals of these incisions are to be well-placed and as small as possible. While much research has been conducted in veterinary medicine regarding access into the abdominal cavity with respect to the different types of ports available (single, multi-port, optical, and so forth) and the number of ports used in each procedure, there hasn't been as much conducted regarding the retroperitoneal space. The retroperitoneal space has been used in human laparoscopy for many decades to access adrenal neoplasms and to aid in nephroureterectomies.[4–7] While this approach is not new in veterinary medicine from an open surgical perspective,[8] it has only recently been discussed as a technique for laparoscopic adrenalectomies.[9,10] The major benefit to retroperitoneal access is the lack of retraction of intra-abdominal organs for dissection. This decreases the chances of iatrogenic injury to those organs and reduces the time spent placing additional ports for retraction.[11] The major disadvantage to retroperitoneal access is the space limitation for maneuverability. Even with insufflation, the space limitations can be challenging. Surgeons also must learn new anatomic landmarks before using this approach and intra-abdominal explore and sampling is also not possible with this technique (**Box 1**).

While human studies have shown a reduction in operation times, blood loss, and postoperative hospitalizations,[4,5] no comparative studies have been performed in veterinary medicine to date. Two experimental veterinary studies have investigated this MIS approach, however, giving us hope that clinical studies are underway. The study by Jeong and colleagues,[9] presented cadaveric and live experimental data on the proper placement of retroperitoneal access ports, the amount of working space established, and the surgical anatomy visualized. Retroperitoneal access was successfully established in all 6 live dogs with animals placed in sternal recumbency with their abdomens suspended and ports placed at the level of the 2nd lumbar vertebrae on the right side and the 3rd lumbar vertebrae on the left side (**Box 2**). The most important anatomic landmark for the retroperitoneum was the transverse process of

---

Box 1
Reported advantages and disadvantages to retroperitoneal access for adrenalectomy

Advantages:

- lack of retraction of intra-abdominal organs for dissection
- decreased iatrogenic injury to organs and
- reduced port placement for retraction
- decreased operative times
- decreased blood loss

Disadvantages:

- limited space for manipulation
- different anatomic views
- Abdominal staging not possible

Box 2
Port placement options for retroperitoneal adrenalectomy

Option 1:

- sternal recumbency with suspended abdomen
- right side: ports placed at a level of 2nd lumbar vertebrae
- left side: ports placed at a level of 3rd lumbar vertebrae
- most important anatomic landmark for the retroperitoneum is the transverse process of the vertebrae.
- 5 to 10 mm Hg insufflation

Option 2:

- sternal recumbency with suspended abdomen
- right side: SILS port between T13 and L1 transverse process
- left side: SILS port between L2 & L3 transverse process
- 5 mm Hg insufflation

---

the vertebrae. The effect on working space with insufflation pressures from 0 to 15 mm Hg in 5 mm Hg increments were assessed via CT scan and the position of retroperitoneal organs was documented by visual inspection with a 0° telescope through the retroperitoneal port. Based on this study, the researchers recommended an insufflation pressure of 5 to 10mmg Hg as this provided adequate working space but did not create peritoneal complications (tearing). Visualization advantages included the ventral retraction of the kidney with the visualization of the renal hilus and adrenal gland.

A second study by Ko and colleagues,[10] investigated the use of retroperitoneal access for adrenalectomy in 8 healthy beagle dogs. This experimental study placed patients in sternal recumbency with abdominal sling and used a SILS port placed between T13 and L1 transverse process on the right and L2 and L3 transverse process on the left (see **Box 2**). An insufflation pressure of 5 mm Hg was used and all patients were able to have adrenalectomies performed successfully. The right adrenal took significantly longer for removal which is consisting of open and transperitoneal laparoscopic techniques. The adrenal gland capsule was found to be damaged in 3 of 8 samples on histologic examination. Future clinical studies will hopefully elucidate the use of this access technique for patients with adrenal tumors so that case-specific selection criteria can be established.

Nephrectomy, nephrotomy

Laparoscopic ureteronephrectomy has been previously reported in veterinary medicine[12] but has not been widely performed or studied. As with all laparoscopic techniques, the advantages of magnification and illumination help surgeons with the delicate dissections required during this procedure. Dissection and ligation of the renal vasculature must be performed carefully as severe hemorrhage can occur and lead to conversion (**Fig. 1**). Realistically the kidney can not be removed from port incisions in most cases, so incision enlargement is necessary but even this incision adjustment leaves patients with smaller incisions than the traditional open approach. Indications for nephrectomy are most commonly related to neoplasia, infection, or calculi obstruction leading to the destruction of renal parenchyma. One recent study by Liu and

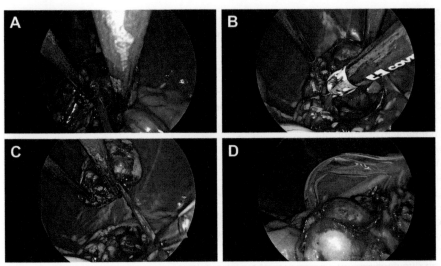

Fig. 1. Laparoscopic photographs of ureteronephrectomy for renal carcinoma. (*A*) Identification of the renal vessels (yellow star) and ureter (yellow *arrow*) at the hilus, (*B*) transection of the renal artery and vein, (*C*) dissection of the ureter from the retroperitoneal space, (*D*) placement of the kidney into a sterile sample retrieval bag. (Photographs courtesy of Dr. Ameet Singh.)

colleagues,[13] investigated the outcome of partial nephrectomy (2/3) on pigs comparing 3 different surgical approaches: laparoscopic, open retroperitoneal, and open laparotomy. This nephron-sparing technique is advantageous in patients with decreased contralateral renal function. Successful partial nephrectomy was performed in all patients, but surgical times were significantly longer for the laparoscopic group (60.71 +-7.34 min) and open laparotomy group (58.57 +- 4.72 min) compared with the open retroperitoneal group (41.4 +-5.33 min). Warm ischemia was performed in all cases and was significantly longer in the laparoscopic group compared with the other 2 surgical groups, but serum markers of stress (C-reactive protein, superoxide dismutase) were significantly lower. The authors concluded that an open retroperitoneal procedure might be best if bilateral procedures must be performed because of the reduced warm ischemia time but that laparoscopic partial nephrectomy should be the first choice in patients suffering from unilateral disease as it created the least stress, a reduction in blood loss and smallest incisions. This procedure is highly complex and should be reserved for experienced laparoscopists with the availability of advanced equipment and comfort with minimally invasive vascular techniques.

A recent case report on the use of laparoscopic ureteronephrectomy in 2 dogs with *Dioctophyme renale* highlights the use of this technique for causes other than neoplasia, bacterial infection, or obstruction.[14] No complications during surgery occurred and both dogs in this report were discharged the following day. Laparoscopic nephrotomy has also been described[15] for the removal of these parasites and calculi and emphasizes the importance of nephron-saving techniques in veterinary medicine. This technique requires dissection around the renal vasculature to temporarily occlude the vessels and should not be undertaken without appropriate experience and equipment. Future randomized controlled studies are hopefully underway to allow rigorous comparison between techniques relating to predetermined outcome measures.

New technologies

Near-infrared fluorescence technology

Near-infrared fluorescence (NIRF) imaging is a relatively new diagnostic technology available to veterinary medicine. The applications of this low-energy technology are still being investigated but to date, it has been used most commonly for biliary, oncologic, thoracic duct, and lymph node mapping. Indocyanine green (ICG) is the most studied dye used in these procedures and seems to be safe in veterinary studies although a standardized dose and regimen have not been established as of yet. The mechanism of action of ICG is not receptor mediated and the ability of the imaging devices to be able to detect the fluorescence is limited to a tissue penetration of 10 to 15 mm. ICG becomes bound to proteins in plasma or lymph fluid and absorbs light in the near-infrared region at 806 nm. Once protein bound, it emits fluorescence (light) at a slightly longer wavelength, with peak emission at 830 nm. Fluorescence imaging devices provide external energy (near-infrared light) for ICG to absorb, resulting in the excitation of ICG molecules. The emitted fluorescence is transferred from the field of view to an image on a monitor. Its visual color is created from microbubbles produced from shaking during product reconstitution, rather than the chemical composition of the dye itself.

One study investigated the use of NIRF for pulmonary tumor detection in 8 client-owned dogs.[16] ICG was administered 24 hours before surgery intravenously at a dose of 5 mg/kg and imaged before, during, and after removal of the affected pulmonary lobe. NIRF imaging identified all tumors in this study and showed high selectivity of cancer tissue from normal. In cases of peritumoral inflammation, ICG was not able to differentiate between inflammatory versus cancerous tissue. No complications occurred associated with the ICG injection, but the authors conclude that more specific receptor-related dyes may be necessary to guide surgical dose as inflammation alone could not be determined. Another study investigated the use of NIRF to detect residual neoplastic cells in wound beds after soft tissue sarcoma in 15 dogs.[17] Animals received 3 mg/kg ICG intravenously 24 hours before surgery and surveillance consisted of scanning the tumor in situ and post-resection, as well as imaging at the wound bed. Ten animals showed no evidence of fluorescence postresection, but one dog did have positive margins on histopathology (sarcoma). Of these 10 dogs, none had local recurrence at > 1-year follow-up. Five dogs had evidence of fluorescence in the wound bed and histopathology of the additionally resected tissue revealed residual tumor cells in 4/5 of these patients giving a sensitivity of 100% (95% confidence interval, CI 0.39–1.00) and a specificity of 90.9% (CI 0.54–0.99) in detecting residual disease at the surgical margins. This study also reported the detection of an overestimation of the tumor margin by NIRF of 3–6 mm from the diffusion of fluorescence light from the primary tumor.

Multiple experimental studies have also illustrated the use of NIRF for sentinel lymph node mapping in dogs.[18–20] The combined results of these studies confirm the usefulness of NIR for sentinel lymph node mapping and 2 recent studies showed that NIRF could be used transcutaneously to track lymphatics to the sentinel lymph node in an oral (**Fig. 2**)and mammary tumor model.[19,20] Time from injection to the visualization of the fluorescence ranged from 4 to 15 minutes in the oral tumor model and 2 to 25 minutes in the cutaneous model making it possible to perform during surgery. Important considerations for imaging accuracy included the injection site, depth of the lymph nodes, positioning of the patient during imaging, and distance of camera to the skin.[19] Other promising applications of NIRF technology in veterinary medicine include

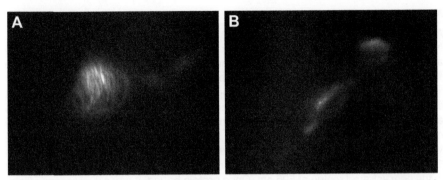

Fig. 2. Near-infrared images after Indocyanine green injection. (*A*) the sentinel lymph node glows bright white when the NIR camera is activated, (*B*) the lymphatic tract. The green color seen in many images is added in postprocessing or is available on advanced laparoscopy equipment.

thoracic duct and cisterna chyli identification to aid in the treatment of chylothorax and biliary tract applications.[21–24] Successful mesenteric lymphangiography with ICG was performed in 8 clinical dogs and aided the identification and ablation of the cisterna chyli.[23] A study in 6 healthy research cats also successfully used a subcutaneous injection of ICG in the perineal region for NIRF imaging during thoracoscopic thoracic duct ligation.[24] Clearly NIRF imaging holds many possibilities for veterinary patients, especially in oncologic fields.

Intraoperative NIRF imaging of the extrahepatic biliary tract to improve the safety of MIS is also under investigation currently for veterinary patients and new protocols are highly anticipated. The use of ICG for the biliary system is logical as ICG is metabolized exclusively by the liver and excreted via the biliary system 15 to 20 minutes after administration with peak levels seen within 30 minutes to 2 hours according to some authors.[25,26] Injuries to the hepatic ducts or common bile duct is the complication most feared by surgeons during cholecystectomy (open or laparoscopic). In human medicine, ICG has been used for many years to highlight the extrahepatic biliary tract anatomy during laparoscopic cholecystectomy. A recent prospective randomized multicenter trial with more than 300 patients in both groups (NIRF vs white light) determined statistically significant improvement in the predissection identification of structures with NIRF when patients were given intravenous ICG 45 minutes before surgery at a dose of 0.05 mg/kg.[25] A recent meta-analysis on the use of NIRF with laparoscopic cholecystectomy also reviewed almost 5000 abstract to report that overall weighted rates for bile duct injury and conversion were 6 and 16/10,000 for patients with NIRF cholangiography versus 25 and 271/10,000 in patients without NIRF cholangiography.[27] An important drawback of NIRF is that currently there are no standardized dose or administration protocols for ICG and NIRF (**Table 1**) leading to challenges with visualization and comparative studies.[26] This work is being performed and human medical sites such as the International Society for Fluorescence Guided Surgery (ISFGS, www.isfgs.org/) does provide members with online resources including suggested protocols for a variety of procedures.

Custom fluorophores, targeting receptors, proteins, and growth factors, have been developed and investigated in murine, feline, and canine models, and show promise for squamous cell carcinomas, fibrosarcomas, and gliomas.[21] The use of receptors-targeted imaging agents can be complicated by the finding that expression of these receptors, proteins or enzymes within a tumor may be heterogeneous. New NIR

Table 1
Published near-infrared fluorescence veterinary protocols by procedure type

Procedure Type	Dose/Route	Timing
Pulmonary tumor detection[16]	5 mg/kg IV	24 h preoperatively
Soft tissue sarcoma[17]	3 mg/kg IV	24 h preoperatively
Sentinel lymph node[18]	0.3 mL gastric submucosa	3–4 h preoperatively gastric cancer model
Sentinel lymph node[19]	0.1 mL (0.5 mg/mL) subdermal	intraoperatively (median time to mammary tumor model fluorescence 5 min (2–25 min), lasted 2 h
Sentinel lymph node[20]	1 mL (0.5 mg/mL) buccal mucosa	intraoperatively (mean time to oral tumor modelfluorescence 8 min (4–15 min), lasted 24 h
Thoracic duct[22]	0.25–0.5 mg/mL mesenteric LN	intraoperatively (fluorescence seen volume to effect <1 min post injection)
	0.5–0.7 mg/mL popliteal LN	intraoperatively (fluorescence seen volume to effect range of <2 min to 25 min postinjection)
Thoracic duct (cat)[23]	1-2 mL (0.25 mg/mL) SQ	intraoperatively (no discussion of time perineal site (massaged) to fluorescence or efficacy of NIRF)
Cisterna chyli[24]	0.02 mg/kg (0.25 mg/mL)	intraoperatively (no discussion of time Jejunal LN, colic LN or to fluorescence but all CC visualized) Mesenteric lymphatic

contrast agents relying on tumor microenvironment pH are also currently being investigated as acidosis in solid tumors seems to be universal. From the clinical perspective, much work needs to be conducted to standardize the dose and timing depending on the proposed use.

Updates on barbed sutures

Barbed suture could be one of the most significant additions to a minimally invasive surgeon's armamentarium after the creation of the vessel-sealing device. The advantages to using this type of suture include a reduction in surgery time, consistent tension along the suture line, and the removal of the need for intracorporeal knot-tying. These sutures can be used laparoscopically or during open procedures and veterinary studies have evaluated their safety and strength.[28–30] Currently there are multiple versions of barbed sutures available on the veterinary market, each with slight differences in the angle, depth, location, and type of barb. It is important to note that suture sizes are labeled differently depending on the manufacturer (**Table 2**). The Quill suture uses the size of the suture before the barbs are cut into it, while the V-Loc uses the size of

Table 2
Various options and differences in available barbed sutures

Name	Suture Size	Barb Type	End of Suture Line
V-Loc™	after barbs cut	Unidirectional dual angle cut	welded loop
Quill™	before barbs cut	Uni/bidirectional Single angle cut	welded loop
STRATAFIX™	after barbs cut	Unidirectional Single angle cut	anchor or loop

the suture after the barbs are created (thus a 0 Quill is equivalent to a 2-0 V-Loc).[31] The Quill suture is double-armed with bidirectional barbs. The V-Loc has unidirectional barbs and a welded loop at the end opposite the needle. The STRATAFIX suture is available in both a Symmetric PDS and Spiral option with an anchor or loop at the end opposite the needle, respectively.

Most MIS veterinary studies relating to barbed suture focus on laparoscopic gastropexy (**Fig. 3**).[29–34] The only prospective randomized control study reported on 30 dogs undergoing laparoscopic gastropexy comparing intracorporeal suturing of 2 lines of traditional PDS suture to the Quill and V-Loc sutures.[31] This study found all gastropexies were intact, determined by ultrasound evaluation, after 6 months but the gastropexy suturing times and total surgical times were significantly lower with barbed suture compared with traditional smooth suture. More recent retrospective studies using barbed sutures (V-Loc) reviewed the use of 1 line (vs 2) of suture, absorbable and nonabsorbable suture types, and the omission of body wall and stomach incisions. Takacs and colleagues,[32] reported on 63 dogs from multiple institutions and found that one line of barbed sutures seemed effective and safe with a follow-up of greater than 6 months. The study by Deroy and colleagues highlighted to strength the adhesion of barbed suture gastropexies by reviewing 21 dogs that underwent incisionless laparoscopic gastropexy with either absorbable or nonabsorbable barbed suture. In these cases, even though no incision was made into the stomach or body wall, postoperative ultrasound performed at a median of 8 months (6–36 mo.) revealed permanent adhesion formation in all dogs.[33] Experimental work comparing different barbed sutures (STRATAFIX vs V-loc) continues as each has inherent advantages and disadvantages.[34]

Other minimally invasive uses for the barbed suture that have been investigated include enterostomy closure, cystopexy, cholecystoduodenostomy (CCD), and hiatal hernia repair.[35–38] The laparoscopic cystopexy and CCD procedures were performed solely on cadavers, therefore, clinical case results are necessary before any recommendations can be made. Laparoscopic cystopexy was feasible with barbed suture but CCD could not be recommended due to anastomotic leakage in 3/5 dogs.[36,37] Laparoscopic enterotomy using the Endo Stitch device with barbed suture has been performed in dogs in a research setting and no leaks were appreciated, and mean bursting strength was equal to conventional suture.[35] The advantage of speed with the Endo Stich and barbed suture coupled with the apparent safety encourage its use for more than just gastropexies. The only study on clinical patients retrospectively reviewed 8 cases of hiatal hernia repaired laparoscopically.[38] While 4/8 dogs required conversion to an open approach and pneumothorax was encountered in 3 dogs, the barbed suture was not the cause of these difficulties and the authors still felt it was the

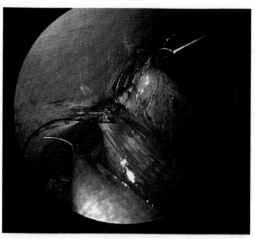

Fig. 3. Laparoscopic photograph of intracorporeally sutured gastropexy with a 0 PDS V-Loc suture. The barbed nature of the suture can be seen to the left of the image and tension is held even though the suture is not being held tight.

best suture choice for this procedure. In the authors' experience, barbed suture has been very useful for hiatal hernia repairs and careful tissue handling and suture placement mitigates the risks involved (**Fig. 4**). Future studies in veterinary medicine need to identify more laparoscopic surgical procedures that might benefit from these sutures and investigate them in controlled clinical prospective studies.

3D-printed ports

As with many aspects of veterinary medicine over the past decade, 3D printing technology has also made its way into the field of laparoscopy. While 3D printing of endo and exoprosthesis and cutting guides has been explored[39–41] found to be very useful, use of this technology on the soft tissue side of surgery has been confined to anatomic modeling and teaching applications.[42] Recently the author investigated the use of 3D printed laparoscopic ports for use in a gastrectomy model in cats. A feline cadaveric model was used to test the 3D printed cannulas and the technique for laparoscopic partial gastrectomy in cats was refined (**Figs. 5** and **6**).[43] 3D printed cannulas facilitated the procedure due to their shortened length thereby allowing easier manipulation of intraabdominal tissues. Cannulas were designed using computer-aided design software (Materialise 3-Matic, 44650 Helm Court, Plymouth, MI 48170 USA). Prototypes were printed with a fused deposition modeling (FDM) 3D printer (Prusa i3 MK3S+, Czech Republic) using PLA material (**Fig. 6**). This material is autoclavable and biocompatible and studies are underway in clinical patients investigating their use. The number of reported ports complications (removal of the port from the abdomen and number of instrument collisions decreased with the use of the shortened 3D printed laparoscopic ports. The benefits of these ports, especially in smaller animals, were their ability to allow for increased working space within the abdomen and less interference between the port and the instruments. Other advantages with 3D printed ports include the ability for institutions to print patient-specific ports depending on the procedure, instruments needed, and the body condition/size of the patient. This in turn may encourage more procedures to be performed on a wider variety of patients with less frustration and more efficiency.

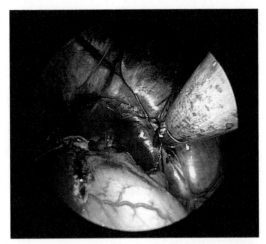

Fig. 4. Laparoscopic photograph of the start of a hiatal hernia repair. The first two bites with a barbed suture (V-Loc) have been performed at the ventral most aspect of the esophageal hiatus. Caudal traction on the stomach is being applied. Mild electrocautery damage is seen on the left lateral liver lobe where the triangular ligament was transected.

A note on NOTES

Natural orifice transluminal endoscopic surgery (NOTES) techniques via gastric or vaginal approaches were developed in human medicine to remove the complications associated with surgical incisions, decrease hospitalization times and reduce pain.[44,45] NOTES procedures in dogs including experimental models and clinical studies on ovariohysterectomy and ovariectomy have been investigated.[46–51] A prospective randomized control study comparing total transvaginal NOTES ovariectomy to hybrid laparoscopic and transvaginal NOTES ovariectomy reported that both techniques were similar with regards to surgery time, complication rate, and pain scores.[50] The biggest difficulty in the total transvaginal NOTES group was noted to be the

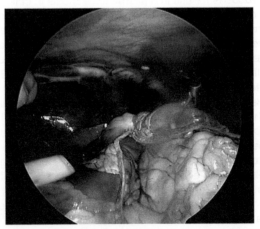

Fig. 5. Laparoscopic photograph after first staple line placed at the fundus for a partial gastrectomy.

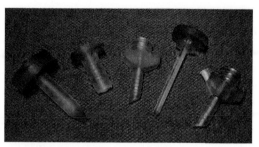

Fig. 6. Autoclavable 3D printed cannulas created in biocompatible, autoclavable resin material (11 mm trocar, 11 mm cannula, 5 mm cannula with no insufflation cannula, 5 mm trocar, and 5 mm cannula with insufflation cannula from left to right).

removal of the ovary from the vagina. Neither procedure was found to have a clear advantage nor additional pain medication was not required in either group postoperatively. A large retrospective study on total transvaginal NOTES ovariectomy in 60 dogs compared results to a historical cohort of 202 dogs undergoing 2-port laparoscopic ovariectomies performed at the same clinic.[51] This study assessed surgical times, intraoperative and postoperative complications, and postoperative owner-perceived comfort and inconvenience. The surgical time for transvaginal NOTES ovariectomy was significantly longer than for laparoscopic ovariectomy (34.3 +- 9.9minuts vs 22.3 +-3.2 minutes) and there were intraoperative complications requiring conversion to abdominal laparoscopy in 3 dogs. There were no postoperative complications reported in the NOTES group and owners of both groups indicated satisfaction with the procedure performed. While NOTES procedures require less postoperative care, as there are no sutures implanted and no exercise restriction needed, they do require experienced laparoscopists and specialized equipment. The limitations of patient and ovary size must also be considered. Future studies still need to demonstrate whether there is more than that can be conducted clinically with this technique and whether there is a true advantage over traditional laparoscopy.

Future directions: robotics

MIS in veterinary medicine still lags behind our human counterparts but advanced techniques are being investigated every day. Most if not all of the procedures commonly conducted on humans were originally tested in an animal model and client-owned patients are beginning to reap the benefits of these advanced techniques. One such area that veterinary surgeons are looking toward in the future is robotics. While it is true that we may be many years away from surgical robots being a routine finding in veterinary operating rooms, the interest is growing, and veterinarians are beginning the work into adapting this technology for our patients. In humans, robotic surgery has been used for urogenital, cardiovascular, orthopedic, oropharyngeal diseases, and recently pediatrics for decades.[52–59] The major advantages to robotic surgery include combining the magnification and illumination of laparoscopy with the versatility of 3-dimensional field of view and enhanced dexterity in instrumentation with improved degrees of freedom and articulation. The limitations to robotics go beyond the cost and physical space requirements (robotic machine and surgeon console) and include a purported steep learning curve and longer operative times. And for veterinary patients, probably more important is the large size of the robotic ports and instruments limiting its use for our smallest animals.

Box 3
Advantages, disadvantages, and possible robotic procedures in veterinary medicine

Advantages:

- Improved visualization (3D) for precise dissection
- Improved dexterity (improved degrees of freedom & articulation)
- Access to smaller anatomic areas

Disadvantages:

- Cost of equipment
- Space needed for equipment
- Longer operative times

Possible Procedures:

- Prostatectomy
- Cholecystectomy
- Cystectomy
- Lung lobectomy
- Abdominal tumor dissection/removal
- Sentinel lymph node dissection/removal (thoracic/abdominal)

Even with these limitations, robotic surgery holds the possibility of advanced procedures in oropharyngeal, urogenital, gastrointestinal, and cardiovascular specialties in veterinary medicine and should be pursued (**Box 3**). To date, most of the studies on robotic techniques in animals are experimental models on prostatic resections, cardiovascular interventions (ablations), laryngectomy, and so forth.[60–63] The only clinical report in a dog relates to a robotic radical prostatectomy for a patient with prostatic carcinoma.[64] This Bernese mountain dog had surgery performed by a physician trained in robotics using a four-arm da Vinci SI robotic system through a transperitoneal approach (**Fig. 7**). A nerve-sparing approach was performed but the patient was not able to urinate 3 days postoperatively when the urinary catheter was removed (**Fig. 8**). The patient required re-catheterization twice more but was able to urinate normally when the urinary catheter was ultimately removed at day 7 postoperatively. While the console time was reported as 120 minutes, the total anesthesia time for the case was not reported. No intraoperative complications were observed but

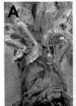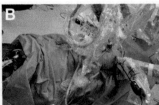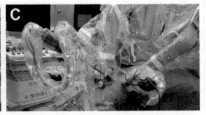

Fig. 7. Positioning of the patient with a DaVinci SI robotic system. (*A*) Patient head at bottom of picture, (*B*) patient head to the left of the picture, (*C*) patient head to the left of the picture. (*Courtesy of* Alexander Schlake.)

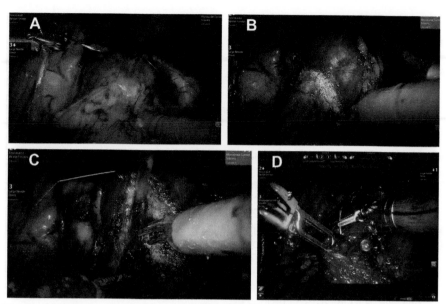

Fig. 8. Intraoperative intracorporeal robotic images from nerve-sparing prostatectomy in a dog. (*A*) Identification of the urinary bladder neck, (*B*) dissection of bladder neck from urethra, (*C*) transection of the posterior prostatic urethra, (*D*) anastomosis of urethra to urinary bladder. (*Courtesy of* Alexander Schlake.)

peritoneal carcinomatosis was diagnosed 43 days after surgery and the patient was euthanized. While this case report does not illustrate a survival benefit of robotic surgery over other readily available management strategies (medical management, urethral stenting, prostatic arterial embolization, or radiation), it does provide evidence that these procedures can be safely performed in certain veterinary populations. Pushing the limits in MIS will allow us to create new surgical procedures and should be encouraged.

CLINICS CARE POINTS

- Retroperitoneal access for adrenalectomy should not be performed in patients needing an abdominal explore for staging and surgeons need a thorough knowledge of anatomy from this view and the space limitations with this technique.

- Laparoscopic nephrectomy and nephrotomy can be considered in certain patients but surgeons must have experience with advanced laparoscopic vascular manipulation and surgery times may be extended.

- Time from injection to the visualization of the NIRF ranges from 4 to 15 minutes in the oral tumor model and 2 to 25 minutes in the cutaneous model but the injection site, depth of the target organ, positioning of the patient, and distance of camera to the target organ must all be considered.

- Barbed suture has been shown to be strong and safe but there are slight differences in the angle, depth, location, and type of barb depending on manufacturer, and suture sizes are labeled differently requiring surgeons to be familiar with the brand before surgical use.

- 3D printed ports allow institutions/practices to print patient-specific ports depending on the procedure, instruments needed, and the body condition/size of the patient encouraging more procedures to be performed on a wider variety of patients.

DISCLOSURE

The author has nothing to disclose.

REFERENCES

1. Mayhew PD, Freeman L, Kwan T, et al. Comparison of surgical site infection rates in clean and clean-contaminated wounds in dogs and cats after minimally invasive versus open surgery: 179 cases (2007–2008). J Am Vet Med Assoc 2012; 240:193–8.
2. Mayhew PD. Recent advances in soft tissue minimally invasive surgery. J Small Anim Pract 2014;55(2):75–83.
3. Jones K, Case JB, Evans B, et al. Evaluation of the economic and clinical feasibility of introducing rigid endoscopy and laparoscopy to a small animal general practice. J Am Vet Med Assoc 2017;250(7).795–800.
4. Ren T, Liu Y, Zhao X, et al. Transperitoneal approach versus retroperitoneal approach: a meta-analysis of laparoscopic partial nephrectomy for renal cell carcinoma. PLoS One 2014;9:e91978.
5. Fan X, Xu K, Lin T, et al. Comparison of transperitoneal and retroperitoneal laparoscopic nephrectomy for renal cell carcinoma: a systematic review and meta-analysis. BJU Int 2013;111:611–21.
6. Constantinides VA, Christakis I, Touska P, et al. Systematic review and meta-analysis of retroperitoneoscopic versus laparoscopic adrenalectomy. Br J Surg 2012;99:1639–48.
7. Nigri G, Rosman AS, Petrucciani N, et al. Meta-analysis of trials comparing laparoscopic transperitoneal and retroperitoneal adrenalectomy. Surgery 2013;153: 111–9.
8. Johnston DE. Adrenalectomy via retroperitoneal approach in dogs. J Am Vet Med Assoc 1977;170:1092–5.
9. Jeong J, Ko J, Lim H, et al. Retroperitoneal laparoscopy in dogs: access technique, working space, and surgical anatomy. Vet Surg 2016;45(S1):O102–10.
10. Ko J, Jeong J, Lee S, et al. Feasibility of single-port retroperitoneoscopic adrenalectomy in dogs. Vet Surg 2018;47(S1):O75–83.
11. Jimenez Pelaez M, Bouvy BM, Dupre GP. Laparoscopic adrenalectomy for treatment of unilateral adrenocortical carcinomas: technique, complications, and results in seven dogs. Vet Surg 2008;37:444–53.
12. Mayhew PD, Mehler SJ, Mayhew KN, et al. Experimental and clinical evaluation of transperitoneal laparoscopic ureteronephrectomy in dogs. Vet Surg 2013;42: 565–71.
13. Liu HF, Meng WJ, Kong XD, et al. Partial (two-thirds) nephrectomy in pigs: a comparison of three surgical approaches. Res Vet Sci 2019;125:459–64.
14. Hart E, Singh A, Peregrine A, et al. Laparoscopic ureteronephrectomy for the treatment of giant kidney worm infection in 2 dogs. Can Vet J 2020;61:1149–54.
15. Brun M. Nephron-sparing laparoscopic nephrotomy in dogs. Abstract. Presented at the World Minimally Invasive Surgery Conference. June 2021, Fort Collins, CO.
16. Holt D, Okusanya O, Judy R, et al. Intraoperative near-infrared imaging can distinguish cancer from normal tissue but not inflammation. PLoS One 2014; 9(7):e103342. https://doi.org/10.1371/journal.pone.0103342.
17. Holt D, Pathasarathy AB, Okusanya O, et al. Intraoperative near-infrared fluorescence imaging and spectroscopy identified residual tumor cells in wounds. J Biomed Opt 2015;20:76002. https://doi.org/10.1117/1.JBO.20.7.076002.

18. Kim H, Lee SK, Kim YM, et al. Fluorescent Iodized emulsion for pre- and intraoperative sentinel lymph node imaging: validation in a preclinical model. Radiology 2015;275:196–204.

19. Favrll I S, Stock E, Hernot S, et al. Sentinel lymph node mapping by near-infrared fluorescence imaging and contrast-enhanced ultrasound in healthy dogs. Vet Comp Oncol 2019;17:89–98.

20. Townsend KL, Milovancev M, Bracha S. Feasibility of near-infrared fluorescence imaging for sentinel lymph node evaluation of the oral cavity in healthy dogs. Am J Vet Res 2018;79:995–1000.

21. Holt D, Singhal S, Selmic LE. Near-infrared imaging and optical coherence tomography for intraoperative visualization of tumors. Vet Surg 2020;49:33–43.

22. Steffey MA, Mayhew PD. Use of direct near-infrared fluorescent lymphography for thoracoscopic thoracic duct identification in 15 dogs with chylothorax. Vet Surg 2018;47:267–76.

23. Morris KP, Singh A, Holt DE, et al. Hybrid single-port laparoscopic cisterna chili ablation for the adjunct treatment of chylothorax disease in dogs. Vet Surg 2019;48:O121–9.

24. Mitchell JW, Mayhew PD, Johnson EG, et al. Video-assisted thoracoscopic thoracic duct sealing is inconsistent when performed with a bipolar vessel-sealing device in healthy cats. Vet Surg 2018;47(S1):O84–90.

25. Dip F, LoMenzo E, Sarotto L, et al. Randomized trial of near-infrared incisionless fluorescent cholangiography. Ann Surg 2019;270:992–9.

26. Vlek SL, van Dam DA, Rubinstein SM, et al. Biliary tract visualization using near-infrared imaging with indocyanine green during laparoscopic cholecystectomy: results of a systematic review. Surg Endosc 2017;31:2731–42.

27. Dip F, Menzo EL, White KP, et al. Does near-infrared fluorescent cholangiography with indocyanine green reduce bile duct injuries and conversions to open surgery during laparoscopic or robotic cholecystectomy? - A meta-analysis. Surgery 2021;169:859–67.

28. Bailey KL, Johnson M, Travers CJ, et al. Biomechanical analysis of unidirectional knotless suture loop weld integrity after passage through a cadaveric body wall. Vet Surg 2019;48:431–6.

29. Arbaugh M, Case JB, Monnet E. Biomechanical comparison of glycomer 631 and glycomer 631 knotless for use in canine incisional gastropexy. Vet Surg 2013;42:205–9.

30. Imhoff DJ, Cohen A, Monnet E. Biomechanical analysis of laparoscopic incisional gastropexy with intracorporeal suturing using knotless polyglyconate. Vet Surg 2014;44(Suppl 1):39–43.

31. Spah CE, Elkins AD, Wehrenberg A, et al. Evaluation of two novel self-anchoring barbed sutures in a prophylactic laparoscopic gastropexy compared with intracorporeal tied knots. Vet Surg 2013;42:932–42.

32. Takacs JD, Singh A, Case JB, et al. Total laparoscopic gastropexy using 1 simple continuous barbed suture line in 63 dogs. Vet Surg 2017;46:233–41.

33. Deroy C, Hahn H, Bismuth C, et al. Simplified minimally invasive surgical approach for prophylactic laparoscopic gastropexy in 21 cases. J Am Anim Hosp Assoc 2019;55:152–9.

34. Scott J, Oramas A, McCoy A, et al. Biomechanical comparison of two barbed sutures in canine gastropexy: a veterinary endoscopic society study. Abstract. Presented at Abstract. Presented at the World Minimally Invasive Surgery Conference. June 2021, Fort Collins, CO.

35. Omotosho P, Yurcisin B, Ceppa E, et al. In vivo assessment of an absorbable and nonabsorbable knotless barbed suture for laparoscopic single-layer enterotomy closure: a clinical and biomechanical comparison against nonbarbed suture. J Laparoendosc Adv Surg Tech A 2011;21:893–7.
36. Alvarez WA, Scharf VF, Case JB. Comparison of laparoscopic and open cystopexy in a cadaveric canine model. Vet Surg 2015;44(Suppl 1):44–9.
37. Díaz-Güemes Martín-Portugués I, Maria Matos-Azevedo A, Enciso Sanz S, et al. Laparoscopic cholecystoduodenostomy in dogs: canine cadaver feasibility study. Vet Surg 2016;45(S1):O34–40.
38. Monnet E. Laparoscopic correction of sliding hiatal hernia in eight dogs: description of technique, complications, and short-term outcome. Vet Surg 2021;50:230–7.
39. Hespel AM, Wilhite R, Hudson J. Invited review-applications for 3D printers in veterinary medicine. Vet Radiol Ultrasound 2014;55:347–58.
40. Worth AJ, Crosse KR, Kersley A. Computer-assisted surgery using 3D printed saw guides for acute correction of antebrachial angular limb deformities in dogs. Vet Comp Orthop Traumatol 2019;32:241–9.
41. Séguin B, Pinard C, Lussier B, et al. Limb-sparing in dogs using patient-specific, three-dimensional-printed endoprosthesis for distal radial osteosarcoma: a pilot study. Vet Comp Oncol 2020;18:92–104.
42. da Silveira EE, da Silva Lisboa Neto AF, Pereira HCS, et al. Canine skull digitalization and three-dimensional printing as an educational tool for anatomical study. J Vet Med Educ 2020;48(6):649–55.
43. Buote, NJ, Porter I, Dakin G. Laparoscopic Partial Gastrectomy with 3D printed cannulas in Feline cadaver specimens. Abstract. Presented at Abstract. Presented at the World Minimally Invasive Surgery Conference. June 2021, Fort Collins, CO.
44. Moris DN, Bramis KJ, Mantonakis EI, et al. Surgery via natural orifices in human beings: yesterday, today, tomorrow. Am J Surg 2012;204:93–102.
45. Tyson MD, Humphreys MR. Urological applications of natural orifice transluminal endoscopic surgery (NOTES). Nat Rev Urol 2014;11:324–32.
46. Freeman LJ, Rahmani EY, Sherman S, et al. Oophorectomy by natural orifice transluminal endoscopic surgery: feasibility study in dogs. Gastrointest Endosc 2009;69:1321–32.
47. Freeman LJ, Rahmani EY, Al-Haddad M, et al. Comparison of pain and postoperative stress in dogs undergoing natural orifice transluminal endoscopic surgery, laparoscopic, and open oophorectomy. Gastrointest Endosc 2010;72:373–80.
48. Freeman L, Rahmani EY, Burgess RC, et al. Evaluation of the learning curve for natural orifice transluminal endoscopic surgery: bilateral ovariectomy in dogs. Vet Surg 2011;40:140–50.
49. Brun MV, Silva MA, Mariano MB, et al. Ovariohysterectomy in a dog by a hybrid NOTES technique. Can Vet J 2011;52:637–40.
50. Linhares MT, Feranti JPS, Coradini GP, et al. Canine ovariectomy by hybrid or total natural orifice transluminal endoscopic surgery: technical feasibility study and pain assessment. Vet Surg 2019;47:O74–82.
51. Arntz G-JHM. Transvaginal laparoscopic ovariectomy in 60 dogs: description of the technique and comparison with 2-portal-access laparoscopic ovariectomy. Vet Surg 2019;48:726–34.
52. Thiel DD, Winfield HN. Robotics in urology: past, present, and future. J Endourol 2008;22:825–30.

53. McGuinness LA, Prasad Rai B. Robotics in urology. Ann R Coll Surg Engl 2018; 100(6 sup):38–44.
54. Truong M, Kim JH, Scheib S, et al. Advantages of robotics in benign gynecologic surgery. Curr Opin Obstet Gynecol 2016;28:304–10.
55. Zhang TWD, Da L. Remote-controlled vascular interventional surgery robot. Int J Med Robotics Comput Assist Surg 2010;6:194–201.
56. Parsley BS. Robotics in orthopedics: a brave new world. J Arthroplasty 2018;33: 2355–7.
57. Liu HH, Li LJ, Shi B, et al. Robotic surgical systems in maxillofacial surgery: a review. Int J Oral Sci 2017;9:63–73.
58. Navarrete-Arellano M. Robotic-assisted minimally invasive surgery in children. In: Kucuk S, editor. Latest developments in medical robotics systems, online. London: IntechOpen Ltd; 2021. p. 1–31. https://doi.org/10.5772/intechopen.96684.
59. Navarrete Arellano M, González FG. Robot-assisted laparoscopic and thoracoscopic surgery: prospective series of 186 pediatric surgeries. Front Pediatr 2019;7:200. https://doi.org/10.3389/fped.2019.00200.
60. Gianduzzo T, Colombo JR, Haber GP, et al. Laser robotically assisted nerve-sparing radical prostatectomy: a pilot study of technical feasibility in the canine model. BJU Int 2008;102:598–602.
61. Faber K, de Abreu AL, Ramos P, et al. Image-guided robot-assisted prostate ablation using water jet-hydrodissection: initial study of a novel technology for benign prostatic hyperplasia. J Endourol 2015;29:63–9.
62. Okumura Y, Johnson SB, Bunch TJ, et al. A systematical analysis of in vivo contact forces on virtual catheter tip/tissue surface contact during cardiac mapping and intervention. J Cardiovasc Electrophysiol 2008;19:632–40.
63. Weinstein GS, O'malley BW Jr, Hockstein NG. Transoral robotic surgery: supraglottic laryngectomy in a canine model. Laryngoscope 2005;115:1315–9.
64. Schlake A, Dell'Oglio P, Devriendt N, et al. First robot-assisted radical prostatectomy in a client-owned Bernese mountain dog with prostatic adenocarcinoma. Vet Surg 2020;49:1458–66.

Updates in Thoracoscopy

Valery Fairfax Scharf, DVM, MS, DACVS

KEYWORDS

- Thoracoscopy • Chylothorax • Pericardiectomy • Lung lobectomy • Mediastinal
- Pneumothorax • Pyothorax • One-lung ventilation

KEY POINTS

- Patient selection for thoracoscopy is critical due to limitations in working space and the need for specialized instrumentation.
- One-lung ventilation and thoracic insufflation may increase working space within the thorax but shouldshould be used with caution to avoid cardiopulmonary complications.
- Thoracoscopic lung lobectomy in large dogs is feasible for masses less than 8 cm in diameter; smaller dogs and cats may require a thoracoscopic-assisted approach.
- Near-infrared fluorescence lymphangiography techniques show promise for facilitating thoracoscopic thoracic duct visualization and dissection.
- Thoracoscopic treatment of persistent right aortic arch is feasible; transection of aberrant left subclavian arteries causing compression of the esophagus should be considered.

  Video content accompanies this article at http://www.vetsmall.theclinics.com.

BACKGROUND

Thoracoscopy is a rapidly expanding field providing surgical treatment of thoracic disease in small animals with the intent of reducing morbidity and improving convalescence in these patients. Given the invasiveness of traditional approaches to the thorax through median sternotomies and intercostal thoracotomies, the thoracoscopic approach has the potential to provide a drastic reduction in incision size, postoperative pain, and length of recovery. Nonetheless, minimally invasive surgery (MIS) of the thorax faces inherent challenges posed by the rigidity of the thoracic wall and the dynamic visual obstruction created by pulmonary excursion. Modified approaches including thoracoscopic-assisted techniques and one-lung ventilation (OLV) have been pursued in small animals in recent years to mitigate these challenges. Similarly, advances in preoperative and intraoperative imaging techniques have helped to promote thoracoscopic surgery in small animals.

Department of Clinical Sciences, NC State University, 1052 William Moore Dr., Raleigh, NC 27607, USA
E-mail address: vfscharf@ncsu.edu

Vet Clin Small Anim 52 (2022) 531–548
https://doi.org/10.1016/j.cvsm.2021.11.005
0195-5616/22/© 2021 Elsevier Inc. All rights reserved.

Fundamentals of thoracoscopy including approaches and techniques for common thoracoscopic procedures have been previously described.[1] Novel approaches and innovations in small animal thoracoscopy are being rapidly developed; thus this article aims to describe recent updates in commonly performed thoracoscopic procedures, including lung lobectomy, pericardiectomy and pericardioscopy, chylothorax treatment, cranial mediastinal mass resection, persistent right aortic arch (PRAA) treatment, and management of pyothorax and primary spontaneous pneumothorax.

IMPROVING THORACOSCOPIC VISUALIZATION

Visualization and exploration within the thorax pose a challenge due to the constant movement of the lungs and the rigidity of the thoracic wall. These limitations may be compounded by the small size of some veterinary patients. Working space in smaller (<15 kg) dogs or cats, barrel-chested breeds, and patients in lateral recumbency may be improved by (1) reduction in tidal volume of up to 50%, (2) selectively ventilating only one lung, or (3) insufflating the thoracic cavity with low levels of carbon dioxide. Selective lung ventilation may also improve visualization; use of OLV, however, may be limited by (1) the need for specialized equipment to visualize and selectively block the desired mainstem bronchus, (2) availability of personnel experienced in placing and maintaining endobronchial blockers, and (3) development of intolerable hypoxemia in some patients. OLV can be established using selective intubation, endobronchial blockers, and double-lumen endobronchial tubes (DLTs). DLTs provide the advantage of allowing the alternation of which lung is ventilated depending on whether fresh gas flow is passed through the tracheal or bronchial lumen (https://www.teleflex.com/usa/en/product-areas/anesthesia/airway-management/endobronchial-tubes/sher-i-bronch/) (**Fig. 1**). OLV with DLT is dependent on correct placement of the DLT, which is traditionally achieved through the use of a small bronchoscope, although blind placement produced correct and complete OLV in an experimental study.[2] Thoracoscopic evaluation of DLT placement may help achieve correct positioning and obviate the need for bronchoscopic visualization.[2]

OLV may also be achieved through the use of an endobronchial blocker. The EZ-blocker (https://www.teleflex.com/usa/en/product-areas/anesthesia/airway-management/endobronchial-blockers/) (**Fig. 2**) is traditionally placed under bronchoscopic

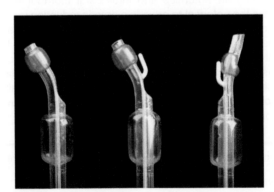

Fig. 1. Three configurations of a double-lumen endobronchial tube used for one-lung ventilation. (*Courtesy of* Philipp D. Mayhew, BVMS, MRCVS, DACVS, University of Davis School of Veterinary Medicine, Davis, California).

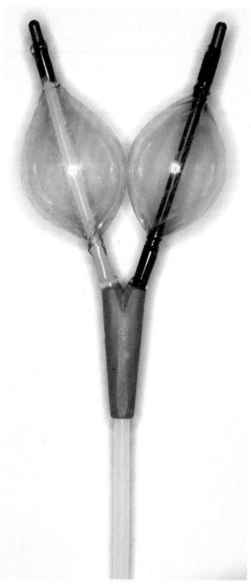

Fig. 2. Endobronchial blocker (EZ-blocker) used for one-lung ventilation. (*Courtesy of* Philipp D. Mayhew, BVMS, MRCVS, DACVS, University of Davis School of Veterinary Medicine, Davis, California).

visualization, although both the EZ-blocker and DLT were able to be placed under fluoroscopic guidance in canine cadavers.[3] Fluoroscopy may, therefore, offer a feasible option for achieving OLV if a small bronchoscope is not available. In the cadaveric study, the EZ-blocker was easier and faster to place than the DLT.[3] A detailed description of the advantages and disadvantages of each OLV technique is beyond the scope of this article; selection of these devices should be based on available equipment, procedure being performed, patient size, and surgeon/anesthesiologist experience.

Insufflation of the thoracic cavity must be performed with caution due to the potential for significant hypoxemia and systemic hypotension. When thoracic insufflation is indicated, carbon dioxide is instilled at low pressures (1–3 mm Hg). Because thoracic insufflation even at low pressures has been associated with cardiopulmonary depression, patients should be carefully monitored and cannulae left open to avoid dangerous increases in intrathoracic pressure.[4] In healthy cats undergoing thoracoscopy, insufflation at 3 and 5 mm Hg was well-tolerated for 30 minutes as long as ventilatory settings were increased to maintain eucapnia and oxygenation.[5] There was no appreciable improvement in working space with 5 mm Hg compared with 3 mm Hg, supporting the clinical recommendation to start with the lowest intrathoracic pressure possible to achieve the necessary visualization.[5] Although OLV also seems to be tolerated in healthy cats, left-sided OLV with thoracic insufflation led to significantly lower oxygen delivery and caused severe desaturation in 2 of 6 cats evaluated in an experimental study.[6]

An alternative to increasing working space within the chest is using a variable angle endoscope to improve maneuverability around pulmonary surfaces and the rigid chest wall (**Fig. 3**). A recent experimental cadaveric study found that the use of a variable endoscope with angulation ranging from 0° to 120° shortened total time for thoracoscopic exploration compared with a fixed 30° endoscope when lungs were ventilated.[7]

THORACOSCOPIC AND THORACOSCOPIC-ASSISTED LUNG LOBECTOMY

Indications for thoracoscopic lung lobectomy include the resection of pulmonary neoplasia and bullous lesions, excision of traumatized, consolidated, or abscessed lung lobes, and peripheral lung biopsy. Benefits of thoracoscopic lung lobectomy include a dramatically reduced incision size (**Fig. 4**). Thoracoscopic lung lobectomy is performed with the patient in lateral recumbency; some partial lobectomies may be performed in dorsal recumbency during exploratory thoracoscopy. Excision of pulmonary neoplasia is the most common indication for thoracoscopic lung lobectomy, although the feasibility of a thoracoscopic approach is often limited by tumor size and patient size.[8] The use of endoscopic gastrointestinal anastomosis (GIA) staplers for thoracoscopic lung lobectomy provides an efficient means of sealing the

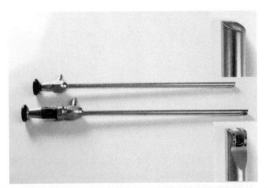

Fig. 3. Image of a fixed-angle (30°) endoscope traditionally used for thoracoscopy (top) versus a variable-angle (0° - 120°) endoscope (bottom) that allows for increased maneuverability around lung surfaces during exploratory thoracoscopy. A magnified view of both endoscope tips is shown in the inset. Angulation of the variable-angle endoscope is controlled by the black knob adjacent to the eyepiece.

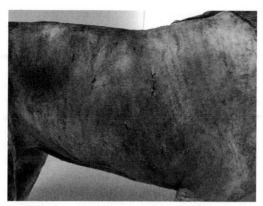

Fig. 4. Postoperative image following thoracoscopic lung lobectomy. One 11.5-mm and three 5.5-mm portals were used to resect a primary lung tumor, facilitating discharge from the hospital 1 day postoperatively.

pulmonary vasculature and bronchus during hilar resection (**Fig. 5**). Endoscopic GIA staplers deploy 6 rows of alternating staples with sharp transection via a blade between the middle rows, leaving 3 row of staples in the patient to achieve hemostasis and pneumostasis. These staplers are relatively large compared with the working room in the thorax of many small animal patients and can be challenging to safely maneuver around the hilus. Use of the 60-mm cartridge length with 3.5 mm staple leg height is most commonly reported in larger (>10 kg) dogs; shorter cartridges were often insufficient to span the length of the hilus and required application of more than one cartridge, increasing procedure time and cost.[9,10] Although initial studies suggest that outcome following thoracoscopic lung lobectomy is comparable to open thoracotomy for primary lung tumors in dogs, conversion to open thoracotomy is reported in 9% to 44% of cases.[8–10] Conversion in dogs is most often due to difficult visualization and may be more likely in smaller dogs and cats.[8–10] Consequently, Mayhew and colleagues recommended selecting tumors < 8 cm diameter or less than 150 cm³ in volume for thoracoscopic lung lobectomy in medium-to large-breed dogs with correspondingly smaller tumors selected for smaller patients undergoing thoracoscopic lung lobectomy.[9]

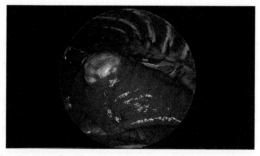

Fig. 5. Intraoperative image of a thoracoscopic lung lobectomy for removal of a primary lung tumor. The endoscopic stapler is positioned along the hilus; visualization is facilitated via one-lung ventilation. (*Courtesy of* Michelle Oblak, DVM, DVSc, DACVS, Ontario Veterinary College, Guelph, Ontario).

Modifications of thoracoscopic lung lobectomy to improve the feasibility of thoracoscopic lung lobectomy in small animals include a thoracoscopic-assisted approach for pulmonary resection in dogs as described by Wormser and colleagues in which an endoscope was inserted approximately 5 to 7 intercostal spaces distant to the site of the pulmonary lesion.[11] Based on the initial thoracoscopic evaluation, a 360° wound retraction device was then placed over the site of planned pulmonary resection to facilitate the exteriorization and resection of the affected lung.[11] Benefits of this technique include improved visualization and access to the pulmonary hilus and ability to introduce GIA or thoracoabdominal staplers in smaller patients for lung transection. Additional clarification of this technique was reported in 2 papers describing port optimization for thoracoscopic-assisted lung lobectomy in canine and feline cadavers.[12,13] The shortest distance from stapler anvil to hilus of the lung lobes in cats and dogs is shown in **Table 1**. This information can be used in planning where to make an intercostal approach when performing thoracoscopic-assisted lung lobectomy.[12,13]

Alternative methods of pulmonary sealing and transection may also facilitate thoracoscopic or thoracoscopic-assisted lung lobectomy in smaller dogs and cats. A comparison of hilar lung lobectomy performed in cat cadavers through a thoracoscopic-assisted approach using either a TA stapler or a resorbable ligation device (LigaTie) found that the LigaTie was more easily placed at the hilus and that lung lobectomies performed with the LigaTie were less likely to leak compared with those performed with the TA stapler.[14] A study in dogs evaluating experimental and clinical use of the LigaTie for lung lobectomy via thoracoscopic-assisted and open thoracotomy found similar ease of placement and effective sealing of pulmonary tissue.[15] Recently, use of a pretied ligature loop through an open thoracotomy was described for total lung lobectomy in 5 clinical canine patients and may also represent a useful alternative to GIA or TA staplers during thoracoscopic or thoracoscopic-assisted lung lobectomy.[16] Nonetheless, use of this device for thoracoscopic total lung lobectomy may be limited by the size of the lung lobe and the ability to pass the lobe through a pretied loop.

Peripheral lung biopsies may be obtained thoracoscopically with the patient in lateral or dorsal recumbency using a pretied ligature loop, an endoscopic stapler, or a vessel sealing device, although studies have shown conflicting evidence regarding whether vessel sealing devices can achieve a pneumostatic seal.[17–19] An evaluation of peripheral lung biopsies performed in fresh canine cadavers using different endoscopic staple configurations found that the both graduated compression stapling devices (medium/thick and vascular/medium) leaked at lower pressures than biopsies obtained with an endoscopic GIA stapler with 2.5-mm staple height.[17]

Table 1
Recommended intercostal space to facilitate the shortest distance from stapler anvil to lung lobe hilus in cats and dogs

Lung Lobe	Intercostal Space (Cat)	Intercostal Space (Dog)
Left cranial	4th, 5th, 6th	4th, 5th
Left caudal	5th, 6th	4th, 5th
Right cranial	4th, 5th	4th, 5th
Right middle	4th, 5th	4th, 5th
Right caudal	5th, 6th	5th, 6th
Accessory	5th, 6th	5th, 6th

One challenge in performing thoracoscopic lung lobectomy for primary lung tumors is the limited sampling of thoracic lymph nodes for the staging of disease. In reports of thoracoscopic and thoracoscopic-assisted lung lobectomy in dogs, lymph nodes were sampled in 0% to 22% of cases.[8–11] A large multi-institutional review of lung tumors treated surgically in dogs found that intrathoracic lymphadenopathy was documented in 94 of 327 dogs with a preoperative computed tomography (CT), and lymph node biopsy was performed in 47 of these 94 dogs (50%).[20] Of those, 53% showed histologic evidence of lymph node metastasis. Of the 89 dogs in which lymph nodes seemed normal visually, 25 (28%) sampled showed histologic evidence of metastasis. Lymph node metastasis is a poor prognostic indicator for survival, further emphasizing the importance of lymph node biopsy at the time of pulmonary tumor resection to allow histologic staging and prognostication.[20] An experimental study by Steffey and colleagues described an approach for the thoracoscopic extirpation of tracheobronchial lymph nodes in normal dogs.[21] Briefly, a 3- or 4-port technique was used with the camera port in ICS 5 and 2 to 3 ports triangulated cranial and caudal to the camera port. A vessel sealing device was used for dissection, and a median percentage surface area of the bisected lymph nodes affected by crush artifact was 20%.[21] Complications included mild to moderate hemorrhage, inability to locate the tracheobronchial lymph nodes, and ability to achieve or maintain OLV.[21] Further evaluation of tracheobronchial lymph node resection in clinical cases is indicated, but current literature suggests that concurrent thoracoscopic or thoracoscopic-assisted sampling of intrathoracic lymph nodes is both feasible and prudent.

PERICARDIAL EFFUSION AND PERICARDIAL AND CARDIAC NEOPLASIA

Thoracoscopic subphrenic pericardiectomy or pericardial window is indicated to palliate pericardial effusion which is most commonly neoplastic or idiopathic.[22,23] Additionally, thoracoscopic evaluation of the intrapericardial space may be useful in visualizing and sampling cardiac and pericardial lesions. Thoracoscopic subphrenic pericardiectomy is described through both a subxiphoid and lateral approach; the lateral approach is more limited in its exposure and should be reserved for patients in which a pericardial window with minimal intrapericardial exploration is desired.[22,23] More commonly, the patient is placed in dorsal recumbency and a subxiphoid port created for the introduction of the endoscope. Intercostal ports in the ventral third of the 5th through 10th intercostal spaces are then created to introduce endoscopic graspers, scissors, and a vessel sealing device. Surgeon preference determines the orientation of these intercostal ports: some prefer to stand at the rear of the patient and operate instruments from bilateral intercostal ports while others prefer to stand alongside the patient and operate through 2 ipsilateral instrument ports. The author prefers to place ports in the ventral third of the 6th through 8th ICS, although placement in the dorsal third of a caudal ICS and middle third of cranial ICS (2nd through 4th) has also been described.[24]

OLV is not necessary in many larger or deep-chested dogs to achieve adequate visualization but may be very helpful in smaller or barrel-chested patients to improve working space and visualization of the lateral aspects of the pericardium.[25] Care should be taken when using a bipolar vessel sealing device near the epicardium due to the potential for electrically induced ventricular fibrillation which can be fatal.[26] The author prefers to reduce the risk of iatrogenic cardiac injury by making initial entry into the pericardium using endoscopic Metzenbaum scissors while grasping the pericardium and using an ultrasonic vessel sealing device to resect pericardial tissue (**Fig. 6**). Because ultrasonic vessel sealing devices use mechanical rather than

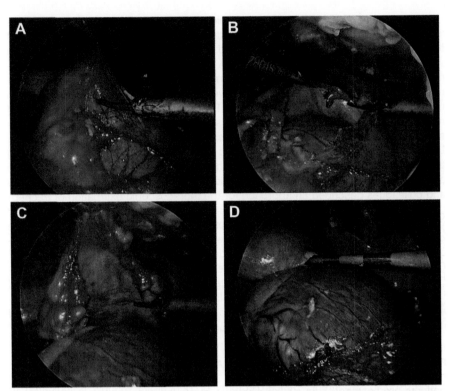

Fig. 6. Intraoperative image of a subphrenic pericardiectomy using an ultrasonic sealing device. (*A*) Initial incision into the pericardium is made using the ultrasonic sealing device or endoscopic Metzenbaum scissors while elevating the pericardium with grasping forceps. (*B*) The pericardium is incised while keeping the oscillating blade a safe distance from the epicardium to avoid thermal injury. (*C*) The initial incision is enlarged while maintaining tension on the ventral pericardium. (*D*) The final size of the pericardial opening is evaluated; if additional length is desired, additional fillet of the pericardium may be performed.

electrical injury to seal tissue, the risk of arrhythmias is reduced. Specimen retrieval bags should be used for the retrieval of biopsied tissue to reduce the risk of port-site metastasis (**Fig. 7**).

The minimum recommended size of the pericardial window is debated and varies by patient size and indication. Larger subphrenic pericardiectomies are indicated when the potential for a restrictive pericardial lesion exists. A study comparing cardiac visualization through an apical pericardial window versus a subphrenic pericardiectomy found that the visualization of intrapericardial structures was significantly improved with the subphrenic pericardiectomy compared with the window.[27] An alternative approach to extensive resection of the subphrenic pericardium which may prove challenging in some dogs is to perform an initial pericardial window followed by fillet or fenestration of the remaining subphrenic pericardium.[28] This can be achieved by grasping the edge of the pericardial window and using endoscopic scissors or a vessel sealing device to create linear incisions from the window's edge through the ventral and lateral pericardium, being careful to visualize and avoid the phrenic nerves.

Outcome for patients with presumptive pericardial effusion treated with thoracoscopic pericardial window or subphrenic pericardiectomy is variable and may depend

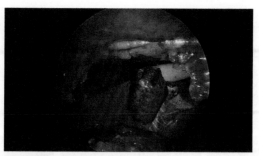

Fig. 7. Pericardium is extracted through an 11.5-mm port using a specimen retrieval bag to minimize the risk of port-site metastasis.

on underlying etiology discovered at the time of surgery.[22,23,29,30] While one study did not find a difference in median survival time between dogs based on histopathological diagnosis alone, other studies have found median survival times ranging from 30 to 76 days with the diagnosis of neoplasia versus 367 to 635 days for dogs with idiopathic pericardial effusion following thoracoscopic treatment.[24,29,30] Similarly, median survival time was significantly shorter for dogs with presumptive pericardial effusion in which pericardioscopy revealed abnormalities versus those with unremarkable pericardioscopic examination (66 days vs an unreached median survival time).[29]

Thoracoscopic resection of right auricular masses may also be performed using a similar approach to that described above for subphrenic pericardiectomy.[31] Small masses toward the tip of the right auricle in large dogs are amenable to thoracoscopic resection; larger masses, those toward the base of the auricle, and those in smaller patients are not good candidates for thoracoscopic resection due to challenges in maneuvering the endoscopic stapler between the mass and the base of the auricle and potential for rapid and fatal hemorrhage.[31] In a retrospective study of 9 dogs undergoing thoracoscopic resection of right auricular masses, one dog was diagnosed with a pyogranulomatous lesion and 8 diagnosed with hemangiosarcoma.[31] Thoracoscopic resection was successful in 8 of 9 dogs; a dog with a mass at the base of the right auricle died intraoperatively due to severe hemorrhage from the staple line.[31] Median survival time for the 8 dogs with hemangiosarcoma was 90 days; the dog with the pyogranulomatous lesion was still alive greater than 3.5 years following surgery.[31]

CHYLOTHORAX

Chylothorax is a challenging disease in both dogs and cats with numerous described techniques for surgical correction. The most commonly performed surgical approaches for chylothorax in small animal patients include thoracic duct ligation, subphrenic pericardiectomy, and cisterna chyli ablation, all of which have been described through open and minimally invasive surgical approaches.

Visualization of the thoracic duct intraoperatively is important for the dissection and ligation of the duct and any branches (**Fig. 8**). Multiple approaches for the intraoperative visualization of the thoracic duct have been described, including preoperative feeding of cream, popliteal or mesenteric lymph node injection with contrast or methylene blue, or injection of diaphragmatic fibers with methylene blue.[32] Recent literature has described several novel approaches for the visualization of the thoracic duct intraoperatively with promising efficacy.[33–36] These include metatarsal pad and regional (metatarsal) subcutaneous injection with a noniodinated contrast agent (iohexol) and ultrasound-guided intrahepatic and popliteal lymph node injection of indocyanine

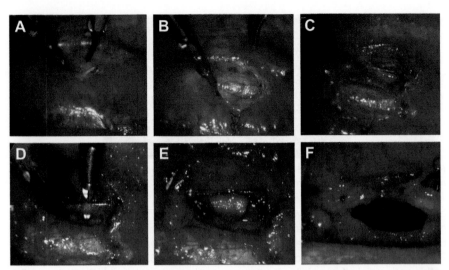

Fig. 8. Intraoperative image of thoracic duct ligation using methylene blue for the visualization of thoracic duct branches. (*A*) Initial dissection of fascia ventral to azygos vein. (*B*) Identification of lateral surface of aorta. (*C*) Two colorized branches of thoracic duct visible dorsal to the aorta. (*D*) Application of endoscopic clips to ventral thoracic duct branch. (*E*) Isolation of dorsal branch of thoracic duct following clipping and transection of ventral branch. (*F*) Dissection continued through mediastinal tissue to evaluate for additional thoracic duct branches.

green (ICG).[33–36] These techniques provide relatively accessible percutaneous or minimally invasive routes for introducing contrast, colorizing, or fluorescence agents and may eliminate the additional time and morbidity of an abdominal incision to access a mesenteric lymph node. Near-infrared fluorescence lymphography (NIRFL) using ICG may provide enhanced visualization compared with traditional methods (**Fig. 9**); in one study, NIRFL identified small lymphatics not visible on CT lymphangiogram in one dog and in 5 of 9 dogs in which methylene blue and ICG were used concurrently, no ducts or fewer ducts were recorded as identifiable by methylene blue than by NIRFL or CT lymphangiogram.[33] Subjectively, the strength of thoracic duct coloration by methylene blue also faded more quickly than NIRFL coloration.[33]

Fig. 9. Intraoperative image demonstrating fluorescence of thoracic duct using indocyanine green. (*Courtesy of* Michelle Oblak, DVM, DVSc, DACVS, Ontario Veterinary College, Guelph, Ontario).

A small cutdown to the distal pole of the popliteal lymph node is recommended for popliteal lymph node injection; a fluorescent signal is noted in the thoracic duct within 1 to 5 minutes of popliteal lymph node injection and within seconds of mesenteric lymph node injection.[33] Concentrations of 0.25 to 0.5 mg/mL and 0.5 to 0.7 mg/mL for mesenteric and popliteal lymph node injection, respectively, are recommended, with dose volume administered to effect until thoracic duct fluorescence is first noted.[33] Similarly, injection of 0.1 mg/kg ICG diluted with sterile NaCl to a total volume of 1.0 mL into hepatic parenchyma over 30 to 60 seconds produced successful NIRFL in a median of 6 minutes and persisted for 20 minutes of observation in an experimental study in Beagles.[34]

Thoracoscopic ligation of the thoracic duct without the use of intraoperative contrast is also feasible. A recent study retrospectively comparing the outcome in a small group of dogs treated with bilateral en bloc thoracic duct ligation using suture versus traditional clipping of the thoracic duct without intraoperative contrast found that clinical improvement was achieved in 92% of dogs surviving surgery.[37] Specifically, bilateral en bloc ligation was associated with a significantly higher rate of long-term remission, decreased anesthesia and operative time, and decreased time till the resolution of pleural effusion compared with traditional clipping of the thoracic duct without the use of an intraoperative contrast agent.[37] Because of the small number of dogs and retrospective nature of this study, additional evaluation is warranted, but thoracoscopic en bloc ligation of the thoracic duct may provide an efficient alternative to thoracic duct ligation using the various colorization and visualization methods previously described.

As thoracoscopic treatment of chylothorax has become more common, increased information regarding long-term outcome with thoracoscopic treatment is more readily available. A multi-institutional retrospective evaluation of thoracoscopic thoracic duct ligation and pericardiectomy for the treatment of chylothorax in 39 dogs found that conversion was required in 1 dog for thoracic duct ligation and 4 dogs for pericardiectomy. Two dogs died intraoperatively from ventricular fibrillation (1) and euthanasia due to severe restrictive pleuritis (1). Resolution of pleural effusion was seen in 95% of dogs that survived the perioperative period, with late recurrence noted at 12 to 19 months postoperatively in 3 dogs.[38]

PERSISTENT RIGHT AORTIC ARCH AND LEFT LIGAMENTUM ARTERIOSUM

Thoracoscopic treatment of PRAA in dogs has been described in several small case series, including one series reporting concurrent ligation of the aberrant left subclavian artery (**Fig. 10**).[39–42] Thoracoscopic correction of PRAA in dogs does not seem to be associated with higher morbidity or mortality compared with open thoracotomy and did not demonstrate notable benefits in surgical time or postoperative complications in a recent study.[42] OLV may be used but has not been shown to improve surgical time, intraoperative complications, or conversion rates compared with thoracoscopic treatment without OLV.[41]

Conversion rates of thoracoscopic PRAA correction range from 0% to 40%.[39–42] Reasons for conversion include poor visualization, hemorrhage, concerns regarding the size of the ligamentum arteriosum, and need to temporarily occlude an aberrant left subclavian.[39–42] Additional challenges include identifying the ligamentum; intraoperative esophagoscopy can aid in ligamentum identification by illuminating the area of constriction for the surgeon. The ligamentum may be ligated and transected using a vessel sealing device, endoscopic hemoclip placement with transection via vessel sealing device or scissors, or intracorporeal ligation and transection. It is

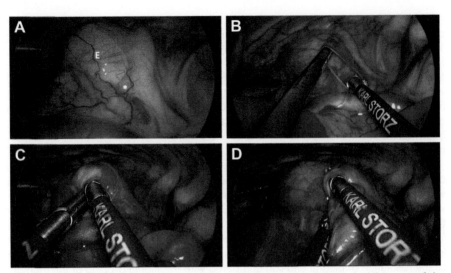

Fig. 10. Intraoperative images of a dog with a persistent right aortic arch. (*A*) Image of the esophageal diverticulum (*E*) and ligamentum arteriosum (*) before dissection. (*B*) Initial dissection to isolate the ligamentum. Dissection of the ligamentum is performed with right angle forceps (*C*) until the tips of the forceps can be visualized (*D*) before sealing and transection of the ligamentum.

imperative to continue the dissection of residual bands of tissue once the ligamentum has been transected to minimize the risk of persistent constriction; care must be taken to avoid accidental perforation of the esophagus during this dissection. Intraoperative esophagoscopy is again useful to help gauge whether additional dissection is warranted. The small size of many patients with PRAA can make dissection challenging despite the use of 3-mm instruments.

Aberrant left subclavian arteries may similarly be ligated and transected thoracoscopically using a vessel sealing device, endoscopic hemoclips, or intracorporeal ligation and division.[39] Whether or not to transect aberrant left subclavian arteries remains controversial. It is the author's opinion that the resolution of regurgitation in 4 of 5 dogs with the transection of the aberrant left subclavian in one study and resolution of recurrent regurgitation following aberrant left subclavian transection 1450 days after initial ligamentum transection in another study support the assertion that the aberrant left subclavian may be a significant contributor to regurgitation and transection should be considered in cases where it may be causing esophageal compression (**Fig. 11**).[39,40] Intraoperative esophagoscopy provides a useful guide for the intraoperative dissection of the ligamentum and remaining bands (**Fig. 12**), and may also aid in assessing the impact of esophageal constriction caused by an aberrant left subclavian (**Fig. 13**).[40]

CRANIAL MEDIASTINAL MASSES

Thymomas and other mediastinal masses are uncommon in dogs and cats but may be resected thoracoscopically (**Fig. 14**).[43–45] OLV facilitates dissection and use of a DLT may be particularly useful to facilitate alternating which lung is ventilated as most mediastinal masses lie on midline and require bilateral dissection. Additionally, a cranial port may be useful to allow the insertion of a finger to facilitate digital dissection and retraction of the mass. Use of carbon dioxide insufflation at 2 to 3 mm Hg has also been described to facilitate thoracoscopic resection of thymoma in a cat.[44]

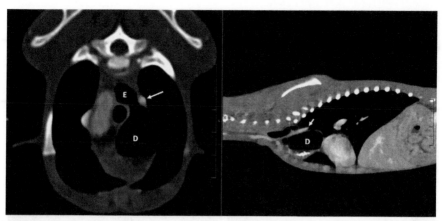

Fig. 11. Transverse and sagittal computed tomography images of a dog with a persistent right aortic arch and aberrant left subclavian. The aberrant left subclavian (*white arrow*) compresses the lateral aspect of the esophagus (E). The esophageal diverticulum (D) is seen ventral to the aberrant left subclavian.

A retrospective study of 18 dogs undergoing thoracoscopic extirpation of cranial mediastinal masses found that conversion was relatively uncommon with 2 of 18 dogs converted to open thoracotomy.[43] The approach in one dog was converted to median sternotomy due to the size of the mass and severe adhesions, whereas emergency intercostal thoracotomy was required in one dog following laceration of the vena cava and severe hemorrhage.[43] Prognosis for dogs undergoing thoracoscopic mediastinal mass resection was relatively guarded, with 72% of dogs surviving to discharge and a median survival time of 20 days for dogs with concurrent myasthenia gravis and megaesophagus.[43]

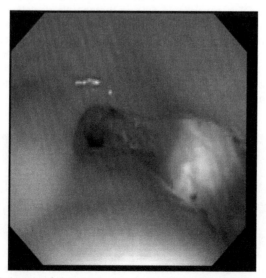

Fig. 12. Endoscopic image of the esophagus during dissection and transection of the ligamentum arteriosum in a dog with a persistent right aortic arch.

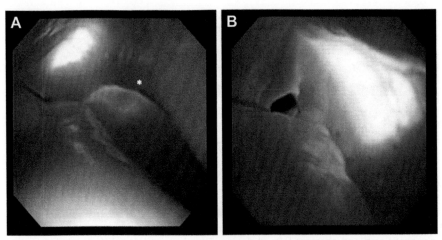

Fig. 13. Intraoperative esophagoscopy of the patient from **Fig. 11.** (*A*) The aberrant left subclavian (*) can be seen before ligation and transection. (*B*) Esophagoscopy shows no additional constriction from the aberrant left subclavian following transection.

PYOTHORAX

Although indications for the surgical management of pyothorax in small animals are controversial, thoracoscopy can be useful in debriding adhesions, lavaging the pleural space and facilitating drainage, optimizing thoracostomy tube placement, and obtaining samples for culture and cytology. Video-assisted thoracic surgery (VATS) may also facilitate the removal of foreign bodies and resection of abscessed pulmonary parenchyma. Indications for the open surgical management of pyothorax include a chronic history or extensive involvement of mediastinal or pulmonary tissue on preoperative CT as severe adhesions and extensive pulmonary and mediastinal involvement will impair thoracoscopic exploration and make efficient treatment using VATS difficult. Thus, preoperative CT is essential in guiding therapeutic decisions for the thoracoscopic management of pyothorax in dogs. In a study of 14 dogs treated with VATS for pyothorax, conversion to an open thoracotomy for the resection of proliferative mediastinal tissue was required in 14% of cases.[46] Penetrating gastric foreign bodies and migrating plant material were identified in 4 dogs, with the remaining 10 diagnosed with idiopathic pyothorax. Clinical signs resolved in all dogs, with one dog developing recurrent pyothorax 17-months postoperatively.[46]

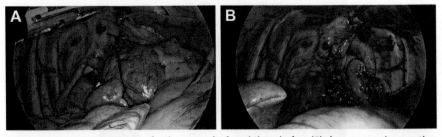

Fig. 14. Intraoperative image of a thymoma before (*A*) and after (*B*) thoracoscopic resection. (*Courtesy of* Michelle Oblak, DVM, DVSc, DACVS, Ontario Veterinary College, Guelph, Ontario).

PRIMARY SPONTANEOUS PNEUMOTHORAX

Thoracoscopic management of primary spontaneous pneumothorax in dogs has historically shown questionable efficacy due to challenges in accurately identifying bullous lesions on preoperative CT and performing thorough pulmonary exploration thoracoscopically.[47] Recent advances in preoperative CT including scanning dogs in both sternal and dorsal recumbency to increase the likelihood of bullae identification may improve efficacy of the thoracoscopic treatment of primary spontaneous pneumothorax.[48] Additionally, use of a variable-angle endoscope to better visualize pulmonary surfaces during exploratory thoracoscopy showed promise in an experimental cadaver study and is currently being evaluated for use in clinical cases of primary spontaneous pneumothorax (Video 1).[7] Due to the potential for multiple and bilateral bullae in dogs with spontaneous pneumothorax, careful bilateral thoracoscopic evaluation of the lungs including the accessory lung lobe should be performed, and surgeons should be prepared to convert to open exploration via median sternotomy if no lesions are noted.[49] If all lesions contributing to pneumothorax can be identified and resected during initial treatment, long-term prognosis for primary spontaneous pneumothorax is good with a low recurrence rate.[49]

SUMMARY

Small animal thoracoscopy continues to develop as a viable and appealing alternative to traditional surgical management of many thoracic diseases in dogs and cats. The relatively high morbidity of open thoracotomies supports the advantages of minimally invasive approaches to thoracic disease despite challenges including limited working space and difficult visualization, particularly in smaller patients. Recent literature reflects numerous adaptations to circumvent these challenges, and continued innovation will allow further refinement of thoracoscopic techniques. As experience increases with thoracoscopic management of the diseases described above, additional information regarding benefits, complications, and outcome associated with thoracoscopic alternatives in larger numbers of dogs and cats will better guide therapeutic decisions.

CLINICS CARE POINTS

- Thoracic insufflation should be limited to 3 mm Hg or less in small animal patients to avoid dangerous cardiopulmonary depression.

- Small and peripheral lung lobe tumors are most amenable to thoracoscopic resection. Tumor diameter of 8 cm is the recommended cut-off for thoracoscopic resection in medium-to large-breed dogs. Larger tumors and tumors in smaller patients may be removed through a thoracoscopic-assisted approach.

- Thoracoscopic pericardial windows may be enlarged using a fillet technique; bipolar vessel sealing devices should be used with caution in proximity to the epicardium due to the risk of electrically-induced arrhythmias.

- Near-infrared fluorescence lymphography of the thoracic duct is performed by injecting 0.25 to 0.5 mg/mL into mesenteric lymph nodes and 0.5 to 0.7 mg/mL into popliteal lymph nodes until thoracic duct fluorescence is first noted, generally within 1 to 5 minutes following popliteal lymph node injection and within seconds of mesenteric lymph node injection.

- Esophagoscopy is a useful intraoperative tool for identifying the ligamentum arteriosum in dogs and cats with PRAA, guiding the extent of dissection of persistent bands, and evaluating the extent of constriction from aberrant left subclavian arteries.

- A chronic history or extensive pulmonary or mediastinal involvement is an indication for open rather than the thoracoscopic management of pyothorax in dogs.

DISCLOSURE

The author is a paid consultant for Storz Veterinary Endoscopy and Johnson and Johnson Medical Devices, Inc.

SUPPLEMENTARY DATA

Supplementary data related to this article can be found online at https://doi.org/10.1016/j.ovsm.2021.11.005

REFERENCES

1. Case JB. Advances in video-assisted thoracic surgery, thoracoscopy. Vet Clin North Am Small Anim Pract 2016;46(1):147–69.
2. Mayhew PD, Culp WTN, Pascoe PJ, et al. Evaluation of blind thoracoscopic-assisted placement of three double-lumen endobronchial tube designs for one-lung ventilation in dogs. Vet Surg 2012;41(6):664–70.
3. Mayhew PD, Chohan A, Hardy BT, et al. Cadaveric evaluation of fluoroscopy-assisted placement of one-lung ventilation devices for video-assisted thoracoscopic surgery in dogs. Vet Surg 2020;49(S1):O93–101.
4. Daly CM, Swalec-Tobias K, Tobias AH. Cardiopulmonary effects of intrathoracic insufflation in dogs. J Am Anim Hosp Assoc 2002;38:515–20.
5. Mayhew PD, Pascoe PJ, Giuffrida MA, et al. Cardiorespiratory effects of variable pressure thoracic insufflation in cats undergoing video-assisted thoracic surgery. Vet Surg 2019;48(S1):O130–7.
6. Mayhew PD, Pascoe PJ, Shilo-Benjamini Y, et al. Effect of one-lung ventilation with or without low-pressure carbon dioxide insufflation on cardiorespiratory variables in cats undergoing thoracoscopy. Vet Surg 2015;44(S1):15–22.
7. Diamond DM, Scharf VF, Chiu KW, et al. A randomized, prospective, comparative trial of a variable-angle versus fixed-angle endoscope for exploratory thoracoscopy in canine cadavers. Vet Surg 2021;50(S1):O17–25.
8. Lansdowne JL, Monnet E, Twedt DC, et al. Thoracoscopic lung lobectomy for treatment of lung tumors in dogs. Vet Surg 2005;34(5):530–5.
9. Mayhew PD, Hunt GB, Steffey MA, et al. Evaluation of short-term outcome after lung lobectomy for resection of primary lung tumors via video-assisted thoracoscopic surgery or open thoracotomy in medium- to large-breed dogs. J Am Vet Med Assoc 2013;243(5).
10. Bleakley S, Duncan CG, Monnet E. Thoracoscopic lung lobectomy for primary lung tumors in 13 dogs. Vet Surg 2015;44(8):1029–35.
11. Wormser C, Singhal S, Holt DE, et al. Thoracoscopic-assisted pulmonary surgery for partial and complete lung lobectomy in dogs and cats: 11 cases (2008–2013). J Am Vet Med Assoc 2014;245(9):1036–41.
12. Singh A, Scott J, Case JB, et al. Optimization of surgical approach for thoracoscopic-assisted pulmonary surgery in dogs. Vet Surg 2019;48(S1):O99–104.
13. Scott JE, Singh A, Case JB, et al. Determination of optimal location for thoracoscopic-assisted pulmonary surgery for lung lobectomy in cats. Am J Vet Res 2019;80(11):1050–4.

14. Nylund AM, Höglund OV, Fransson BA. Thoracoscopic-assisted lung lobectomy in cat cadavers using a resorbable self-locking ligation device. Vet Surg 2019; 48(4):563 9.

15. Ishigaki K, Höglund OV, Asano K. Resorbable self-locking device for canine lung lobectomy: a clinical and experimental study. Vet Surg 2021;50(S1):O32–9.

16. Cronin AM, Pustelnik SB, Owen L, et al. Evaluation of a pre-tied ligature loop for canine total lung lobectomy. Vet Surg 2019;48(4):570–7.

17. Imhoff DJ, Monnet E. Inflation pressures for ex vivo lung biopsies after application of graduated compression staples. Vet Surg 2016;45(1):79–82.

18. Mayhew PD, Culp WTN, Pascoe PJ, et al. Use of the ligasure vessel-sealing device for thoracoscopic peripheral lung biopsy in healthy dogs. Vet Surg 2012; 41(4):523–8.

19. Marvel S, Monnet E. Ex vivo evaluation of canine lung biopsy techniques. Vet Surg 2013;42(4):473–7.

20. McPhetridge JB, Scharf VF, Regier PJ, et al. Distribution of histopathological types of primary pulmonary neoplasia in dogs and outcome of affected dogs: 340 cases (2010-2019). J Am Vet Med Assoc 2021;1–10.

21. Steffey MA, Daniel L, Mayhew PD, et al. Video-assisted thoracoscopic extirpation of the tracheobronchial lymph nodes in dogs. Vet Surg 2015;44(S1):50–8.

22. Case JB, Maxwell M, Aman A, et al. Outcome evaluation of a thoracoscopic pericardial window procedure or subtotal pericardectomy via thoracotomy for the treatment of pericardial effusion in dogs. J Am Vet Med Assoc 2013;242(4): 493–8.

23. Jackson J, Richter KP, Launer DP. Thoracoscopic partial pericardiectomy in 13 dogs. J Vet Intern Med 1999;13:529–33.

24. Michelotti KP, Youk A, Payne JT, et al. Outcomes of dogs with recurrent idiopathic pericardial effusion treated with a 3-port right-sided thoracoscopic subtotal pericardiectomy. Vet Surg 2019;48(6):1032–41.

25. Dupré GP, Corlouer J, Bouvy B. Thoracoscopic pericardectomy performed without pulmonary exclusion in 9 dogs. Vet Surg 2001;30(1):21–7.

26. Studer N, Reves VV, Rytz U, et al. Suspected electrically induced ventricular fibrillation during thoracoscopic partial pericardectomy in two dogs. Vet Rec Case Rep 2019;7:1–5.

27. Skinner OT, Case JB, Ellison GW, et al. Pericardioscopic imaging findings in cadaveric dogs: Comparison of an apical pericardial window and sub-phrenic pericardectomy. Vet Surg 2014;43(1):45–51.

28. Barbur LA, Rawlings CA, Radlinsky MG. Epicardial exposure provided by a novel thoracoscopic pericardectomy technique compared to standard pericardial window. Vet Surg 2018;47(1):146–52.

29. Carvajal JL, Case JB, Mayhew PD, et al. Outcome in dogs with presumptive idiopathic pericardial effusion after thoracoscopic pericardectomy and pericardioscopy. Vet Surg 2019;48(S1):O105–11.

30. Atencia S, Doyle RS, Whitley NT. Thoracoscopic pericardial window formanagementof pericardial effusion in 15 dogs. J Small Anim Pract 2013;54(11):564–9.

31. Ployart S, Liebermann S, Doran I, et al. Thoracoscopic resection of right auricular masses in dogs: 9 cases (2003-2011). J Am Vet Med Assoc 2013;242(2):237–41.

32. Bayer BJ, Dujowich M, Krebs AI, et al. Injection of the diaphragmatic crus with methylene blue for coloration of the canine thoracic duct. Vet Surg 2014;43(7): 829–33.

33. Steffey MA, Mayhew PD. Use of direct near-infrared fluorescent lymphography for thoracoscopic thoracic duct identification in 15 dogs with chylothorax. Vet Surg 2018;47(2):267–76.

34. Korpita MF, Mayhew PD, Steffey MA, et al. Thoracoscopic detection of thoracic ducts after ultrasound-guided intrahepatic injection of indocyanine green detected by near-infrared fluorescence and methylene blue in dogs. Vet Surg 2021;1–10. https://doi.org/10.1111/vsu.13682.

35. Lin L, Chiu H, Nishimura R, et al. Computed tomographic lymphangiography via intra-metatarsal pad injection is feasible in dogs with chylothorax. Vet Radiol Ultrasound 2020;61(4):435–43.

36. Kim K, Cheon S, Kang K, et al. Computed tomographic lymphangiography of the thoracic duct by subcutaneous iohexol injection into the metatarsal region. Vet Surg 2020;49(1):180–6.

37. Kanai H, Furuya M, Hagiwara K, et al. Efficacy of en bloc thoracic duct ligation in combination with pericardiectomy by video-assisted thoracoscopic surgery for canine idiopathic chylothorax. Vet Surg 2020;49(S1):O102–11.

38. Mayhew PD, Steffey MA, Fransson BA, et al. Long-term outcome of video-assisted thoracoscopic thoracic duct ligation and pericardectomy in dogs with chylothorax: A multi-institutional study of 39 cases. Vet Surg 2019;48(S1):O112–20.

39. Regier PJ, Case JB, Fox-Alvarez WA. Ligation of the ligamentum arteriosum and aberrant left subclavian artery in five dogs in which persistent right aortic arch had been diagnosed. Vet Surg 2021;50(S1):O26–31.

40. Townsend S, Oblak ML, Singh A, et al. Thoracoscopy with concurrent esophagoscopy for persistent right aortic arch in 9 dogs. Vet Surg 2016;45(S1):O111–8.

41. Marvel SJ, Hafez A, Monnet E. Thoracoscopic treatment of persistent right aortic arch in dogs with and without one lung ventilation. Vet Surg 2021.

42. Nucci DJ, Hurst KC, Monnet E. Retrospective comparison of short-term outcomes following thoracoscopy versus thoracotomy for surgical correction of persistent right aortic arch in dogs. J Am Vet Med Assoc 2018;253(4):444–51.

43. MacIver MA, Case JB, Monnet EL, et al. Video-assisted extirpation of cranial mediastinal masses in dogs: 18 cases (2009–2014). J Am Vet Med Assoc 2017;250(11):1283–90.

44. Griffin MA, Sutton JS, Hunt GB, et al. Video-assisted thoracoscopic resection of a noninvasive thymoma in a cat with myasthenia gravis using low-pressure carbon dioxide insufflation. Vet Surg 2016;45(S1):O28–33.

45. Mayhew PD, Friedberg JS. Video-assisted thoracoscopic resection of noninvasive thymomas using one-lung ventilation in two dogs. Vet Surg 2008;37(8):756–62.

46. Scott J, Singh A, Monnet E, et al. Video-assisted thoracic surgery for the management of pyothorax in dogs: 14 cases. Vet Surg 2017;46(5):722–30.

47. Case JB, Mayhew PD, Singh A. Evaluation of video-assisted thoracic surgery for treatment of spontaneous pneumothorax and pulmonary bullae in dogs. Vet Surg 2015;44(S1):31–8.

48. Dickson R, Scharf VF, Nelson NC, et al. Computed tomography in two recumbencies aides in the identification of pulmonary bullae in dogs with spontaneous pneumothorax. Vet Radiol Ultrasoun 2020;61(6):641–8.

49. Dickson R, Scharf VF, Michael AE, et al. Surgical management and outcome of dogs with primary spontaneous pneumothorax: 110 cases (2009–2019). J Am Vet Med Assoc 2021;258(11):1229–35.

Updated Concepts in Oncologic Surgery: Apocrine Gland Anal Sac Adenocarcinoma and Mast Cell Tumors

Megan Ann Mickelson, DVM, DACVS-SA, ACVS Fellow, Surgical Oncology

KEYWORDS

- Surgical oncology • Tumor staging • Apocrine gland anal sac adenocarcinoma
- Mast cell tumors • Surgical margins

KEY POINTS

- Comprehensive cancer centers using a multidisciplinary approach to veterinary patients with cancer can achieve superior patient outcomes.
- Aggressive locoregional control via anal sacculectomy and metastectomy for metastatic lymph nodes, including repeat lymphadenectomies for recurrent disease, provides the best possible outcome for dogs with apocrine gland anal sac adenocarcinomas (AGASACA).
- The role of adjuvant radiation therapy and chemotherapy for AGASACA needs to be better defined, although both are biologically justified therapies.
- Full preoperative staging for dogs without negative prognostic factors for cutaneous mast cell tumors (MCTs) may not be indicated in every case before wide surgical excision, and therapeutic advantages to lymph node extirpation are being further evaluated.
- Recommended surgical margins for wide surgical excision of cutaneous MCTs are evolving.

INTRODUCTION

Regarding oncology patients, surgery remains critical in the overall treatment plan and offers the opportunity to cure cancer more often than any other treatment modality.[1] For human patients with cancer, 60% are cured by surgery alone,[2] emphasizing the critical role surgeons play. Use of multiple modalities for individual veterinary patients with cancer is more common in recent decades with the implementation of comprehensive cancer centers. Comprehensive oncology encourages the assessment of patients with cancer as a "whole," using a multidisciplinary approach to incorporate multiple modalities, including

Assisant Professor, Small Animal Surgical Oncology, University of Missouri, College of Veterinary Medicine, Department of Veterinary Medicine and Surgery, 900 East Campus Drive, Columbia, MO 65201, USA
E-mail address: Megan.mickelson@missouri.edu

Vet Clin Small Anim 52 (2022) 549–580
https://doi.org/10.1016/j.cvsm.2021.12.008
0195-5616/22/© 2021 Elsevier Inc. All rights reserved.
vetsmall.theclinics.com

surgery, radiation therapy (RT), chemotherapy, immunotherapy, and/or interventional approaches to achieve superior patient outcomes.[3] A comprehensive approach includes careful consideration of owner goals when determining diagnostic and therapeutic plans. Surgical oncologists recognize and understand alternative and adjuvant therapy options, along with associated complications.[3,4] In human patients, outcomes improve with treatment by specialized oncologic surgeons in cancer centers,[1] likely due to added knowledge from additional specialty-focused training.

Early communication is imperative to establish the surgical dose that aligns with owner expectations (curative-intent, cytoreduction, or palliation), and streamline adjuvant therapy expectations postoperatively. Surgical oncologists critically evaluate when surgery may not be the best treatment modality. For human patients with cancer, 60% have RT incorporated in their oncologic treatment plan[5]; thus, the best locoregional approach to minimize morbidity, while considering tissue injury from neoadjuvant or adjuvant RT, should be determined.[3] Rarely, neoadjuvant chemotherapy may be applied, for example, to "down-stage" a mast cell tumor (MCT),[3] and surgical timing planned to avoid chemotherapeutic nadirs impacting wound healing.

Knowledge of tumor biology facilitates staging diagnostics, while considering paraneoplastic syndromes and underlying comorbidities.[3,4] Staging results may impact the surgical plan, altering surgical dose (eg, palliation for advanced metastatic disease) or incorporating additional procedures (eg, lymphadenectomy).[1]

Precise, advanced imaging has become commonplace in veterinary medicine with computed tomography (CT) readily available at most specialty hospitals. Use of CT and magnetic resonance imaging (MRI) has increased over historic use of abdominal ultrasound and radiographs.[4] While considered standard in humans, even positron emission tomography (PET)/CT has become more available within veterinary medicine for whole-body staging.[6] Abdominal ultrasound remains commonly used as a screening modality given increased availability, lower cost, ease and efficiency of use, and ability to obtain image-guided samples.[6] However, sedated CTs, rather than fully anesthetized, can be performed with the advent of more rapid data acquisition machines.[7] Thoracic CT offers increased sensitivity for pulmonary metastasis compared with standard radiographs.[8] While MRI offers superior tumor soft-tissue detail with local invasion into surrounding structures compared with CT, outside of neuroimaging, CT remains standard due to longer data acquisition times under general anesthesia for MRI.[6] Advanced imaging modalities allow the evaluation of three-dimensional reconstructions that aid preoperative planning with better evaluation of local anatomy, including structures involved in the tumor, measurement of surgical margins, and determination of tissues available for reconstruction. Use of PET/CT, most commonly labeled with radiopharmaceutical ^{18}F-fluorodeoxyglucose (FDG) provides functional anatomic information along with metabolic information for the primary tumor, allowing the detection of possible metastatic lesions with FDG uptake for cancer staging.[9] PET/CT is increasingly being assessed for tumor staging and monitoring of veterinary patients with cancer for various cancers, but currently remains limited in availability and costly.[9–11]

This chapter focuses on updates in staging, treatment, alternative therapies, and adjuvant therapy for apocrine gland anal sac adenocarcinomas (AGASACA) and MCTs.

APOCRINE GLAND ANAL SAC ADENOCARCINOMA
Background

AGASACA account for 17% of perianal neoplasms[12] and 2% of skin and subcutaneous neoplasms in dogs.[13] AGASACA is most common in middle-to-older age dogs (9–

11 years)[12–18] with breed predispositions in spaniels, German Shepherd dogs, and Dachshunds.[13–16,19] Patients most commonly present with unilateral masses, but bilateral simultaneous masses and/or temporally separate bilateral masses are reported in 14% of cases.[13,16,20–22] Common presenting clinical signs are associated with complete or partial fecal obstruction from the primary mass or metastatic disease, and signs related to underlying paraneoplastic syndromes. Clinical signs include local pain and discomfort, ribbon-like stools, hematochezia, tenesmus, scooting, perianal licking, lethargy, anorexia, and hindlimb weakness or lameness.[14] Polyuria, polydipsia, hyporexia, weight loss, and vomiting can be associated with hypercalcemia which is commonly seen with AGASACA.[14,15,23] Up to 47% are incidentally found on rectal examination.[15,16] Overall tumor behavior is considered locally aggressive and highly metastatic.

Staging

Metastasis is reported in 46% to 96% of dogs at presentation, with 26% to 89% to locoregional lymph nodes, and 0% to 42% to distant sites.[14,15,23,24] Distant metastatic sites vary widely including liver, spleen, lungs, bone and, less commonly, other organs.[12,14,15,17,18,20,25–29] Locoregional lymph nodes, including sublumbar (internal and external medial iliacs) and sacral lymph nodes are the most commonly involved sites of metastatic disease.[12,14,15,17,18,20,25–29] Presence of metastasis is not dependent on primary tumor size, such that small primary anal sac tumors may have large metastatic lymph nodes.[16,23] Rarely, patients can have distant metastasis without locoregional lymph node involvement.[24] Paraneoplastic syndromes accompanying AGASACA include hypercalcemia (16%–53%)[14–16,21,30] due to parathyroid hormone-related protein (PTHrp)[30] and hypertrophic osteopathy.[31] Hypercalcemia can occur with metastatic lesions and/or local recurrence and can be serially monitored after the initial treatment.[30] Complete preoperative staging includes multiple diagnostics as seen in **Box 1**.

Abdominal radiographs may reveal ventral colonic deviation with significant lymphadenomegaly or rare metastatic bone lesions, but cannot assess organ parenchyma nor identify smaller lymph node metastasis sufficiently.[24] Abdominal ultrasound is more sensitive,[32] but cannot visualize under the pelvis to fully assess the sacral lymphocenter.[24]ve CT or MRI ha multiple advantages as they can detect enlarged lymph nodes missed on abdominal ultrasound along with increased numbers of enlarged lymph nodes.[33–35] Advanced imaging also allows the assessment of resectability and relative risk of lymphadenectomy. The surgeon can further evaluate

---

Box 1
AGASACA staging

Physical examination *(focus on rectal for size of mass, LN palpation)*

Blood work - Complete blood count, Chemistry

iCa *(if indicated from Chemistry)*

Urinalysis

Cytology of mass *(typically neuroendocrine,[24] rules out inflammation and other tumor types)*

Imaging thorax (CT preferred over thoracic radiographs)

Imaging abdomen (CT or MRI preferred over abdominal radiographs or abdominal ultrasound)

Other *(consider SLN mapping techniques)*

vascular association, size, possible invasion into epaxial musculature, depth within the pelvic canal, and consistency of the lymph node (cystic vs solid). With CT commonly performed for the staging of the abdomen, including the thoracic cavity is recommended for more sensitive detection of pulmonary metastasis (**Fig.** 1A–C).[8,24] PET/CT, whereby available, can also be performed for whole-body staging and has advantages of providing not only the anatomic location of possible metastasis but also the metabolic function of the primary tumor (**Figs. 2**A and B).

Sentinel lymph node (SLN) mapping, has been evaluated for AGASACA staging in multiple studies. Indirect computed tomography lymphography (ICTL) is a feasible technique to identify the SLN and lymphatic drainage in 92% of cases.[36] ICTL is most commonly performed using peritumoral or peri-scar injections with iohexol, followed by serial CT scans. Lymph nodes do not always drain ipsilaterally from the primary

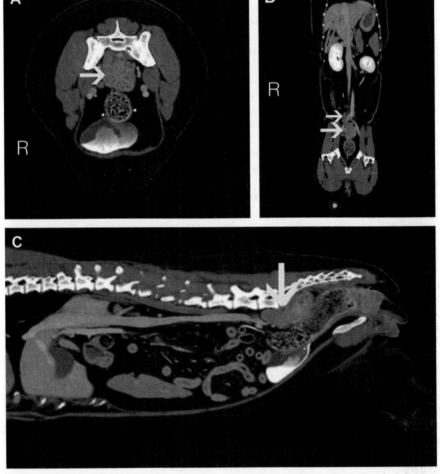

Fig. 1. Dog with AGASACA with sublumbar lymphadenopathy (yellow *arrow*). (*A*) Transverse postcontrast CT scan. (*B*) Coronal postcontrast CT demonstrating anatomic location with close association with the terminal branches of the aorta and caudal vena cava. (*C*) Sagittal postcontrast CT demonstrating significant ventral deviation of the colon.

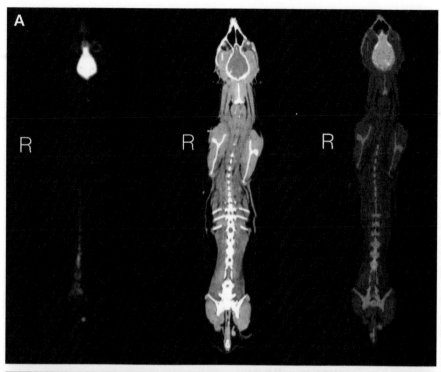

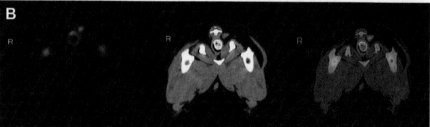

Fig. 2. Dog with recurrent AGASACA in the left perianal region that has intense uptake (avidity), representing increased metabolic activity, but is minimally contrast-enhancing. (*A*) Coronal images from left to right: PET imaging, corresponding postcontrast CT, and (PET)/CT. (*B*) Axial images from left to right: PET, corresponding postcontrast CT, and (PET)/CT. There is normal uptake in the proximal femur bilaterally.

tumor and commonly involve multiple lymphocenters.[36] The sacral lymph node was identified as the SLN in 25%-37.5% of dogs.[36,37] A pilot study using lymphoscintigraphy in normal dogs was successful in all dogs with intramural anal sac injection being superior to peritumoral. Importantly, the inguinal lymph node was identified as the SLN in one dog.[37] Intraoperative SLN mapping techniques may have significant benefit during abdominal exploratory for lymphadenectomy to ensure all SLNs are removed.

Surgery

While multiple treatment options exist for AGASACA, surgery is the mainstay treatment of locoregional control via anal sacculectomy (**Table 1**).[17,20,25] Preoperative treatment of hypercalcemia should be pursued, if indicated,[24] to increase patient

Table 1
AGASACA treatment options

AGASACA Treatment Modalities	
Surgery	Anal sacculectomy • OST 529–1205 d[17,18,20,23] + Lymphadenectomy, as indicated • OST 293–448 d[17,18,20,23] Metastectomy and/or revision surgery for recurrent disease, as indicated • Median additional survival time 283–374 d[20,27]

Radiation therapy	Definitive-intent primary therapy and/or adjuvant therapy to gross measurable disease
	• Intensity-modulated RT (IMRT), with or without prior surgery[38]
	  • 73% acute side effects, no late side effects
	• Stereotactic body RT (SBRT)[39]
	  • N = 12 dogs, gross disease or adjuvant following Incomplete excision primary ± lymph nodes
	  • PFS 549 d
	  • MST 991 d
	  • Late side effect: rectal stricture (n = 1)
	Adjuvant therapy to microscopic disease
	• No significant difference survival times[15]
	• N = 15 dogs, RT to primary site ± lymph nodes with adjuvant mitoxantrone chemotherapy, median OST 956 d[23]
	Palliative-intent measurable gross disease
	• Improves clinical signs up to 63%[21,30,40,41]
	• RT side effects mild, infrequent[40]
	• PFI 10–11 mo[18,21,30,42]
	• MST 8–15 mo[18,21,30,42]

Chemotherapy	Injectable
	• Unclear evidence in the gross disease setting
	• Antitumor effects reported with carboplatin, cisplatin, actinomycin D, melphalan, mitoxantrone[14,19,23,25,29,43]
	• No significant difference MST or disease progression vs surgery alone[15,20]
	• Benefit with adjuvant carboplatin postoperatively[14]
	Toceranib phosphate
	• Failure with prior therapy, durable response 10–47 wk[44,45]
	• Late-stage disease without lymphadenectomy may improve survival
	  • PFI 354 d, MST 356 d
	• Dogs with or without surgery, with or without adjuvant chemotherapy[46]
	  • 21% PR, those with response had longer OST and PFS
	• No significant difference in disease progression vs surgery alone[47]

Electrochemo therapy	Primary line of treatment with bleomycin[41] • N = 9 dogs with/without chemotherapy • MST 365 d • Median time to progression 303 d • 60% PR • Limited local side effects Adjuvant with bleomycin postoperatively[41] • N = 1 dog Adjuvant with cisplatin postoperatively[48] • N = 1 dog, 2 courses of ECT • CR 18 mo • No local toxicity

Abbreviations: Overall survival time (OST), Median survival time (MST), Progression free survival (PFS), Progression free interval (PFI), Partial response (PR), Complete response (CR)

stability for general anesthesia. Incomplete or narrow excision occurs in up to 73% of cases due to the anatomy of the perineal region and lack of natural barriers for margins[28]; however, local recurrence is not associated with completeness of histopathologic margins (**Box 2**).[16,23]

Lymphadenectomy should be standard-of-care for those with metastatic locoregional lymph nodes, as survival is significantly improved with removal.[15,18,27] Surgery, however, can be technically challenging given proximity and association of lymph nodes with terminal branches of the caudal vena cava and aorta. This coupled with possible invasion into epaxial musculature, creates a risk for intraoperative hemorrhage, potentially requiring blood products.[50] With cystic lymph nodes, the surgeon risks rupture during dissection potentially seeding tumor cells. Lymph node omentalization for the palliation of obstructive, nonresectable disease is reported with a good clinical outcome and survival 18 months postoperatively.[51] Surgical complications occur in 0% to 12% of AGASACA lymphadenectomy cases, mostly associated with intraoperative hemorrhage or unresectable lymph nodes.[17,20,27,40] Careful, tedious dissection using digital palpation often allows avoiding a pelvic osteotomy for sacral lymph node dissection, but is often considered "blind" dissection.[50] Hypercalcemia can be seen with lymph node metastasis and typically resolves postoperatively within 1 to 2 days of lymphadenectomy.[52] While rare, some patients can become hypocalcemic postoperatively, potentially requiring treatment.[53,54] Hypercalcemia is associated with recurrent disease and can be used as a potential marker during patient surveillance.[52]

Optical coherence tomography (OCT) can be used for real-time surgical margin evaluation intraoperatively, which could have significant benefit for a tumor whereby marginal surgery is the goal, by default. In a veterinary study, ex vivo specimens were evaluated to identify areas of concern for the pathologist along the margin, demonstrating the ability to characterize postoperative AGASACA samples[55]; however, considering historical data that states incomplete margins do not influence survival,[18,23,28] it is unclear if OCT will be used for AGASACA.

Ample evidence exists to support additional surgery for recurrent disease, including lymphadenectomy procedures with new or recurrent lymph node metastasis. Recurrent lymph node metastasis occurs in up to 42% of cases,[27] with median additional survival time of 283 days[27] or 374 days[20] following recurrent metastectomy for

Box 2
Anal sacculectomy complications

Anal Sacculectomy Complications	
Overall complications	Low, 0%–24%[17,20,27]
Local recurrence	Recent literature < 20%[27,49]; historic up to 45%[14,16,17,20,23,27,49]
Dehiscence	
Surgical site infection	Up to 12%[49]
Intraoperative hemorrhage	
Tenesmus	
Fecal incontinence, temporary or permanent	Rare, *higher risk with greater circumference presumed*
Rectal perforation	Up to 7%; *associated with 19x increased risk postoperative complications*[49]
Rectocutaneous fistula formation	

progressive disease, compared with 47 days for dogs not treated for recurrent or metastatic disease. Splenectomy can also be considered for dogs with splenic metastasis with unknown impact on patient outcomes.[23] Owners supportive of clinician restaging recommendations are more likely to pursue treatment of progressive disease.[56]

Adjuvant Electrochemotherapy

Adjuvant electrochemotherapy (ECT) or primary ECT without surgery using cisplatin (complete remission for 18 months) or bleomycin (median survival time 365d, median time to progression 303d) is reported in small numbers of dogs, with limited local side effects.[41,48]

Radiation Therapy

Primary radiation therapy for AGASACA is reserved for inoperable tumors, nonresectable metastatic disease, or those for which the owner does not wish to pursue surgical treatment, and/or elects palliation. For RT alone, response in gross measurable disease ranges from 38% to 75% with various protocols.[21,29,30,42] RT for palliative-intent with AGASACA is well-defined. In cases where lymph node metastasis measured greater than 4.5 cm, hypofractionated RT has shown better outcomes compared with surgery.[21] Adjuvant RT in a microscopic disease setting for AGASACA is not well-defined at this time, but consideration is reasonable given the planned marginal excision nature of anal sacculectomy.[24] Further controlled, cohort studies are needed to better evaluate RT and its potential clinical benefit for microscopic disease clinical scenarios: local perianal use only, local perianal and gross lymph node enlargement, or local perianal and lymphatic bed.[24]

Adjuvant Chemotherapy

A recent retrospective revealed 80% of owners were given recommendations for treatment following initial surgery for AGASACA; however, only 49% of owners elected some form of adjuvant therapy, and only 66% pursued some form of re-staging to monitor disease progression.[56] Overall adherence rates for treatment (34%) and re-staging (21%) were very low,[56] potentially impacting patient outcomes. Adjuvant chemotherapy tends to be recommended due to the tumor biology of metastatic risk and increased disease progression when lymph node metastasis is present[17]; however, no survival advantage is clear in the literature to-date.

Prognostic Factors/Outcomes

Various negative prognostic indicators have been reported (**Table 2**). Stage is significantly associated with patient outcomes in AGASACA dogs with or without metastasis, especially with respect to lymph node metastasis.[17,20,23] Shorter disease-free intervals (DFI) are associated with dogs with lymph node metastasis (134–197 days) compared with those without (529–760 days).[16,20,23] Size of the locoregional lymph nodes (>4.5 cm) is another negative prognostic factor[18] and not surprisingly, distant metastases are associated with worse patient outcomes.[15,18] Vascular and lymphatic invasion seen on histopathology are associated with local recurrence a median of 374 days postoperatively,[49] and vascular invasion alone is predictive of metastatic disease at presentation.[57]

Even with these factors, long-term survival outcomes are absolutely possible for dogs with AGASACA. Median survival times (MSTs) range from 386 to 1205 days,[18] with a 1-year survival rate of 65% and 2-year survival rate of 29%.[15] Overall survival

Table 2
AGASACA prognostic factors

AGASACA Negative Prognostic Factors	
Clinical signs at presentation	More likely to have lymph node metastasis[23]
Size	primary tumor >2.5 cm[17,57]
Stage	Lymph node metastasis, distant metastasis
Histopathologic features[22,23,26,57]	Solid pattern Lymphovascular invasion Necrosis
Type of treatment elected	No surgery[15,18] or no treatment at all[18]
+/− Paraneoplastic hypercalcemia	Inconsistent in literature[15,23,26]

time (OST) with lymph node metastasis is 293 to 448 days versus 529 to 1205 days without.[17,18,20,23] MST with distant metastasis is 71 to 219 days.[15,18]

Feline Apocrine Gland Anal Sac Adenocarcinomas

AGASACA is rare in cats, making up only 0.5% of skin and subcutaneous tumors.[58] Cats are older (median 13 years) when they present with these tumors, and Siamese cats are predisposed.[58] Clinical signs are typically associated with local disease, including perianal ulceration, irritation, pain, and discharge in 85%[59]; hence feline AGASACA is commonly misdiagnosed early on as an anal sac abscess. Lymph node metastasis occurs in up to 20% of cats,[59] with distant metastasis rarely reported to the diaphragm, lung, and liver.[59,60] Paraneoplastic hypercalcemia occurs in only 11% of cats.[58,59] Known negative prognostic factors in cats include local recurrence and a higher nuclear pleomorphic score on histopathology.[59]

Cats treated with surgery, with or without adjuvant therapy, have an MST of 260 days,[59] with 1-year survival rates of 42%, 2-year survival rates of 27%, and 3-year survival rates of 18%.[59] Disease progression within 6 months despite adjuvant curative-intent RT and carboplatin has been reported in cats.[60]

MAST CELL TUMORS
Background

Mast cell tumors are considered the most common cutaneous tumor in dogs and second most common in cats.[61,62] They tend to present in middle-to-older age dogs (8–9 years) with English bulldogs, boxers, Boston terriers, pugs, Labrador retrievers, Golden retrievers, cocker spaniels, schnauzers, Staffordshire terriers, beagles, Rhodesian ridgebacks, Weimaraners, and Chinese shar-peis overrepresented.[63–67]

Most of the cases present with solitary masses on the trunk or perineal region (50%), limbs (40%), or head/neck region (10%), with 14% of dogs having multiple masses on initial presentation.[68–71] Solitary cutaneous lesions vary in appearance. Some masses are focal, slow-growing, alopecic lesions, while others display significant inflammation or ulceration and rapid increase in size, along with size fluctuation.[72,73] Dogs with advanced disease may have clinical signs attributed to systemic diseases, such as vomiting, diarrhea, peripheral edema and bruising, fever, or collapse.[72] A local "Darier sign" characterized by erythema, edema, and wheal formation represents degranulation and a local anaphylactic response (**Fig. 3**).[74]

All MCTs are considered locally aggressive, while high-grade MCTs have a propensity to metastasize. Metastasis is typical to the locoregional lymph nodes prior to prior to distant sites including spleen, liver, and bone marrow.[73]

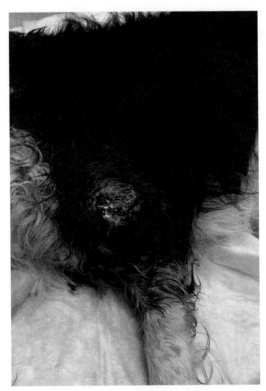

Fig. 3. Dog with a large, firm, fixed, ulcerated MCT with a Darier sign including erythema, bruising, and edema extending down the forelimb and axillary region. This MCT was found to be a grade II/low-grade MCT on histopathology.

Staging

For patients without negative prognostic factors that have a curative-intent surgical option, full diagnostic staging preoperatively may not be indicated (**Box 3**).[72,75] While cytologic grading could be helpful to guide preoperative staging recommendations,[76–78] an incisional biopsy for histopathologic grade may be useful for those without wide surgical options or multiple negative prognostic factors to guide treatment recommendations.[73,79] CT or MRI may be indicated for surgical planning (**Fig. 4**A–C). Although not performed regularly, primary tumors are well-marginated on MRI.[80] PET/CT has also been evaluated for whole-body staging in dogs with MCTs using [18]FDG, as well as for potential correlation to grade (**Fig. 5**A–D).[81,82] PET/CT identified lymph node metastasis and previously undetected distant metastasis.[81] A pilot study in dogs using [18]FDG PET/CT revealed a significant correlation between standard uptake volume maximum and histopathologic grade of MCTs[82] that could be beneficial in guiding treatment options.

Routine cytology of spleen and liver for staging is controversial, given conflicting literature results. One study showed resident mast cells within liver and spleen were normal and complicated interpretation.[83] Other studies reported that normal echogenicity on ultrasound is unlikely to yield metastatic mast cells on cytology.[84,85] Using CT to evaluate for liver and splenic metastasis in dogs with MCTs, the appearance of the liver was not correlated to cytologic metastasis, while multifocal hypoattenuating

| **Box 3** |
| **MCT staging** |
| *MCT complete staging* |
| Physical examination *(focus on mass palpation, lymph node palpation)* |
| Blood work - Complete blood count, Chemistry |
| Urinalysis |
| Cytology of mass |
| Locoregional lymph node cytology and/or SLN mapping |
| Abdominal ultrasound |
| +/− Cytology of liver and spleen |
| +/− Thoracic radiographs *(comorbidity assessment or sternal lymphadenopathy)* |
| +/− Advanced imaging for surgical planning |

splenic lesions were more often consistent with splenic metastasis.[86] However, considering the decrease in survival time associated with distant metastasis, cytology may be justified regardless of appearance on ultrasound or advanced imaging in patients with negative prognostic factors.[85–87] In the author's opinion, cytology of liver and spleen is indicated in patients with known negative prognostic indicators, historical high-grade MCTs or multiple prior MCTs, or for owners wanting all staging before surgical excision.

Lymph node size does not correlate with histopathologic or cytologic evidence of metastasis, as there has been confirmed metastasis in 50% of palpably normal lymph nodes.[88,89] Lymph node cytology can be complicated as individual mast cells are normally present in up to 24% of lymph nodes in normal dogs.[90] Clusters or aggregates of mast cells are considered necessary for a diagnosis of cytologic metastatic lymph node,[91] representing lymph nodes that should be extirpated along with wide excision of the primary tumor. Cytologic detection of lymph node metastasis has proven to be much lower (5%) than histopathologic (45%), and confirmation of lymph node metastasis can significantly influence adjuvant treatment recommendations.[92,93] Appearance of metastatic lymph nodes on MRI is consistent with the increased size of heterogeneous intensity on T2-W images compared with normal lymph nodes, but no imaging findings were statistically significant between groups.[80] With ICTL, the SLN enhancement pattern is not correlated with the presence of lymph node metastasis, and histopathology is necessary.[94]

SLN mapping is increasingly being used for MCT staging; however, it remains inconsistently performed, likely given the increased time, cost, and specialized equipment associated with its use. The author recommends SLN mapping be offered in every case; however, it is considered more heavily for masses located on the head/neck or trunk and in cases with existing negative prognostic factors. Preoperative lymphoscintigraphy along with intraoperative lymphoscintigraphy and blue dye was first described for SLN mapping in dogs with MCTs.[93] Importantly, the locoregional anatomic lymph node does not correlate to the SLN in up to 63% of cases.[88,92,93,95] ICTL can be used preoperatively in dogs with MCTs with successful SLN identification in 90% to 100% of cases (**Figs. 6**A and B).[92,94] No additional SLNs were identified using intraoperative methylene blue dye that had not been identified on preoperative ICTL.[94] Contrast-enhanced ultrasound (CEUS) is a feasible technique for SLN mapping in dogs with MCTs, with successful SLN identification in 95% of cases.[95] Even

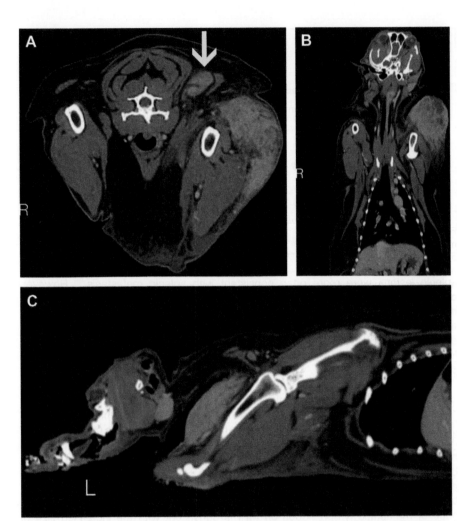

Fig. 4. Post-contrast CT scan of the dog pictured in **Fig. 3** used for staging and evaluation of margins for surgical planning for a grade II/low-grade MCT with left superficial cervical metastasis. (*A*) Axial CT image showing the enlarged and heterogenous superficial cervical lymph node (yellow *arrow*) and fat stranding consistent with cellulitis and edema. (*B*) Coronal CT image with visible fat stranding caudal to the tumor. (*C*) Sagittal CT image demonstrating the association of the mass along the proximal limb and humerus.

with masses in similar anatomic locations, identified SLNs vary,[95] supporting the need for SLN mapping to guide appropriate node dissection for MCTs.

Surgery

Wide surgical excision is standard-of-care for curative-intent treatment of MCTs without evidence of distant metastasis. Recommended surgical margins historically consist of 3 cm lateral margins and a single fascial plane deep.[72,96] This recommendation has been challenged recently with multiple studies evaluating less aggressive lateral margins (**Table 3**).[96–99,101] More recently, the use of proportional margins has been described, whereby the lateral surgical margin measurement equals the largest

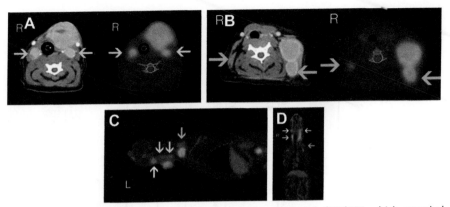

Fig. 5. Dog with a grade II MCT in the ventral neck staged with (PET)/CT, which revealed metastasis to the medial retropharyngeal (yellow *arrows*), deep cervical (blue *arrows*), and superficial cervical lymph nodes (green *arrows*). (*A*) Axial postcontrast CT image and corresponding (PET)/CT demonstrating the primary cervical mass and deep cervical lymph node metastases. (*B*) Axial postcontrast CT scan and corresponding (PET)/CT demonstrating the superficial cervical lymph node metastasis. (*C*) Sagittal (PET)/CT image and (*D*) Coronal (PET)/CT image revealing the primary mass and multiple high intensity (avid) lymph nodes.

diameter of the mass. Chu and colleagues[100] compared modified proportional margins to traditional wide excision (3 cm lateral margins) for grade I/II (low-grade) MCTs and found comparable rates of complete excision (93% vs 92%).

Further evaluation using the metric approach with fixed lateral margins has been evaluated. Another study evaluating MCTs less than 3.1 cm in diameter found no local recurrence with lateral margins of greater than 1 cm and deep margins greater than 4 mm.[102] Most of the tumors (95.7%) were Patnaik grade I and II and 4% of dogs developed metastasis unassociated with the histopathologic margin.[102] Edema surrounding the masses was not associated with outcome,[102] which is important for surgeons given that measuring metric lateral margins from the gross tumor versus the Darier sign has not been evaluated. When resecting grade II MCTs less than 4 cm in diameter using 2 to 3 cm wide margins, 95% were histopathologically complete

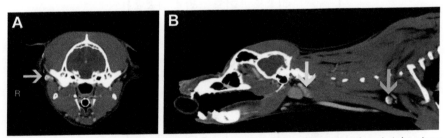

Fig. 6. Dog with incompletely excised grade III/ high-grade MCT on the dorsal right pinna with ICTL performed via peri-scar injection for SLN mapping before scar revision via pinnectomy. (*A*) Axial postcontrast image 3-min postinjection ICTL demonstrating contrast uptake within the ipsilateral parotid lymph node (blue *arrow*). (*B*) Sagittal postcontrast 3-min postinjection ICTL demonstrating contrast uptake in the ipsilateral medial retropharyngeal (yellow *arrow*) and superficial cervical lymph nodes (green *arrow*). All three lymph nodes were confirmed metastatic on histopathology following lymph node extirpation.

Table 3
MCT surgical margins

Surgical Margin	Tumor Size	Grades Included	Completeness Histopathology	Local Recurrence	Follow-up (Median)
Proportional	Tumors up to 6 cm (max at 4 cm margins)[97]	Patnaik I and II (95%) Kiupel low (90%)	85%	2% (n = 1)	420 d
	Tumors <2.6 cm[98]	Kiupel low	92%[a]	0%	976 d
Modified proportional (maximum lateral margin of 2 cm)	Tumors <8.5 cm[99]	Kiupel low and high grade	95%	3% (0% low grade; 25% high grade)	533 d
	Tumors <7 cm[100]	Patnaik I and II (Kiupel low grade)	93%	Not assessed	Not applicable
Metric 1 cm	Tumors <5 cm[96]	Patnaik I and II	100% grade I 75% grade II	Not assessed	Not applicable
Metric 2 cm	Tumors <5 cm[96]	Patnaik I and II	100%	Not assessed	Not applicable
	Tumors <3.1 cm[101]	Patnaik I and II	91%	0%	Not reached >538 d

[a] Complete or close.

or close and 5% had local recurrence.[103] A prospective study with 50 low-grade (grade I/II) and 2 high-grade (grade III) tumors with a maximum diameter of 1.7 cm reported local recurrence in only 4% of cases despite 1/3 having less than 2 cm lateral gross margins obtained in surgery.[104] Interestingly, completeness of histopathologic excision has not been associated with tumor size[96,99] nor Kiupel grade,[99] and there is no association between the width of histologic tumor-free margin and local recurrence.[104,105]

A recent systematic review of literature regarding MCT margin recommendations concluded 2 cm lateral margins and a single deep fascial plane is acceptable for cutaneous grade I/II MCTs measuring less than 4 cm given low overall rates of incomplete excision and local recurrence.[106] Rates of incomplete resection using lateral margins of 1-, 2-, or 3-cm were 0% to 31.6%, 0% to 10.5%, and 0% to 1.7%, respectively.[106] This may be especially helpful when margins are limited by anatomy, for instance on the extremities (**Figs. 7**A and B). Grade is unknown preoperatively unless an incisional biopsy has been performed; thus, clinical suspicion and negative prognostic factors should be considered in surgical decision-making. Grade III MCTs are still expected to behave aggressively and are associated with more difficult complete excision and higher local recurrence rates.[63,73,105,107] More conservative lateral margins cannot be justified for grade III MCTs at this time without further assessment of patient outcomes.

Subcutaneous MCTs are difficult to assess for surgical margins, as the overlying skin typically moves freely over the top of the mass itself (**Figs. 8**A and B). A prospective, randomized, blinded clinical study assessed intersurgeon agreement for planned 3 cm lateral metric margins measuring from the gross tumor edge for subcutaneous MCTs and soft tissue sarcomas and found 95% of surgeons would actually obtain 2.4 to 3.6 cm lateral margins.[108] This finding emphasizes potentially unacceptable variation in individual margin measurement related to human surgeon error during intraoperative margin planning, which is difficult to control.

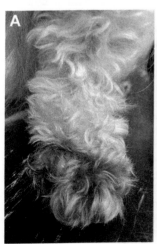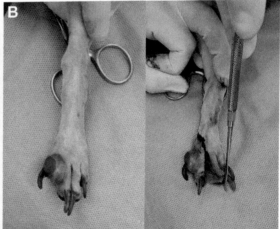

Fig. 7. (*A*) Photograph of dog with ulcerated MCT between digits 2 and 3 on the left pelvic limb. This patient had left popliteal lymph node metastasis at presentationat. (*B*) Preoperative photographs: Left-The mass is ulcerated and inflamed; Right-Proportional margins are marked for excision via partial foot amputation. Final histopathology demonstrated complete excision.

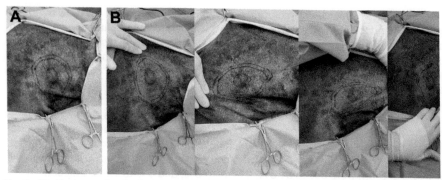

Fig. 8. (*A*) Photograph of subcutaneous MCT with proportional (2.5 cm) and 3 cm standard wide excision lateral margins marked for comparison. (*B*) The surgeon is demonstrating variation in the positioning of the mass for the deep plane. When the dog is standing, the mass is loose within the skin folds of the caudal neck, while it is positioned over the jugular vein with the patient in lateral recumbency.

Lymph node extirpation is not only diagnostic but also prognostic, aiding in adjuvant therapy recommendations. Lymph node extirpation is recommended, as the removal of metastatic lymph nodes in dogs with grade II MCTs is associated with prolonged survival time compared to those without.[109] Increased time to disease progression (median not reached vs 170 days) and a prolonged tumor-specific survival time (2213 vs 360 days) were confirmed in dogs with primary surgery, lymph node extirpation, and adjuvant therapy compared with those without lymph node removal in stage II MCTs.[110] If lymph node metastasis is treated with either surgery or RT, dogs have a prolonged survival time compared with untreated dogs.[111] With limited morbidity associated with peripheral lymphadenectomy for experienced surgeons, knowledge that adjuvant chemotherapy is more effective in the face of microscopic disease, and potential for a survival advantage, lymph node extirpation should be recommended along with primary tumor excision any time metastatic disease is confirmed.

Intraoperative frozen sections are considered standard-of-care in human oncologic surgery, but the technique remains impractical in veterinary medicine.[112] A focus on intraoperative imaging for the assessment of surgical margins and residual disease is increasing within veterinary surgical oncology.[113–115] Near-infrared fluorescence (NIRF) imaging is being evaluated for its use intraoperatively to guide the surgeon in the assessment of surgical margins real-time. It consists of injecting an imaging agent, usually the day before surgery, that will experience proteolytic activation in vivo and preferentially accumulate within cancerous tissue.[113] A handheld device is used intraoperatively to assess for residual disease within the tumor bed by measuring fluorescence intensity ratios.[113] A pilot study using a cathepsin-activated NIRF probe in dogs with soft tissue sarcomas and MCTs confirmed tumor fluorescence using the imaging agent with positive residual fluorescence in the tumor bed correlated to incomplete foci on surgical margins.[114] There were no adverse events in any patients.[114] The imaging agent, LUM-15, for canine MCTs is able to correctly differentiate cancerous tissue from noncancerous tissue using fluorescence confirmed histopathologically in 92% of cases (92% sensitivity and specificity).[113] With respect to the identification of residual tumor foci, imaging correlates well with surgeon impression.[113] Transient hypersensitivity with facial erythema occurred in 53% of patients in this study, all of which responded to diphenhydramine.[113] An additional pilot study using indocyanine green (ICG) as the imaging agent for dogs with various tumor types, including MCTs, had an overall sensitivity and specificity of 72% and 80%, respectively, for residual neoplastic foci in the tumor bed.[115] NIRF may not be readily available at many institutions currently and additional prospective clinical trials for dogs with MCTs are indicated to evaluate the potential benefit for improved patient outcome.

A pilot study using OCT proved the technique to be feasible in dogs with MCTs to identify suspicious areas ex vivo at the resected margin of tumors to draw further attention for the pathologist during histopathologic sectioning.[116] The sensitivity and specificity for incomplete margins was 90% and 56%, respectively,[116] and may hold promise for increasing the accuracy of surgical margin assessment, as well as intraoperative confidence to proactively obtain additional margins.

Adjuvant Therapy

Adjuvant therapy for completely excised low grade and grade I/II MCTs is not recommended, while adjuvant chemotherapy is indicated for completely excised high grade and grade III MCTs given the high metastatic rate.[73] The mainstay treatment of an incompletely excised MCT is scar revision surgery with larger margins, if amenable **(Table 4)**.[73]

Alternative Treatments

In one study, adjuvant ECT with cisplatin following incomplete excision of MCTs was performed with 78% having no local recurrence after a median of 1 year.[128] Local transient MCT degranulation occurred in 32% of these patients within 10 minutes of treatment.[128] An 85% response rate with median time to recurrence of 53 months was reported using ECT with intralesional bleomycin following incomplete excision of MCTs.[129] A retrospective, multi-institutional study evaluated ECT in 4 clinical scenarios: single therapy in the gross disease setting, intraoperative ECT to the tumor bed following marginal excision, ECT following incomplete excision 2 to 4 weeks postoperatively, or ECT following local recurrence with complete remission (CR) noted in 80%, 91%, 93%, and 64%, respectively.[130] ECT is especially useful in the adjuvant therapy setting, especially for tumors that are located on extremities whereby wide excision cannot be achieved, but it is unlikely to achieve long-term control comparable to adjuvant RT. In a retrospective study of dogs with MCTs treated with surgical excision or ECT with cisplatin, CR was obtained in 62.5% of ECT cases with a longer time to recurrence compared with surgically excised masses (not reached vs 31.5 months) **(Fig. 9)**.[131]

Tigilanol tiglate is a novel therapeutic Protein kinase C activator labeled for the intratumoral treatment of nonmetastatic, nonresectable cutaneous MCTs or subcutaneous MCTs distal to the elbow or hock, measuring less than 8 cm³ overall tumor volume.[132] This drug works by causing a local inflammatory response and tumor necrosis via tumor cell death and impact on tumor vasculature.[133–135] In a controlled clinical trial, 75% of dogs treated with a single injection achieved CR by day 28, increasing to 88% after retreatment for nonresponders. When efficacious, a wound forms and the tumor sloughs; therefore, 95% of cases that experienced CR developed a wound compared with 5% of dogs in the sham control group.[134] For those that developed wounds, 89% reached the maximum wound size by day 7 postinjection.[135] Cases without wounds did not have a clinical response, confirming efficacy is related to wound area posttumor slough.[135] Time to full wound healing was variable, with only 57% healed by day 28 and 96% by day 84.[135] Overall, 99% of the wounds healed by second intention. The majority of these wounds were not bandaged, and prophylactic antibiotics were prescribed in 42%.[134] Size of the wound surface that develops is related to tumor volume, with larger wounds in larger tumor volumes.[134] In a study

Table 4
MCT adjuvant treatment recommendations

MCT Adjuvant Treatment Recommendations			
Clinical Scenario	**Tumor Grade**	**Local Recurrence**	**Recommendation**
Complete excision	Grade I and II (low grade)	5%–11% local recurrence[63,103,117]	Active surveillance
	Grade III (high grade)		Adjuvant chemotherapy
Incomplete excision	Grade I and II (low grade)	27% local recurrence[118] • Associated with shorter survival times • Relapse earlier (12 vs 24 mo)	Scar revision • 84% no evidence residual disease on recut histopathology[119] • 27% residual disease, not associated with local recurrence[120] Adjuvant RT (if scar revision not possible) • Good long-term control[121–125] • Scar revision or adjuvant RT longer survival times and longer time to local recurrence[119] • Grade II adjuvant surgical revision, chemotherapy, RT no difference survival time, local recurrence or metastasis[126] Adjuvant ECT (if scar revision not possible)
	Grade III (high grade)	35% local recurrence[127]	Scar revision Adjuvant RT (if scar revision not possible)[127] • Median remission 27 mo, MST 28 mo • 1-y survival 71% Adjuvant ECT (if scar revision or RT not possible) Adjuvant chemotherapy
With lymph node metastasis (Stage II disease)	All grades		Wide excision with lymph node extirpation Adjuvant chemotherapy

with 1-year long-term follow-up, 89% of dogs remained tumor free, with 11% experiencing local recurrence, all within the first 6 months.[133] Besides the complications of wound care, which should not be understated, a significant downside of this treatment is the absence of a histopathologic grade, imperative to determine prognosis and adjuvant therapy recommendations.[64] Tigilanol tiglate offers another potential local treatment option for MCTs, but standard-of-care treatment with surgery ± adjuvant RT and/or chemotherapy should remain the primary recommendation for patients with MCT.

Prognostic Factors

MCTs remain a very difficult neoplasm to provide detailed information regarding survival times and outcomes. Many prognostic factors have been identified, making it challenging to predict an individual patient's MCT behavior (**Table 5**). Cases with

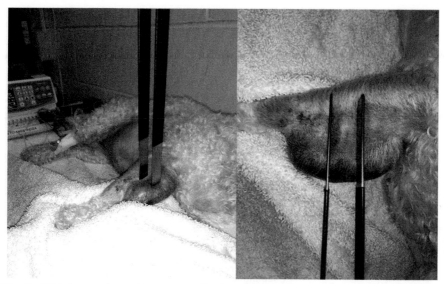

Fig. 9. ECT being performed in a dog with a large MCT on the right cranial antebrachium. The owner declined limb amputation. (*Images courtesy of* Dr. Lindsay Donnelly, DVM, MS, DACVIM (Oncology).)

cytologic evidence of metastasis to the lymph nodes have shorter MSTs, with grade III MCTs being more likely to have lymph node metastasis.[91] Cases with lymph node metastasis have a higher risk of death and local recurrence.[149] Median OST is 1020 days among all stages of tumors, with MST not reached for stage I, 203 days, 164 days, and 15 days for stages II, III, and IV, respectively.[157]

Histopathologic grade has been consistently thought to be the most important prognostic factor for MCTs.[63,64,91,111,121,149–151] High-grade/grade III MCTs are more likely to metastasize in up to 55% to 96% of cases and generally carry a poor prognosis, with survival being less than 1 year.[61,111,162] Recently, better outcomes of up to 28 months[127] and 34 months[163] have been reported, however. Unfortunately, even some low-grade/grade II tumors will have metastasis at diagnosis and this will affect overall survival.[64,109,137,151,164–168] Additional characterization of lymph node metastasis using a histopathologic classification scheme identified that higher classification lymph nodes with more extensive nodal mast cells had shorter DFIs and survival times.[169] Mitotic index[152] and histopathologic proliferation markers can be used to further evaluate behavior in grade II MCTs, with higher values associated with higher tumor grades.[136,153–156] Increased receptor tyrosine kinase protein (KIT) expression via immunohistochemistry is associated with increased risk of local recurrence and decreased survival.[157–161]

A recent study separated MCT dogs with overall low-risk versus high-risk, with at least one known negative prognostic factor, and found MST of 899 days for high-risk dogs compared with MST not being reached for low-risk dogs.[75] Many factors should be considered when evaluating an individual patient with MCT, most importantly stage and histopathologic grade.

Feline Mast Cell Tumor

In cats, MCTs comprise 20% of all cutaneous tumors,[62] most commonly located in the head and neck region followed by trunk, limbs, oral cavity, and other various

Table 5
MCT prognostic factors

	MCT Prognostic Factors
Age	Older dogs have shorter DFIs[117,136]
Breed	*Brachycephalic dogs, boxers predisposed to low grade Boxers, Golden retrievers, Labrador retrievers increased risk for multiple cutaneous MCTs[61,67,72,137–140]
Sex	Males have shorter survival times with chemotherapy Female dogs increased risk of multiple cutaneous MCTs[68,137,141]
Tumor location[121,143,144]	*Subcutaneous may be less aggressive than cutaneous[142] Mucocutaneous Perineal Oral Preputial Scrotal Inguinal Axillary Digital Subungual Muzzle
Tumor size	>3 cm or >5 cm[127,137,145]
Tumor growth behavior	Rapid growth[75,137]
Local recurrence[118,146]	
Presence of clinical signs[147,148]	
Treatment elected[72]	
Stage[75,91,111,121,143,149]	Lymph node metastasis distant metastasis
Grade[63,64,91,111,121,145,150,151]	Grade III High grade
Histopathologic factors	DNA aneuploidy[136] Mitotic index (>5 per 10 high power field)[152] DNA proliferation markers[136,153–156] • argyrophilic nucleolar organizer regions (agNOR) • percent positive proliferating-cell nuclear antigen (PCNA) • Ki67 KIT expression[157–161]

locations.[62,170,171] Masses are usually single, raised, white-to-pink, alopecic masses, 25% of which are ulcerated.[72] Up to 20% of cats have multiple masses.[61] There are 2 main types of cutaneous MCTs in cats. "Mastocytic, typical," similar to MCTs in dogs, is further characterized as compact (well-differentiated) versus diffuse (poorly differentiated), with compact behaving in benign fashion.[171–173] The second type, "histiocytic, atypical" MCTs, regress spontaneously within 2 years of appearance[174,175] and are found in young, Siamese cats, most often with multiple, simultaneous lesions.[174] Staging recommendations remain the same as with dogs. Visceral forms, primarily splenic and gastrointestinal, are found in cats, hence evaluation for splenic and GI disease is important.[172]

Treatment of cutaneous MCTs may not require as wide of margins as with dogs; however, no literature regarding margins specific to feline MCTs is published.[72] No association between completeness of resection and local recurrence or metastasis has been reported in studies on feline MCTs.[172,173] Systemic spread occurs postoperatively in up to 22% of cats,[170] with local recurrence in up to 36%.[171–173,175,176] Local control with strontium-90 irradiation has also been reported, achieving long-term tumor control and MST over 3 years, but this treatment is hindered by a shallow treatment zone (considered most effective for depths of <4 mm).[177] Splenectomy is indicated for primary splenic MCT and complete resolution of simultaneous cutaneous MCTs may occur postoperatively.[178] Additional organ involvement at the time of splenectomy has no impact on survival,[179] and despite possible systemic spread, MST up to 19 months is reported following splenectomy.[180,181]

The role of adjuvant chemotherapy in cats remains unclear,[178] with less response to prednisone in cats compared with dogs.[72,180] Lomustine,[182] and toceranib phosphate[183] have been reported with evidence of clinical benefit, but no controlled studies demonstrating survival advantage exist.[178]

As most feline MCTs are considered more benign,[176] no reliable grading scheme has been developed to-date[184] and histopathologic grading as done for canine MCTs is not associated with prognosis in cats.[185] High MI > 5/10hpf is the variable most associated with survival in cats, and no additional histopathologic features have shown consistency with prognosis.[175,176,186,187]

CLINICS CARE POINTS

- Canine AGASACA should be treated aggressively initially with surgery for removal of the primary mass via anal sacculectomy, along with lymphadenectomy to address metastatic lymph nodes.

- Patients with AGASACA can live for an extended period of time following aggressive surgical treatment.

- Wide resection of MCTs is still indicated as standard-of-care; however, the use of modified proportional margins is gaining favor in low-grade (Grade I and II) MCTs.

- Individual patient prognostic factors should be heavily considered when determining whether full preoperative staging is indicated and in assessing patient outcomes for MCTs.

DISCLOSURE

The author has nothing to disclose.

REFERENCES

1. Ehrhart N, Culp WTN. Principles of surgical oncology. In: Kudnig ST, Seguin B, editors. Veterinary surgical oncology. 1st edition. Ames: John Wiley and Sons, Inc; 2012. p. 3–13.
2. Poston GJ. Is there a surgical oncology?. In: Poston GJ, Beauchamp RD, Ruers TJM, editors. Textbook of surgical oncology. 1st edition. London: Informa Healthcare; 2007. p. 1–4.
3. Banks TA. Multimodal therapy. In: Kudnig ST, Seguin B, editors. Veterinary surgical oncology. 1st edition. Ames: John Wiley and Sons, Inc; 2012. p. 15–33.
4. Farese JP, Liptak JM, Withrow SJ. Surgical oncology. In: Vail DM, Thamm DH, Liptak JM, editors. Withrow & MacEwen's small animal clinical oncology. 6th edition. St. Louis: Elsevier, Inc; 2020. p. 164–73.
5. Paoloni M, Khanna C. Translation of new cancer treatments from pet dogs to humans. Nat Rev Cancer 2008;8:147–56.

6. Mattoon JS, Bryan JN. The future of imaging in veterinary oncology: learning from human medicine. Vet J 2013;197:541–52.

7. Oliveira CR, Ranallo FN, Pijanowski GJ, et al. The VetMousetrap: a device for computed tomographic imaging of the thorax of awake cats. Vet Radiol Ultrasound 2011;52:41–52.

8. Nemanic S, London CA, Wisner ER. Comparison of thoracic radiographs and single breathhold helical CT for detection of pulmonary nodules in dogs with metastatic neoplasia. J Vet Intern Med 2006;20:508–15.

9. Randall EK. PET-Computed Tomography in veterinary medicine. Vet Clin Small Anim 2016;46:515–33.

10. Lawrence J, Rohren E, Provenzale J. PET/CT today and tomorrow in veterinary cancer diagnosis and monitoring: Fundamentals, early results and future perspectives. Vet Comp Oncol 2010;8:163–87.

11. LeBlanc AK, Daniel GB. Advanced imaging for veterinary cancer patients. Vet Clin Small Anim 2007;37:1059–77.

12. Berrocal A, Vos JH, van den Ingh TS, et al. Canine perineal tumours. J Vet Med Ser A 1989;36:739–49.

13. Goldschmidt MH, Zoltowski C. Anal sac gland adenocarcinoma in the dog: 14 cases. J Small Anim Pract 1981;22:119–28.

14. Bennett PF, DeNicola DB, Bonney P, et al. Canine anal sac adenocarcinomas: clinical presentation and response to therapy. J Vet Intern Med 2002;16:100–4.

15. Wiliams LE, Gliatto JM, Dodge RK, et al. Carcinoma of the apocrine glands of the anal sac in dogs: 113 cases (1985-1995). J Am Vet Med Assoc 2003;223: 825–31.

16. Ross JT, Scavelli TD, Matthiesen DT, et al. Adenocarcinoma of the apocrine glands of the anal sac in dogs: a review of 32 cases. J Am Anim Hosp Assoc 1991;27:349–55.

17. Potanas CP, Padgett S, Gamblin RM. Surgical excision of anal sac apocrine gland adenocarcinomas with and without adjunctive chemotherapy in dogs: 42 cases (2005-2011). J Am Vet Med Assoc 2015;246:877–84.

18. Polton GA, Brearly MJ. Clinical stage, therapy, and prognosis in canine anal gland carcinoma. J Vet Intern Med 2007;21:274–80.

19. Polton GA, Mowat V, Lee HC, et al. Breed, gender and neutering status of British dogs with anal sac gland carcinoma. Vet Comp Oncol 2006;4:125–31.

20. Wouda RM, Borrego J, Keuler NS, et al. Evaluation of adjuvant carboplatin chemotherapy in the management of surgically excised anal sac apocrine gland adenocarcinoma in dogs. Vet Comp Oncol 2016;14:67–80.

21. White RAS, Gorman NT. The clinical diagnosis and management of rectal and pararectal tumours in the dog. J Small Anim Pract 1987;28:87–107.

22. Bowlt KL, Friend EJ, Delisser P, et al. Temporarily separated bilateral anal sac gland adenocarcinomas in four dogs. J Small Anim Pract 2013;54:432–6.

23. Turek MM, Forrest LJ, Adams WM, et al. Postoperative radiotherapy and mitoxantrone for anal sac adenocarcinoma in the dog 15 cases (1991-2001). Vet Comp Oncol 2003;1:94–104.

24. Liptak JM, Turek MM. Cancer of the gastrointestinal tract: section H-Perianal tumors. In: Vail DM, Thamm DH, Liptak JM, editors. Withrow & MacEwen's small animal clinical oncology. 6th edition. St. Louis: Elsevier, Inc; 2020. p. 468–91.

25. Emms SG. Anal sac tumours of the dog and their response to cytoreductive surgery and chemotherapy. Aust Vet J 2005;83:340–3.

26. Meuten DJ, Segre GV, Capen CC, et al. Hypercalcemia in dogs with adenocarcinoma derived from apocrine glands of the anal sac. Lab Invest 1983;48:428–34.

27. Barnes DC, Demetriou JL. Surgical management of primary, metastatic and recurrent anal sac adenocarcinoma in the dog: 52 cases. J Small Anim Pract 2017;58:263–8.

28. Pradel J, Berlato D, Dobromylskyj M, et al. Prognostic significance of histopathology in canine anal sac gland adenocarcinomas: preliminary results in a retrospective study of 39 cases. Vet Comp Oncol 2018;16:518–28.

29. Meier V, Polton G, Cancedda S, et al. Outcomes in dogs with advanced (stage 3b) anal sac gland carcinoma treated with surgery or hypofractionated radiation therapy. Vet Comp Oncol 2017;15:1073–86.

30. Rosol TJ, Capen CC, Danks JA, et al. Identification of parathyroid hormone-related protein in canine apocrine adenocarcinoma of the anal sac. Vet Pathol 1990;27:89–95.

31. Giuliano A, Salguero R, Dobson J. Metastatic anal sac carcinoma with hypercalcemia and associated hypertrophic osteopathy in a dog. Open Vet J 2015;4:48–51.

32. Llabrés-Díaz FJ. Ultrasonography of the medial iliac lymph nodes in the dog. Vet Radiol Ultrasound 2004;45:156–65.

33. Palladino S, Keyerleber M, King R, et al. Utility of computed tomography versus abdominal ultrasound examination to identify iliosacral lymphadenomegaly in dogs with apocrine gland adenocarcinoma of the anal sac. J Vet Intern Med 2016;30:1858–63.

34. Pollard RE, Fuller MC, Steffey MA. Ultrasound and computed tomography of the iliosacral lymphatic centre in dogs with anal sac carcinoma. Vet Comp Oncol 2017;15:299–306.

35. Anderson CL, MacKay CS, Roberts GD, et al. Comparison of abdominal ultrasound and magnetic resonance imaging for detection of abdominal lymphadenopathy in dogs with metastatic apocrine gland adenocarcinoma of the anal sac. Vet Comp Oncol 2015;13:98–105.

36. Majeski SA, Steffey MA, Fuller M, et al. Indirect computed tomographic lymphography for iliosacral lymphatic mapping in a cohort of dogs with anal sac gland adenocarcinoma: a technique description. Vet Radiol Ultrasound 2017;58:295–303.

37. Linden DS, Cole R, Tillson DM, et al. Sentinel Lymph node mapping of the canine anal sac using lymphoscintigraphy: a pilot study. Vet Radiol Ultrasound 2018;60:346–50.

38. Sterman A, Butler JR, Chamber A, et al. Post-operative complications following apocrine gland anal sac adenocarcinoma resection in dogs. Vet Comp Oncol 2021;19(4):743–9.

39. Liptak JM. Anal sac adenocarcinoma: clinical stage and management options. Oral presentation at: American College of Veterinary Surgeons Surgical Summit, 2018. Phoenix, AZ. p.427-430.

40. Hoelzler MG, Bellah JR, Donofro MC. Omentalization of cystic sublumbar lymph node metastasis for long-term palliation of tenesmus and dysuria in a dog with anal sac adenocarcinoma. J Am Vet Med Assoc 2001;219:1729–31.

41. McQuown B, Keyerleber MA, Rosen K, et al. Treatment of advanced canine anal sac adenocarcinoma with hypofractionated radiation therapy: 77 cases (1999-2013). Vet Comp Oncol 2017;15:840–51.

42. Hause WR, Stevenson S, Meuten DJ, et al. Pseudohyperparathryoidism associated with adenocarcinomas of anal sac origin in four dogs. J Am Anim Hosp Assoc 1981;17:373–9.

43. Olsen JA, Sumner JP. Clinical hypocalcemia following surgical resection of apocrine gland anal sac adenocarcinomas in 3 dogs. Can Vet J 2019;50:591–5.

44. Saba C, Ellis A, Cornell K, et al. Hypocalcemia following surgical treatment of metastatic anal sac adenocarcinoma in a dog. J Am Anim Hosp Assoc 2011; 47:e173–7.

45. Dornbusch JA, Selmic LE, Huang P, et al. Optical coherence tomography imaging of excised canine apocrine gland anal sac adenocarcinoma tumours. Vet Comp Oncol 2021;19(4):759–62.

46. Chambers AR, Skinner OT, Mickelson MA, et al. Adherence to follow-up recommendations for dogs with apocrine gland anal sac adenocarcinoma: a multicentre retrospective study. Vet Comp Oncol 2020;18:683–8.

47. Spugnini EP, Dotsinsky I, Mudrov N, et al. Adjuvant electrochemotherapy for incompletely excised anal sac carcinoma in a dog. In Vivo 2008;22:47–50.

48. Valenti P, Menicagli F, Baldi A, et al. Evaluation of electrochemotherapy in the management of apocrine gland anal sac adenocarcinomas in dogs: a retrospective study. Open Vet J 2021;11:100–6.

49. McDonald C, Looper J, Greene S. Response rate and duration associated with 4Gy 5 fraction palliative radiation protocol. Vet Radiol Ultrasound 2012;53: 358–64.

50. Korner M, Staudinger C, Meier V, et al. Retrospective assessment of radiation toxicity from a definitive-intent, moderately hypofractionated image-guided intensity-modulated protocol for anal sac adenocarcinoma in dogs. Vet Comp Oncol 2021;1–12.

51. Swan M, Morrow D, Grace M, et al. Pilot study evaluating the feasibility of stereotactic body radiation therapy for canine anal sac adenocarcinomas. Vet Radiol Ultrasound 2021;62(5):621–9.

52. Hammer AS, Couto CG, Ayl RD, et al. Treatment of tumor-bearing dogs with actinomycin D. J Vet Intern Med 1994;8:236–9.

53. London C, Mathie T, Stingle N, et al. Preliminary evidence for biologic activity of Toceranib phosphate (Palladia®) in solid tumours. Vet Comp Oncol 2012;10: 194–205.

54. Elliott JW. Response and outcome following Toceranib phosphate treatment for stage four anal sac apocrine gland adenocarcinoma in dogs: 15 cases (2013-2017). J Am Vet Med Assoc 2019;254:960–6.

55. Heaton CM, Fernandes AFA, Jark PC, et al. Evaluation of Toceranib for treatment of apocrine gland anal sac adenocarcinoma in dogs. J Vet Intern Med 2020;34: 873–81.

56. Yamazaki H, Tanaka T, Mie K, et al. Assessment of postoperative adjuvant treatment using Toceranib against adenocarcinoma in dogs. J Vet Intern Med 2020; 34:1272–81.

57. Schlag AN, Johnson T, Vinayak A, et al. Comparison of methods to determine primary tuomour size in canine apocrine gland anal sac adenocarcinoma. J Sm Anim Pract 2020;61:185–9.

58. Shoieb AM, Hanshaw DM. Anal sac gland carcinoma in 64 cats in the United Kingdom (1995-2007). Vet Pathol 2009;46:677–83.

59. Amsellem PM, Cavanaugh RP, Chou PY, et al. Apocrine gland anal sac adenocarcinoma in cats: 30 cases (1994-2015). J Am Vet Med Assoc 2019;254: 716–22.

60. Elliott JW, Blackwood L. Treatment and outcome of four cats with apocrine gland carcinoma of the anal sac and review of the literature. J Feline Med Surg 2011; 13:712–7.

61. Bostock DE. Neoplasms of the skin and subcutaneous tissues in dogs and cats. Br Vet J 1986;142:1–19.

62. Miller MA, Nelson SL, Turk JR, et al. Cutaneous neoplasia in 340 cats. Vet Pathol 1991;28:389–95.

63. Murphy S, Sparkes AH, Smith KC, et al. Relationships between the histological grade of cutaneous mast cell tumours in dogs, their survival and the efficacy of surgical resection. Vet Rec 2004;154:743–6.

64. Patnaik AK, Ehler WJ, MacEwen EG. Canine cutaneous mast cell tumor: morphologic grading and survival time in 83 dogs. Vet Pathol 1984;21:469–74.

65. Peters JA. Canine mastocytoma: excess risk as related to ancestry. J Natl Cancer Inst 1969;42:435–43.

66. White CR, Hohenhaus AE, Kelsey J, et al. Cutaneous MCTs: associations with spay/neuter status, breed, body size, and phylogenetic cluster. J Am Anim Hosp Assoc 2011;47:210–6.

67. McNiel EA, Prink AL, O'Brien TD. Evaluation of risk and clinical outcome of mast cell tumours in pug dogs. Vet Comp Oncol 2004;4:2–8.

68. Mullins MN, Dernell WS, Withrow SJ, et al. Evaluation of prognostic factors associated with outcome in dogs with multiple cutaneous mast cell tumors treated with surgery with and without adjuvant treatment: 54 cases (1998-2004). J Am Vet Med Assoc 2006;228:91–5.

69. Van Pelt DR, Fowler JDD, Leighton FA. Multiple cutaneous mast cell tumors in a dog: a case report and brief review. Can Vet J 1986;27:259–63.

70. Cohen D, Reif SS, Brodey RS. Epidemiological analysis of the most prevalent sites and types of canine neoplasia observed in a Veterinary hospital. Cancer Res 1974;34:2859–68.

71. Hottendorf GH, Nielsen SW. Pathologic survey of 300 extirpated canine mastocytomas. Zentralbl Veterinarmed A 1967;14:272–81.

72. London CA, Thamm DH. Mast cell tumors. In: Vail DM, Thamm DH, Liptak JM, editors. Withrow & MacEwen's small animal clinical oncology. 6th edition. St. Louis: Elsevier, Inc; 2020. p. 382–403.

73. Ryan S, Wouters EGH, van Nimwegen S, et al. Skin and subcutaneous tumors. In: Kudnig ST, Seguin B, editors. Veterinary surgical oncology. 1st edition. Ames: John Wiley and Sons, Inc; 2012. p. 55–85.

74. Tams TR, Macy DW. Canine mast cell tumors. Comp Cont Ed Pract Vet 1981;27: 259–63.

75. Fejos C, Troedson K, Ignatenko N, et al. Extensive staging has no prognostic value in dogs with low-risk mast cell tumors. Vet Comp Oncol 2021;1-11. https://doi.org/10.1111/vco.12773.

76. Camus MS, Priest HL, Koehler JW, et al. Cytologic criteria for mast cell tumor grading in dogs with evaluation of clinical outcome. Vet Pathol 2016;53: 1117–23.

77. Hergt F, von Bomhard W, Kent MS, et al. Use of a 2-tier histologic grading system for canine cutaneous mast cell tumors on cytology specimens. Vet Clin Pathol 2016;45:477–83.

78. Scarpa F, Sabattini S, Bettini G. Cytological grading of canine cutaneous mast cell tumors. Vet Comp Oncol 2016;14:245–51.

79. Shaw T, Kudnig ST, Firestone SM. Diagnostic accuracy of pretreatment biopsy for grading cutaneous mast cell tumours in dogs. Vet Comp Oncol 2018;16: 214–9.

80. Pokorny E, Hecht S, Sura PA, et al. Magnetic resonance imaging of canine mast cell tumors. Vet Radiol Ultrasound 2012;53:167–73.

81. Leblanc AK, Jakoby BW, Townsend DW, et al. 18FDG-PET imaging in canine lymphoma and cutaneous mast cell tumor. Vet Radiol Ultrasound 2009;50: 215–23.

82. Griffin LR, Thamm DH, Selmic LE, et al. Pilot study utilizing Fluorine-18 fluoro-deoxyglucose-positron emission tomography/computed tomography for glycolytic phenotyping of canine mast cell tumors. Vet Radiol Ultrasound 2018;59: 461–8.

83. Finora K, Leibman NF, Fettman MJ, et al. Cytological comparison of fine-needle aspirates of liver and spleen of normal dogs and of dogs with cutaneous mast cell tumours and an ultrasonographically normal appearing liver and spleen. Vet Comp Oncol 2006;4:178–83.

84. Sato AF, Solano M. Ultrasonographic findings in abdominal mast cell disease: a retrospective study of 19 patients. Vet Radiol Ultrasound 2004;45:51–7.

85. Stefanello D, Valenti P, Faverzani S, et al. Ultrasound-guided cytology of spleen and liver: a prognostic took in canine cutaneous mast cell tumor. J Vet Intern Med 2009;23:1051–7.

86. Hughes JR, Szladovits B, Drees R. Abdominal CT evaluation of the liver and spleen for staging mast cell tumors in dogs yields nonspecific results. Vet Radiol Ultrasound 2019;60:306–15.

87. Book AP, Fidel J, Wills T, et al. Correlation of ultrasound findings, liver and spleen cytology, and prognosis in the clinical staging of high metastatic risk canine mast cell tumors. Vet Radiol Ultrasound 2011;52:548–54.

88. Ferrari R, Marcanato L, Buracco P, et al. The impact of extirpation of non-palpable/normal-sized regional lymph nodes on staging of canine cutaneous mast cell tumours: A multicentre retrospective study. Vet Comp Oncol 2018; 16:505–10.

89. Mutz ML, Boudreaux BB, Royal A, et al. Cytologic comparison of the percentage of mast cell s in lymph node aspirate samples from clinically normal dogs versus dogs with allergic dermatologic disease and dogs with cutaneous mast cell tumors. J Am Vet Med Assoc 2017;251:421–8.

90. Bookbinder PF, Butt MT, Harvey HJ. Determination of the number of mast cells in lymph node, bone marrow, and buffy coat cytologic specimens from dogs. J Am Vet Med Assoc 1992;200:1648–50.

91. Krick EL, Billings AP, Shofer FS, et al. Cytological lymph node evaluation in dogs with mast cell tumours: association with grade and survival. Vet Comp Oncol 2009;7:130–8.

92. Lapsley J, Hayes GM, Janvier V, et al. Influence of locoregional lymph node aspiration cytology vs. sentinel lymph node mapping and biopsy on disease stage assignment in dogs with integumentary mast cell tumors. Vet Surg 2021;50:133–41.

93. Worley DR. Incorporation of sentinel lymph node mapping in dogs with mast cell tumors: 20 consecutive procedures. Vet Comp Oncol 2014;12:215–26.

94. Grimes JA, Secrest SA, Wallace ML, et al. Use of indirect computed tomography lymphangiography to determine metastatic status of sentinel lymph nodes in dogs with a pre-operative diagnosis of melanoma or mast cell tumour. Vet Comp Oncol 2020;18:818–24.

95. Fournier Q, Thierry F, Longo M, et al. Contrast-enhanced ultrasound for sentinel lymph node mapping in the routine staging of canine mast cell tumours: A feasibility study. Vet Comp Oncol 2021;19:451–62.

96. Simpson AM, Ludwig LL, Newman SJ, et al. Evaluation of surgical margins required for complete excision of cutaneous mast cell tumors in dogs. J Am Vet Med Assoc 2004;224:236–40.

97. Pratschke KM, Atherton MJ, Sillito JA. Evaluation of a modified proportional margins approach for surgical resection of mast cell tumors in dogs: 40 cases (2008-2012). J Am Vet Med Assoc 2013;243:1436–41.

98. Fulcher RP, Ludwig LL, Bergman PJ, et al. Evaluation of a two-centimeter lateral surgical margin for excision of grade I and grade II cutaneous mast cell tumors in dogs. J Am Vet Med Assoc 2006;228:210–5.

99. Itoh T, Kojimoto A, Uchida K, et al. Long-term postsurgical outcomes of mast cell tumors resected with a margin proportional to the tumor diameter in 23 dogs. J Vet Med Sci 2021;83:230–3.

100. Saunders H, Thomson MJ, O'Connell K, et al. Evaluation of a modified proportional margin approach for complete surgical excision of canine cutaneous mast cell tumours and its association with clinical outcome. Vet Comp Oncol 2021;19(4):604–15.

101. Chu ML, Hayes GM, Henry JG, et al. Comparison of lateral surgical margins of up to two centimeters with margins of three centimeters for achieving tumor-free histologic margins following excision of grade I or II cutaneous mast cell tumors in dogs. J Am Vet Med Assoc 2020;256:567–72.

102. Schultheiss PC, Gardiner DW, Rao S, et al. Association of histologic tumor characteristics and size of surgical margins with clinical outcome after surgical removal of cutaneous mast cell tumors in dogs. J Am Vet Med Assoc 2011; 232:1464–9.

103. Seguin B, Leibman NF, Bregazzi VS, et al. Clinical outcome of dogs with grade-II mast cell tumors treated with surgery alone: 55 cases (1996-1999). J Am Vet Med Assoc 2001;218:1120–3.

104. Milovancev M, Townsend KL, Tuohy JL, et al. Long-term outcomes of dogs undergoing surgical resection of mast cell tumors and soft tissue sarcomas: a prospective 2-year-long study. Vet Surg 2020;49:96–105.

105. Donnelly L, Mullin C, Balko J, et al. Evaluation of histological grade and histologically tumour-free margins as predictors of local recurrence in completely excised canine mast cell tumours. Vet Comp Oncol 2013;13:70–6.

106. Selmic LE, Ruple A. A systematic review of surgical margins utilized for removal of cutaneous mast cell tumors in dogs. BMC Vet Res 2020;16:5.

107. Monteiro B, Boston S, Monteith G. Factors influencing complete tumor excision of mast cell tumors and soft tissue sarcomas: a retrospective study in 100 dogs. Can Vet J 2011;52:1209–14.

108. Ranganathan B, Milovancev M, Mehrkens L, et al. Intersurgeon agreement in determining 3 cm surgical margins of subcutaneous tumors in dogs. Vet Surg 2021;50(8):1573–8.

109. Baginski H, Davis G, Bastian RP. The prognostic value of lymph node metastasis with grade 2 MCTs in dogs: 55 cases (2001-2010). J Am Anim Hosp Assoc 2014;50:89–95.

110. Marconato L, Polton G, Stefanello D, et al. Therapeutic impact of regional lymphadenectomy for stage II cutaneous mast cell tumours. Vet Comp Oncol 2018;16:580–9.

111. Hume C, Kiupel M, Rigatti L, et al. Outcome of dogs with grade III mast cell tumors: 43 cases (1997-2007). J Am Anim Hosp Assoc 2011;47:37–44.

112. De Boer E, Harlaar NJ, Taruttis A, et al. Optical innovations in in surgery. Br J Surg 2015;102:e56–72.

113. DeWitt SB, Eward WC, Eward CA, et al. A novel imaging system distinguishes neoplastic from normal tissue during resection of soft tissue sarcomas and mast cell tumors in dogs. Vet Surg 2016;45:715–22.

114. Eward WC, Mito JK, Eward CA, et al. A novel imaging system permits real-time in vivo tumor bed assessment after resection of naturally occurring sarcomas in dogs. Clin Orthop Relat Res 2013;471:834–42.

115. Favril S, Abma E, Stock E, et al. Fluorescence-guided surgery using indocyanine green in dogs with superficial solid tumours. Vet Rec 2020;187(7). https://doi.org/10.1136/vr.104445.

116. Dornbusch JA, Cocca C, Jennings R, et al. The feasibility and utility of optical coherence tomography directed histopathology for surgical margin assessment in canine mast cell tumours. Vet Comp Oncol 2021;19(4):616–23.

117. Michels GM, Knapp DW, DeNicola DB, et al. Prognosis following surgical excision of canine cutaneous mast cell tumors with histopathologically tumor-free versus nontumor-free margins: a retrospective study of 31 cases. J Am Anim Hosp Assoc 2002;38:458–66.

118. Seguin B, Besancon MF, McCallan JL, et al. Recurrence rate, clinical outcome, and cellular proliferation indices as prognostic indicators after incomplete surgical excision of cutaneous grade II mast cell tumors: 28 dogs (1994-2002). J Vet Intern Med 2006;20:933–40.

119. Kry KL, Boston SE. Additional local therapy with primary re-excision or radiation therapy improves survival and local control after incomplete or close surgical excision of mast cell tumors in dogs. Vet Surg 2014;43:182–9.

120. Vincenti S, Findji L. Influence of treatment on the outcome of dogs with incompletely excised grade-2 mast cell tumors. Schweiz Arch Tierheilkd 2017;159:171–7.

121. Karbe GT, Davis E, Runge JT, et al. Evaluation of scar revision after inadequate primary excision of cutaneous mast cell tumors in 85 dogs (2000-2013). Vet Surg 2021;50:807–15.

122. Turrel JM, Kitchell BE, Miller LM, et al. Prognostic factors for radiation treatment of mast cell tumor in 85 dogs. J Am Vet Med Assoc 1988;193:936–40.

123. LaDue T, Price GS, Dodge R, et al. Radiation therapy for incompletely resected canine mast cell tumors. Vet Radiol Ultrasound 1988;39:57–62.

124. Al-Sarraf R, Mauldin GN, Patnaik AK, et al. A prospective study of radiation therapy for the treatment of grade 2 mast cell tumors in 32 dogs. J Vet Intern Med 1996;10:376–8.

125. Frimberger AE, Moore AS, LaRue SM, et al. Radiotherapy of incompletely resected, moderately differentiated mast cell tumors in the dog: 37 cases (1989-1993). J Am Anim Hosp Assoc 1997;33:320–4.

126. Poirier VJ, Adams WM, Forrest LJ, et al. Radiation therapy for incompletely excised grade II canine mast cell tumors. J Am Anim Hosp Assoc 2006;42:430–4.

127. Hahn KA, King GK, Carreras JK. Efficacy of radiation therapy for incompletely resected grade-III mast cell tumors in dogs: 31 cases (1987-1998). J Am Vet Med Assoc 2004;224:79–82.

128. Spugnini EP, Vincenzi B, Citro G, et al. Evaluation of cisplatin as an electroche-motherapy agent for the treatment of incompletely excised mast cell tumors in dogs. J Vet Intern Med 2011;25:407–11.

129. Spugnini EP, Vincenzi B, Baldi F, et al. Adjuvant electrochemotherapy for the treatment of incompletely resected canine mast cell tumors. Anticancer Res 2006;26:4585–9.

130. Lowe R, Gavazza A, Impellizeri JA, et al. The treatment of canine mast cell tumors with electrochemotherapy with or without surgical excision. Vet Comp On-col 2017;15:775–84.

131. Kodre V, Cemazar M, Pecar J, et al. Electrochemotherapy compared to surgery for treatment of canine mast cell tumours. In Vivo 2009;23:55–62.

132. EMA. European medicines Agency-STELFONTA summary of product Charac-teristics (SmPC). 2020. Available at: https://www.ema.europa.eu/en/documents/product-information/stelfonta-epar-product-information_en.pdf. October 5, 2020.

133. Jones PD, Campbell JE, Brown G, et al. Recurrence-free interval 12 months af-ter local treatment of mast cell tumors in dogs using intratumoral injection of ti-gilanol tiglate. J Vet Int Med 2021;35:451–5.

134. De Ridder TR, Campbell J, Burke-Schwarz C, et al. Randomized controlled clin-ical study evaluating the efficacy and safety of intratumoral treatment of canine mast cell tumors with tigilanol tiglate (EBC-46). J Vet Intern Med 2021;35:415–29.

135. Reddell P, De Ridder TR, Morton JM, et al. Wound formation, wound size, and progression of wound healing after intratumoral treatment of mast cell tumors in dogs with tigilanol tiglate. J Vet Intern Med 2021;35:430–41.

136. Simoes JP, Schoning P, Butine M. Prognosis of canine mast cell tumors: a com-parison of three methods. Vet Pathol 1994;31:637–47.

137. Bostock DE. The prognosis following surgical removal of mastocytomas in dogs. J Small Anim Pract 1973;14:27–41.

138. O'Connell K, Thomson M. Evaluation of prognostic indicators in dogs with mul-tiple, simultaneously occurring cutaneous mast cell tumours: 62 cases. Vet Comp Oncol 2011;11:51–62.

139. Mochizuki H, Motsinger-Reif A, Bettini C, et al. Association of breed and histo-pathological grade in canine mast cell tumours. Vet Comp Oncol 2017;15:829–39.

140. Thamm DH, Mauldin EA, Vail DM. Prednisone and vinblastine chemotherapy for canine mast cell tumor—41 cases 1992-1997). J Vet Intern Med 1999;13:491–7.

141. Kiupel M, Webster JD, Miller RA, et al. Impact of tumour depth, tumour location and multiple synchronous masses on the prognosis of canine cutaneous mast cell tumours. J Vet Med A Physiol Pathol Clin Med 2005;52:280–6.

142. Gieger TL, Theon AP, Werner JA, et al. Biologic behavior and prognostic factors for mast cell tumors of the canine muzzle: 24 cases (1990-2001). J Vet Intern Med 2003;17:687–92.

143. Smiech A, Slaska B, Lopuszynski W, et al. Epidemiological assessment of the risk of canine mast cell tumours based on the two-grade malignancy classifica-tion. Acta Vet Scand 2018;60:70.

144. Thompson JJ, Pearl DL, Yager JA, et al. Canine subcutaneous mast cell tumor: characterization and prognostic indices. Vet Pathol 2011;48:156–68.

145. Ginn PE, Fox LE, Brower JC, et al. Immunohistochemical detection of p53 tumor-suppressor protein is a poor indicator of prognosis for canine cutaneous mast cell tumors. Vet Pathol 2000;37:33–9.

146. O'Keefe DA. Canine mast cell tumors. Vet Clin North Amer Sm Anim Pract 1990; 20:1105–15.

147. O'Keefe DA, Couto CG, Burke-Schwartz C, et al. Systemic mastocytosis in 16 dogs. J Vet Intern Med 1987;1:75–80.

148. Murphy S, Sparkes AH, Blunden AS, et al. Effects of stage and number of tumours on prognosis of dogs with cutaneous mast cell tumours. Vet Rec 2006; 158:287–91.

149. Blackwood L, Murphy S, Buracco P, et al. European consensus document on mast cell tumours in dogs and cats. Vet Comp Oncol 2012;10:e1–29.

150. Horta RS, Lavelle GE, Monteiro LN, et al. Assessment of canine mast cell tumor mortality risk based on clinical, histologic, immunohistochemical, and molecular features. Vet Pathol 2018;55:212–23.

151. Hillman LA, Garrett LD, de Lorimier LP, et al. Biological behavior of oral and perioral mast cell tumors in dogs: 44 cases (1996-2006). J Am Vet Med Assoc 2010;237:936–42.

152. Stefanello D, Buracco P, Sabattini S, et al. Comparison of 2- and 3-category histologic grading systems for predicting the presence of metastasis at the time of initial evaluation in dogs with cutaneous mast cell tumors: 386 cases (2009-2014). J Am Vet Med Assoc 2015;246:765–9.

153. Thamm DH, Turek MM, Vail DM. Outcome and prognostic factors following adjuvant prednisone/vinblastine chemotherapy for high-risk canine mast cell tumour: 61 cases. J Vet Med Sci 2006;68:581–7.

154. Moore AS, Frimberger AE, Taylor D, et al. Retrospective outcome evaluation for dogs with surgically excised, solitary Kiupel high-grade, cutaneous mast cell tumours. Vet Comp Oncol 2020;18:402–8.

155. Miller RL, Van Lelyveld S, Warland J, et al. A retrospective review of treatment and response of high-risk mast cell tumours in dogs. Vet Comp Oncol 2016; 14:361–70.

156. Moraino SJ, Lima SF, Hume KR, et al. Association of prognostic features and treatment on survival time of dogs with systemic mastocytosis: a retrospective analysis for 40 dogs. Vet Comp Oncol 2018;16:E194–201.

157. Bae S, Milovancev M, Bartels C, et al. Histologically low-grade, yet biologically high-grade, canine cutaneous mast cell tumours: A systemic review and meta-analysis of individual participant data. Vet Comp Oncol 2020;18:580–9.

158. Lejeune A, Skorupski KA, Frazier S, et al. Aggressive local therapy combined with systemic chemotherapy provides long-term control in grade II stage 2 canine mast cell tumour: 21 cases (199-2012). Vet Comp Oncol 2013;13: 267–80.

159. Olsen JA, Thomson M, O'Connell K, et al. Combination vinblastine, prednisolone and toceranib phosphate for treatment of grade II and III mast cell tumours in dogs. Vet Med Sci 2018;4:237–51.

160. Weishaar KM, Thamm DH, Worley DR, et al. Correlation of nodal mast cells with clinical outcome in dogs with mast cell tumour and a proposed classification system for the evaluation of node metastasis. J Comp Pathol 2014;151:329–38.

161. Romansik EM, Reilly CM, Kass PH, et al. Mitotic index is predictive for survival for canine cutaneous mast cell tumors. Vet Pathol 2007;44:335–41.

162. Gil da Costa RM. C-kit as a prognostic and therapeutic marker in canine cutaneous mast cell tumours: from laboratory to clinic. Vet J 2015;205:5–10.

163. Scase TJ, Edwards D, Miller J, et al. Canine mast cell tumors: correlation of apoptosis and proliferation markers with prognosis. J Vet Intern Med 2006;20: 151–8.

164. Maglennon GA, Murphy S, Adams V, et al. Association of Ki67 index with prognosis for intermediate-grade canine cutaneous mast cell tumours. Vet Comp Oncol 2008;6:268–74.

165. Bergman PJ, Craft DM, Newman SJ, et al. Correlation of histologic grading of canine mast cell tumors with Ki67/PCNA/AgNOR/c-Kit scores: 38 cases (2002-2003). Vet Comp Oncol 2004;2:98.

166. Kiupel M, Webster JD, Kaneene JB, et al. The use of KIT and tryptase expression patterns as prognostic tools for canine cutaneous mast cell tumors. Vet Pathol 2004;41:371–7.

167. Giantin M, Vascellari M, Morello EM, et al. c-KIT messenger RNA and protein expression and mutations in canine cutaneous mast cell tumors: correlations with post-surgical prognosis. J Vet Diagn Invest 2012;24:116–26.

168. Webster JD, Yuzbasiyan-Gurkan V, Thamm DH, et al. Evaluation of prognostic markers for canine mast cell tumors treated with vinblastine and prednisone. BMC Vet Res 2008;4:32.

169. Thompson JJ, Yager JA, Best SJ, et al. Canine subcutaneous mast cell tumors: cellular proliferation and KIT expression as prognostic indices. Vet Pathol 2011; 48:169–81.

170. Carpenter J, Andrews L, Holzworth J. Tumors and tumor-like lesions. In: Holzworth J, editor. Diseases of the cat: medicine and surgery. Philadelphia: WB Saunders; 1986. p. 406–596.

171. Buerger RGm Scott DW. Cutaneous mast cell neoplasia in cats: 14 cases (1975-1985). J Am Vet Med Assoc 1987;190:1440–4.

172. Litster AL, Sorenmo KU. Characterisation of the signalment, clinical and survival characteristics of 41 cats with mast cell neoplasia. J Feline Med Surg 2006;8: 177–83.

173. Molander-McCrary H, Henry CJ, Potter K, et al. Cutaneous mast cell tumors in cats: 32 cases (1991-1994). J Am Anim Hosp Assoc 1998;34:281–4.

174. Chastain CB, Turk MA, O'Brien D. Benign cutaneous mastocytomas in two litters of Simese kittens. J Am Vet Med Assoc 1988;193:959–60.

175. Wilcock BP, Yager JA, Zink MC. The morphology and behavior of feline cutaneous mastocytomas. Vet Pathol 1986;23:320–4.

176. Johnson TO, Schulman FY, Lipscomb TP, et al. Histopathology and biologic behavior of pleomorphic cutaneous mast cell tumors in fifteen cats. Vet Pathol 2002;39:452–7.

177. Turrel JM, Farrelly J, Page RL, et al. Evaluation of strontium 90 irradiation in treatment of cutaneous mast cell tumors in cats: 35 cases (1992-2002). J Am Vet Med Assoc 2006;228:898–901.

178. Evans BJ, O'Brien D, Allstadt SD, et al. Treatment outcomes and prognostic factors of feline splenic mast cell tumors: a multiinstitutional retrospective study of 64 cases. Vet Comp Oncol 2018;16:20–7.

179. Kraus KA, Clifford CA, Davis GJ, et al. Outcome and prognostic indicators in cats undergoing splenectomy for splenic mast cell tumors. J Am Anim Hosp Assoc 2015;51:231–8.

180. Feinmehl R, Matus R, Maludin GN, et al. Splenic mast cell tumors in 43 cats (1975-1992). Proc Annu Conf Vet Cancer Soc 1992;12:50 (abstract).

181. Liska WD, MacEwen EG, Zaki FA, et al. Feline systemic mastocytosis: a review and results of splenectomy in seven cases. J Am An Hosp Assoc 1979;15: 589–97.

182. Rassnik KM, Williams LE, Kristal O, et al. Lomustine for treatment of mast cell tumors in cats: 38 cases (1999-2005). J Am Vet Med Assoc 2008;232:1200–5.

183. Berger EP, Johannes CM, Post GS, et al. Retrospective evaluation of toceranib phosphate (Palladia) use in cats with mast cell neoplasia. J Feline Med Surg 2018;20:95–102.

184. Sabattini S, Bettini G. Prognostic value of histologic and immunohistochemical features in feline cutaneous mast cell tumors. Vet Pathol 2012;47:643–53.

185. Buss MS, Mollander H, Potter K, et al. Predicting survival and prognosis in cats with cutaneous mastocytomas of varying histological grade. Proc Annu Conf Vet Cancer Soc 1996;16:56–7 (abstract).

186. Melville K, Smith KC, Dobromylskyj MJ. Feline cutaneous mast cell tumours: a UK-based study comparing signalment and histological features with long-term outcomes. J Feline Med Surg 2015;17:486–93.

187. Lepri E, Ricci G, Leonardi L, et al. Diagnostic and prognostic features of feline cutaneous mast cell tumours: a retrospective analysis of 40 cases. Vet Res Comm 2003;27:707–9

Printed and bound by CPI Group (UK) Ltd, Croydon, CR0 4YY

03/10/2024

01040471-0008